# Emergency Ophthalmology

# ERRATA

We regret the typographical errors and the omission of a section on Capsule Opacification in Chapter 12.

| | |
|---|---|
| p.5, line 2 | for "N4.8" read **N48** |
| p.11, line 1 | for "clot" read **dot** |
| p.55, line 18 | for "Tregonema" read **Treponema** |
| p.65, in box | for "pararteritis" read **polyarteritis** |
| p.90, fig 4.6 | for "???" read **FH = Family history, PH = Previous history** |
| p.163, line 23 | for "Abdominal" read **Abnormal** |
| p.169, fig 7.4 *and* p.180, line 30 | for "medical rectus" read **medial rectus** |
| p.278, line 28 | the "Management" refers to the management of capsule opacification which has unfortunately been omitted |
| p.282, line 6 | for "posterior" read **anterior synechiae** |
| p.302, line 11 | for "venous bleeding" read **venous beading** |
| p.304, fig 13.12 | arrow after "Positive risk factors" should point towards "Diagnose open angle glaucoma" |

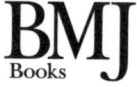

# Emergency Ophthalmology

**A symptom based guide to diagnosis and early management**

H Cheng, MA, FRCS, FRCOph
Consultant, Radcliffe Infirmary NHS Trust, Oxford

M A Burdon, BSc, MRCP, FRCOph
Senior Registrar, National Hospital for Nervous Diseases
and
St Thomas' Hospital, London

S A Buckley, BSc, MB, FRCOph
Senior Registrar, King's College Hospital, London

C Moorman, FRCS, FRCOph
Senior Registrar, Radcliffe Infirmary NHS Trust, Oxford

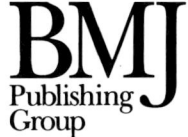

© BMJ Publishing Group 1997

All rights reserved. No part of this publication may be reproduced, stored in a retrieval system, or transmitted, in any form or by any means, electronic, mechanical, photocopying, recording and/or otherwise, without the prior written permission of the publishers.

First published in 1997
by the BMJ Publishing Group, BMA House, Tavistock Square,
London WC1H 9JR

**British Library Cataloguing in Publication Data**

A catalogue record for this book is available from the British Library

ISBN 0-7279-0861-8

Typeset by Apek Typesetters, Nailsea, Bristol
Printed and bound by Craft Print Pte Ltd, Singapore

# Contents

*Preface* vii

*Acknowledgments* ix

1 Introduction: history taking and methods of examination 1

2 Visual loss 22

3 Transient visual loss 65

4 Flashes and floaters 77

5 Red eye 92

6 Trauma 132

7 Diplopia 159

8 Headache 187

9 Pain 211

10 Swellings around the eye 223

11 Contact lens problems 256

12 Postoperative complications 270

13 Coincidental findings 294

*Appendices* 305

*Further reading* 318

*Index* 321

# Preface

Why another textbook of ophthalmology when there are so many already? Traditionally, most textbooks, presumably for ease of classification, have arranged their material either anatomically or according to some disease classification which has little bearing on the symptomatology. A patient usually consults a doctor because of a set of symptoms. Therefore, it would be helpful to have a symptom oriented book that deals with the common complaints.

It is not our intention to produce an exhaustive account of all the disease processes that could give rise to a particular symptom, but only the common and important ones that are likely to present to an accident and emergency department.

Before choosing the symptoms we audited our accident and emergency department for three months, in addition to making use of the results of another audit carried out at the Oxford Eye Hospital just before and after the implementation of the Health and Medicines Act 1988 (over a 15 week period). The choice of symptoms is based partly on the outcome of these two audits and partly on what we consider to be important symptoms that may pose a problem to the junior doctor.

The frequency of presentation is only one facet of a condition's importance. Thus we found that foreign bodies and corneal abrasions comprised the largest single category of cases using the A&E department, but all will agree that such cases do not pose a problem in diagnosis by and large. On the other hand, although an aneurysm of the posterior communicating artery presenting acutely in the eye department is rare, it is important to recognise it because of the serious implications for the individual. Where possible, life or sight threatening conditions that are likely to present acutely in an eye department are mentioned. For such cases, by their very nature, the ultimate management lies outside the A&E department, and the treatment of such cases is not dealt with in detail. The emphasis of the book is to help the trainee to

## PREFACE

recognise certain groups of conditions and to start investigations that may pinpoint the diagnosis. Where possible we have adopted an algorithmic approach so that there is a logical progression of steps to be taken. Some chapters do not lend themselves to a graphic display of the algorithms involved and we have not slavishly displayed them in every chapter. We have also allowed some overlap and repetition to avoid interrupting the flow of the text.

The high prevalence of contact lens wear reflects a social trend and is an index of the general acceptance of such devices. The frequency of acute problems caused by contact lenses mirrors their ready availability and the lack of supervised aftercare. Patients often present at unsocial hours and, because of the acute and severe symptoms, attending doctors need to have an understanding of the underlying problems and ways of management. Hence there is a section devoted to contact lenses which may seem disproportionately large for a general textbook of this nature.

In our audit, somewhat surprisingly, a significant proportion of patients presented with postoperative problems soon after surgery. The presenting problems were mostly trivial, but it is useful for novices to know a few of the common operations and their chief complications so they have an idea of the relative importance of each set of symptoms.

Finally, a chapter of common conditions is presented which includes those that do not fit naturally into the sections grouped by symptoms, for example, diabetic retinopathy and raised intraocular pressure, because of their importance or relative frequency.

At the inception of the book, the main contributors were directly involved in the work of the A&E department. The authors are therefore in touch with what is relevant and we hope that the contents and approach offered will be of help to those working in the emergency room, especially those newly starting their career in ophthalmology.

H Cheng, MA Burdon,
SA Buckley, and C Moorman

# Acknowledgments

We wish to thank our partners without whose forbearance this book could not have been written.

Many colleagues have generously allowed us to use their illustrations; Mr JJ Kanski for Figs 1.11b and 1.12; Mr JF Salmon for Fig 1.11a; Mr SN Cox for Figs 5.1–5.4, 5.6, 5.7, 5.9–5.11, 5.16, 5.18–5.21, 5.23–5.26 and 5.28, 10.1, 10.5, 11.1 and 11.3–11.7; Ms Sue Ford for Figs 5.17; Ms S Wheatcroft for Fig 4.1 and Fig 11.9; Miss Patsy Terry for Fig 11.2; and Mr J Elston for Fig 2.16 and Fig 13.5.

We are indebted to Sylvia Barker for the line drawings, and Paul Parker and the Medical Illustration Department of the Radcliffe Infirmary for some excellent photographs.

We also wish to thank Sue Reynolds for helpful comments on Chapter 7 and Miss Patsy Terry for help with Chapter 11.

# 1 Introduction: history taking and methods of examination

It is one of the paradoxes of medical practice that trainees who are often new to the specialty, and also the least experienced, may be seeing the most serious and acute conditions by having to staff the accident and emergency department (A&E) as "frontline troops". As a result of the crowded curriculum most doctors, when they graduate, will have had only brief exposure to ophthalmology. This book aims to introduce the trainee to some general principles in the practice of ophthalmology starting with history taking and techniques of examination. In each chapter that describes the major symptoms, the scope of the problem is briefly outlined and the relevant features of signs and symptoms that distinguish one condition from another are reiterated. The chief aim is to enable the trainee to manage at a practical level, by arriving at a probable diagnosis, and to institute initial steps in management.

## History taking

Few organs lend themselves to inspection in the way that the eye does and tnere is a temptation to bypass history taking especially when pressed for time. Good history taking will, however, often lead to the correct diagnosis before an examination is made. Useful information is rarely given spontaneously, and the examiner will have to ask directly about certain symptoms. At the start of every chapter, the relevant and important symptoms are emphasised, but the essential working framework of all history taking is based on the following systematic approach.

- Define the complaint, for example, what does the patient actually mean by double vision? Is it truly double or just blurred?
- Define the severity of the complaint and whether there is loss of normal function, that is, how has it affected the patient's life and does it prevent normal activities?
- How long has the patient had symptoms and are they worsening?
- Determine rapidity and mode of onset.
- Has the patient had similar problems before? Typically certain conditions are recurrent such as iritis and herpes simplex.
- Are there any problems with the fellow eye? While concentrating on the symptomatic eye it is easy to overlook the fellow eye. Many conditions tend to be bilateral, such as retinal degenerations, glaucoma, and expressions of general disease.
- Ascertain if there is involvement of other systems of the body. Eye symptoms may express ocular manifestations of systemic disease, for example, Graves' disease, systemic hypertension, diabetes mellitus.
- In trying to make a provisional diagnosis bear in mind the classification used in normal clinical practice (in box).

---

**General aetiological classification in clinical practice**

Congenital
Acquired
  Trauma
  Inflammation
    Infection
    Allergy
    Others
  Toxic: including medications
  Tumour
    Benign or malignant
    Primary or secondary
  Metabolic
  Vascular
  Degenerative

---

Examination will either provide more clues to fit the provisional diagnosis, or it may produce evidence to refute it, so always keep an open mind.

# Examination of visual function

The assessment of vision needs to take into account the different aspects of vision. The chief components of vision are "visual acuity", "visual field", and "colour vision".

## Visual acuity measurements

### Distance visual acuity in adults

A commonly used method of measuring visual acuity is to use the Snellen chart which is designed to be read from a distance of 6 metres. It consists of up to nine rows of capital letters, with each row of letters becoming progressively smaller. The lines are designated as 6/60, 6/36, 6/24, 6/18, 6/12, 6/9, 6/6, 6/5, and 6/4 from top to bottom. An eye with 6/6 acuity implies that the height of the letters of the 6/6 line would subtend an angle of 5' (5 minutes of an arc) at the fovea, with each bar of the letter (for example, E) subtending an angle of 1'. This test is therefore based on using 1' of arc as the minimum resolving power of the eye.

In a statement of visual acuity, for example, 6/24, the numerator of the visual acuity measurement refers to the distance from which the chart is read, that is, 6 metres. The denominator refers to the distance from the chart in metres when the size of the letter will subtend an angle of 5' on the retina and be seen by a normal sighted person, that is, 24 metres. The same principle applies for all the other visual acuity lines.

When patients are unable to see the top letter at 6 metres, they are moved nearer the board until the top letter is visible. This distance is then used as the numerator. For example, if the top letter can only be seen when the person is 3 metres from the board the vision is 3/60.

The notation for recording acuities worse than 1/60 are as follows:

- CF for counting fingers vision at a specified distance (for example, 1 metre or 1 foot)
- HM for detection of hand movements
- PL for light perception only (document if the patient can localise the direction of light in the four quadrants of visual field)
- NPL for no light perception.

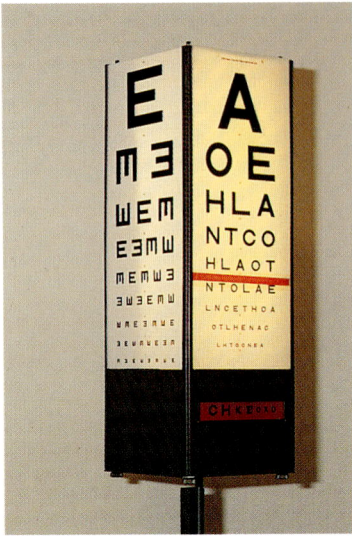

Figure 1.1   Snellen test types.

When there is a language problem, the Snellen "E" chart can be used. Rows of capital letters E can be oriented in four different directions. The patient is given a cardboard cut out of the letter E and asked to hold it in the same orientation as the letter that the examiner points to on the Snellen chart (Fig 1.1).

### *Distance visual acuity in children*

Distance visual acuity in young children may have to be recorded with both eyes open because a young child or infant will often object to having one eye occluded. If there is asymmetry in response, that is, if the child objects only to one being covered and not the other, that may be significant in itself. In young children of around three years or more, single letters of varying size are held up for the child to identify (Sheridan–Gardiner cards). The children can either say what the letters are or identify them by pointing to the same letter on a master board held in front of them (Fig 1.2).

For younger children tests involve identifying pictures or preferential looking. In an A&E setting, however, the easiest way to find out if a very young infant can see anything at all is to determine if he or she will fix and follow a brightly coloured moving target or the light of a pen torch. Be careful not to make a noise which will alert the infant.

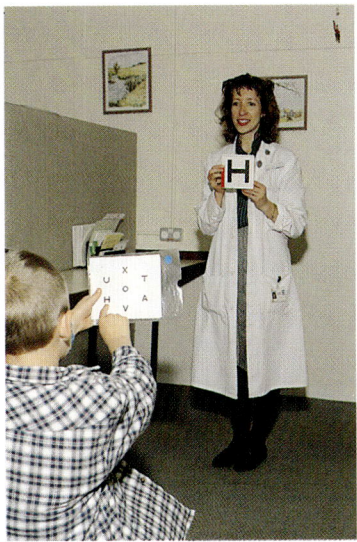

Figure 1.2 The Sheridan–Gardiner test.

## Measurement of near visual acuity

Near acuity is measured using standard print varying from small print defined as N 4·5 to the largest print defined as N 4·8. The near vision is recorded as the smallest type that can be read comfortably in a good light at a given distance.

## Corrected visual acuity

Visual acuity should be measured with the patient wearing corrective distance spectacles, and recorded as the "corrected visual acuity". Visual acuity measurements without spectacles are recorded as "unaided visual acuity". Similarly the patient's corrective reading spectacles should be worn when testing near vision.

## Pinhole visual acuity

Use the pinhole when vision is less than 6/6 with spectacles, or if there are none. This test is based on the same principle as the pinhole camera; theoretically it allows only a single ray of light to pass through the eye. Therefore, a clear image should be formed regardless of the position of the back of the camera or the refraction of the eye. This test is not only useful in patients with refractive errors who do not have corrective spectacles, but it also overcomes, to a certain extent, optical imperfections caused by media opacities such as early cararact. Vision is recorded as the "pinhole visual acuity".

In practice, however, a narrow pencil of light comes through the pinhole rather than a single ray, so with large refractive errors (that is, outside the −4 dioptres to +4 dioptres (D) range), the image would still be blurred and 6/6 vision may not be achieved.

## Other tests of central vision
### Colour vision

Colour vision is a function of the cones in the central retina and extends out to 25–30° of the visual field. In the periphery, all colour perception is absent.

Pathology in the macular area, causing colour deficiency, is usually associated with a marked loss of acuity. By contrast, inflammatory or compressive lesions of the optic nerve typically cause loss of colour perception even when acuity is only mildly reduced.

There are several ways of assessing colour vision some of which tend to be time consuming, for example, the Farnsworth–Munsell "100 hue" test. In the A&E setting, Ishihara pseudoisochromatic plates are the most convenient for detecting red–green colour confusion. Ishihara plates are made of a matrix of coloured dots arranged so that a number is visible in the centre, although not to those with defective colour vision (Fig 1.3). The number of plates seen correctly is recorded, and divided by the total number of plates shown to the patient. The first plate has an orange number on a blue background which can be seen by anyone with 6/60 acuity or better and shows the patient what to expect in

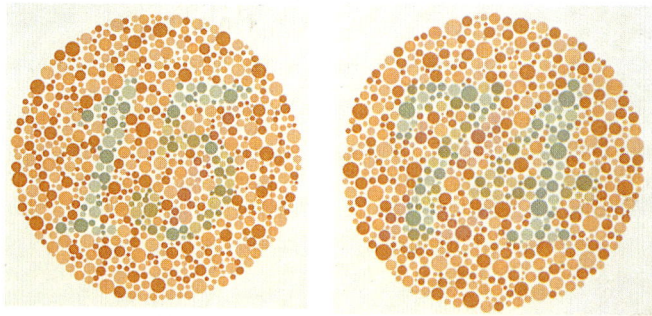

Figure 1.3    Ishihara isochromatic plates for testing colour blindness.

# HISTORY TAKING AND EXAMINATION METHODS

succeeding plates. By comparing one eye against the other, possible pathological changes in colour perception can be detected.

A simpler but subjective way of detecting colour desaturation is to hold up a bright red object to the patient's good eye, stating that this object has a redness graded 10 out of 10. The patient then looks at the object with the poor eye only and gives a subjective grading of how much the colour appears washed out compared with the good eye, for example, 5 out of 10.

## Amsler grid

The Amsler grid is used for detection of distortion of central vision and is a test of macular function. This is a 20 × 20 grid of 5 mm squares with a central fixation dot. While looking at the fixation dot, the patient is asked to view it (wearing reading spectacles if necessary) with each eye in turn to identify any areas in which the lines are distorted or missing.

## Visual fields

### Terms used in describing visual fields

| | |
|---|---|
| **Homonymous field defects** | Defects affecting the same side of the visual field in each eye |
| **Heteronymous field defects** | Defects affecting the opposite side of the visual field in each eye |
| **Congruity** | The degree to which the field loss in each eye corresponds and shows similarity |
| **Scotoma** | An abnormal area of visual field, surrounded by normal visual field |
| **Absolute defect** | No stimulus seen at all |
| **Relative defect** | A limited number of stimuli seen depending on size of target and light intensity |

## The visual pathway

An appreciation of the anatomy of the visual pathway is important in understanding the visual field (Fig 1.4).

The first stage in the visual pathway is the retinal photoreceptors—the rods and cones. Visual information then

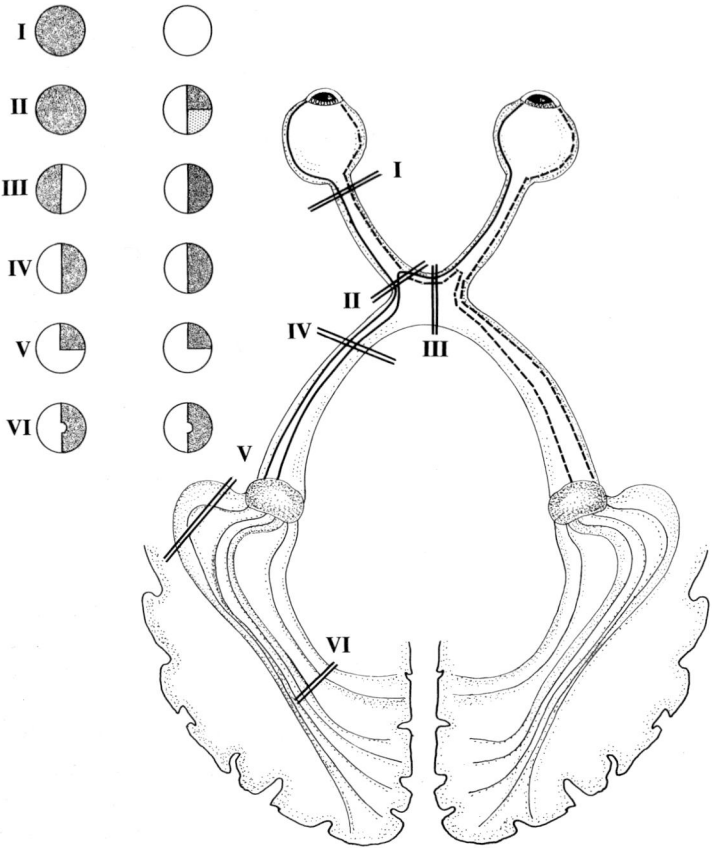

Figure 1.4 The visual pathway, showing field defects corresponding to lesions at different points of the pathway.

passes via the retinal ganglion cells, the axons of which form the inner nerve fibre layer. Axons from the macular area and the nasal retina can pass directly into the optic nerve. Ganglion cell axons from the temporal retina, however, have to arch around the macular fibres to enter either the superior or the inferior pole of the optic nerve. The anatomical arrangement of the nerve fibre layer creates a horizontal division. This results in the nerve fibre layer of the superior half of the retina passing into the superior half of the disc, and that of the inferior retina into the inferior half of the disc. A lesion of the nerve fibre layer on the peripheral retina will cause a pattern of field loss which will tend to respect the *horizontal* meridian.

## HISTORY TAKING AND EXAMINATION METHODS

The optics of the eye are such that the image formed on the retina is inverted and reversed. The temporal retina detects visual information from the nasal visual field and the nasal retina from the temporal visual field. The information from each eye passes down the optic nerves which meet in the cranial cavity at the optic chiasma.

The fibres from the nasal retina cross in the optic chiasma, with the fibres from the inferior nasal retina crossing first and passing slightly forward in the contralateral optic nerve (Wilbrand's knee) before continuing posteriorly towards the lateral geniculate body. Lesions involving the posterior optic nerve may also involve Wilbrand's knee, causing a superotemporal field defect in the contralateral eye in addition to loss of vision in the ipsilateral eye. Pathology involving the central chiasma will result in a bitemporal hemianopia. Chiasmal lesions are frequently slow growing so these defects are usually asymmetrical and incomplete.

In the optic tract, the contralateral nasal fibres are accompanied by the ipsilateral temporal fibres, so the information being carried is from the contralateral visual *field*. Therefore lesions of the visual system posterior to the chiasma produce homonymous loss of visual field in the two eyes. Within the optic tracts this loss is typically an *incongruous homonymous hemianopia*.

After synapsing in the lateral geniculate bodies, the visual pathways continue as the optic radiations. Those fibres relaying information from the inferior retina loop around the anterior horn of the lateral ventricles within the temoral lobes, whereas those from the superior retina have a more direct route through the parietal lobes to each occipital lobe. Involvement of the temporal lobe will produce a hemianopia mostly affecting the superior field, whereas parietal lobe lesions will preferentially affect the inferior visual field.

In the occipital cortex, the macular retina is represented at the tips of each lobe and the peripheral retina along their medial surfaces. The superior retina is represented above, and the inferior retina below the calcarine fissures. An occipital lobe lesion is recognised by a *congruous homonymous hemianopia*. The macular representation or the temporal crescent (the most peripheral 30° of the visual field which is represented monocularly) may be spared or solely involved. Hypotheses for the phenomenon of macular sparing include binocular representation and dual blood supply.

## Methods of documenting the visual field

**Confrontation techniques** Done properly, confrontation techniques will give valuable clinical information.

The patient is positioned in front of the examiner about 1 metre away. One eye is occluded and the steps outlined below are then followed.

1. Step 1: the patient is asked to fix on the examiner's nose and is then asked whether any part of the face is missing or blurred. This is a crude but effective way of assessing the integrity of the central visual field.
2. Step 2: ask the patient to fix on the examiner's eye directly opposite. The examiner then holds up between one and five fingers in each quadrant of the patient's visual field, approximately 20° from fixation, and the patient is asked to count the fingers while still looking at the examiner's eye.
3. Step 3: if fingers cannot be counted in a particular quadrant, the patient is asked whether hand movement can be seen, and the abnormal area mapped out by moving the hand.
4. Step 4: if the patient is able to count fingers in all quadrants, the field should be further examined using a red target such as a hat pin. The examiner first places the red target in the middle of the patient's visual field and asks the patient to identify its colour. The target is then held in each quadrant of the patient's visual field, abut 10° from fixation, and the patient is asked to say if the target appears equally red in each quadrant.

Colour confrontation can be very sensitive in detecting bitemporal hemianopias before other more formal methods, with decreased colour perception on either side of the vertical meridian. As colour is processed maximally at fixation, colour should always be brighter centrally than peripherally, so colour confrontation is also useful in identifying central and centrocaecal defects.

In mapping out the field, the *extent* of a field defect can be mapped by moving the red target out from the centre of any scotoma detected. The periphery of the field can be mapped by bringing the red target in from the periphery towards the centre, approached from the four quadrants.

**Central field examination with the Amsler grid** The central 10° of the field can be assessed subjectively with an Amsler grid.

The patient is asked, when fixing on the central clot, whether the grid is broken or distorted. The test needs a cooperative and observant patient.

**Mechanical or computerised perimetry** A variety of mechanical or computerised perimeters is available for accurate assessment of the visual fields. Although they may not always be necessary to localise a lesion, they are often required to quantify the degree of field loss so that disease progression or response to treatment can be monitored.

### Pupillary reaction

The only completely *objective* test of visual function is the assessment of the pupillary reaction to light.

Ideally, before assessing the reactivity of the pupils to light, pupillary size should be recorded under both bright and dim illumination. Any difference in the pupil size is termed anisocoria.

When the anisocoria is greater in darkness than in light, this is the result of failure of the small or miotic pupil to dilate in low illumination and indicates a sympathetic paresis. When the anisocoria is greater in light than in darkness, the failure of the larger pupil to constrict in response to the brighter illumination indicates a parasympathetic paresis. If the difference in pupil size is the same in both lighting conditions, a diagnosis of essential anisocoria, which is of no neurological significance, can be made.

#### *The relative afferent pupillary response*

The anatomy of the pupillary light reflex pathway is such that both pupils respond equally to a light shone in one eye, that is, there is a direct response to the light in the illuminated eye and an identical consensual response in the non-illuminated eye. The amplitude of the response is normally the same whichever eye is illuminated and any difference between them (assuming an intact efferent arc) indicates a problem with the afferent arc of the pathway (Fig 1.5).

The "swinging light test" is used to detect a relative afferent pupillary defect (RAPD) between the two eyes. The test is performed as follows:

1 The test is performed in reduced lighting, to help maximise pupil response.

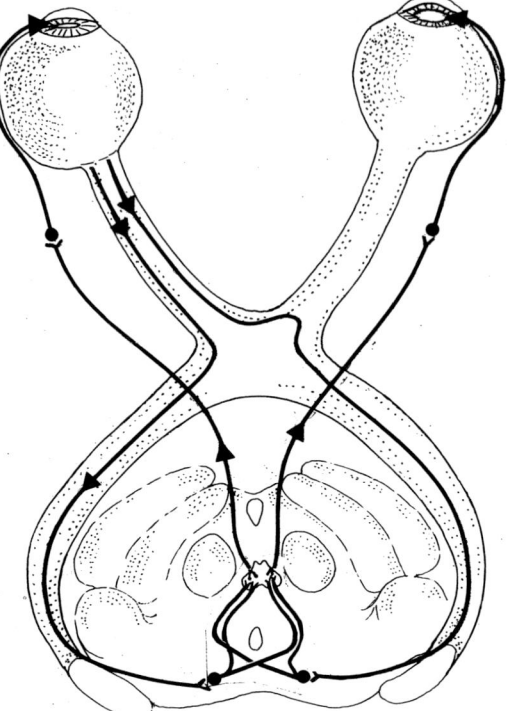

Figure 1.5 The pupillary pathway.

2 Distance fixation is maintained to prevent accommodation induced miosis as part of the near response.
3 A light is swung from one eye to the other, leaving the light in position for 1–2 seconds to observe pupillary responses. A bright light maximises any potential relative difference between the two eyes, and makes an afferent pupil defect easier to detect but a light of low intensity may be more sensitive.

For example, if a patient has a right optic nerve atrophy, when the light is shone into the left eye both pupils will constrict, but when shone shortly afterwards into the right eye, both pupils will dilate. The damage to the afferent pathway on the right side reduces the nerve signals to the efferent arc, so that despite the light intensity being the same, the pupil response to light is reduced on the defective side.

Subtle afferent pupil defects may be confused with hippus, where a natural oscillation of the pupil size is observed when a light is shone on the eye.

The RAPD is not affected by media opacities that cause light scatter but do not prevent light from reaching the retina. Therefore the swinging light test can be used in the presence of a cataract or vitreous haemorrhage. If one pupil is unreactive as a result of damage to nerve III, trauma, or pharmacological preparations, it is still possible to examine for an RAPD by observing the unaffected pupil alone.

## Notes on the use of ophthalmic instruments

### The slitlamp (biomicroscope)

The slitlamp consists of a binocular microscope mounted horizontally and lit by a light source which can provide diffuse light or slit beams; both the height and the width of these, as well as the angle of incidence, can vary. There are also filters that vary the wavelength. Thus it is possible to examine the surface, make optical sections, or focus on some point within the eye; with the help of additional lenses, it is even possible to see the fundus. Learning to use the slitlamp properly is best done by hands on experience but some points are worth highlighting.

#### *Direct illumination*

Examination of the surface: slanting diffuse illumination with a wide slit is useful for examining the superficial layers of the cornea and tear film. It is possible to reduce luminance to gain patient cooperation.

To obtain a thin optical slice of the anterior part of the eye, use a narrow beam positioned obliquely (Fig 1.6).

#### *Specular reflection*

When a wide beam of light passes through the optical media of the eye, most of the light is transmitted, although at each optical interface a small proportion will be reflected back. If the angle of illumination is adjusted it allows the image from the deeper layers to be seen. At a critical angle, where the relatively intense reflection from the epithelial surface has been reduced sufficiently, it is possible to see the cellular pattern of the corneal endothelium (Fig 1.7).

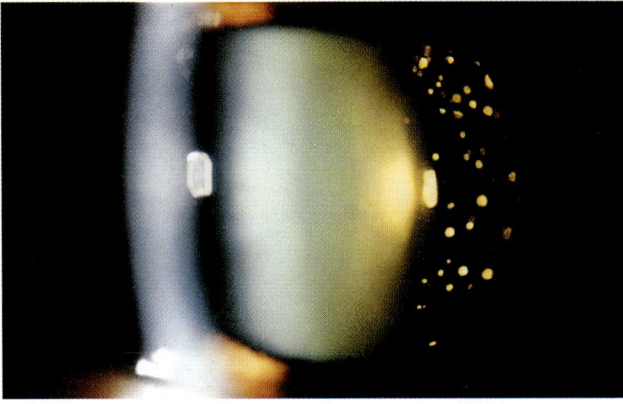

Figure 1.6   The slitlamp beam positioned obliquely to give an optical section of the anterior segment of the eye. The beam also shows scintillating bodies in the anterior vitreous from asteroid hyalosis.

### *Scleral scatter*

The beam needs to be offset by unlocking the centre locking screw. The slit beam is displaced laterally so that the light falls onto the limbus while the microscope is focused centrally. The feature to be studied will be viewed in relief with light transmitted through the cornea, for example, subtle opacities and corneal oedema.

### *Retroillumination*

Again the beam needs to be offset; light can be reflected from the iris or retina to illuminate the cornea from behind. This allows the detection of both epithelial or endothelial changes and changes within the lens (Figs 1.8 and 1.9).

### *Examination of the anterior chamber*

Aqueous humour in the anterior chamber is normally optically clear. In ocular inflammation, circulating "cells" and "flare" appear resembling dust and smoke seen in the beam of a projector in the cinema. "Flare" refers to the light scatter caused by proteins in colloidal solution leaked from inflamed iris vessels. "Cells" are cellular aggregates in suspension forming scintillating particles and subject to the convection movements of the aqueous humour. Aggregates of macrophages and white cells can also

# HISTORY TAKING AND EXAMINATION METHODS

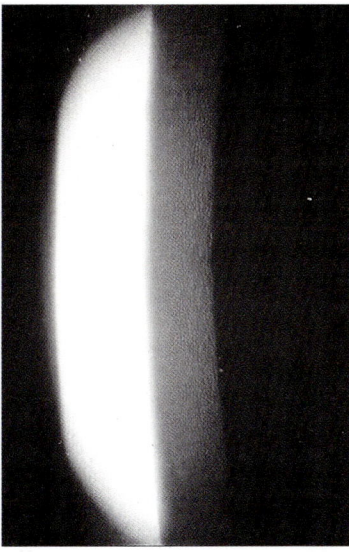

Figure 1.7 Specular reflection: the secondary beam reflected from the posterior surface of the cornea shows the endothelial mosaic (just to the right of the bright main beam).

accumulate on the back of the inferior cornea as keratic precipitates (KPs) (Fig 1.10).

As a result of the effect of gravity, deposits of blood (hyphaema) (see Fig 6.1 in Chapter 6) and white blood cells (hypopyon) (see Fig 5.7 in Chapter 5) in the anterior chamber will have a fluid level in front of the iris.

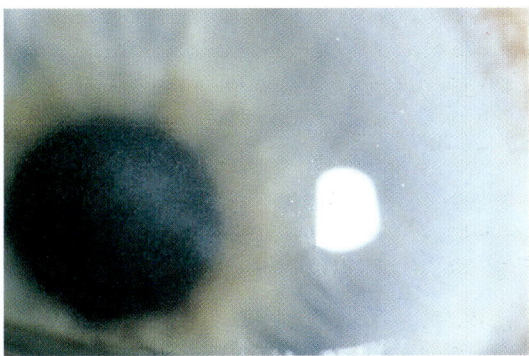

Figure 1.8 Retroillumination: the beam reflected from the iris shows deep corneal opacities.

# EMERGENCY OPHTHALMOLOGY

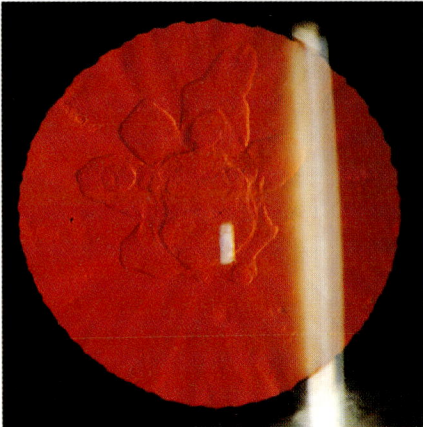

Figure 1.9 Retroillumination: the beam reflected from the choroid shows lens irregularities and vacuoles against the red reflex.

**Grading of cells in the anterior chamber** The number of cells in the anterior chamber is graded from 0 to +4 depending on the number seen in the field of a slit beam 3 mm long and 1 mm wide (Table 1.1).

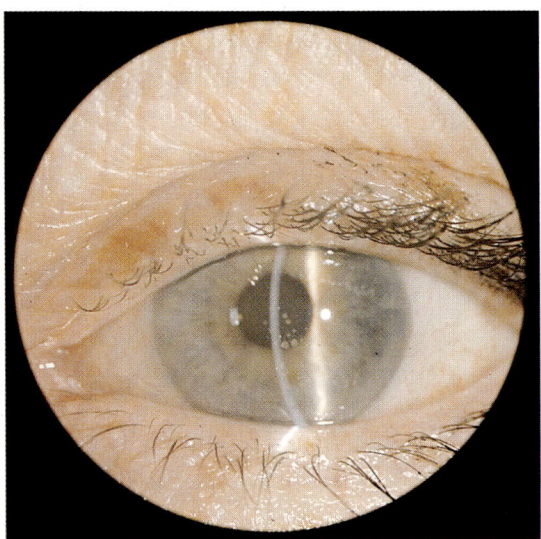

Figure 1.10 Image obtained with the slit beam, showing a deep anterior chamber and keratic precipitates (KPs) from granulomatous uveitis.

Table 1.1  Grading of cells

| Cells per field | Grade | Numerical grades |
|---|---|---|
| 0 | 0 | 1 |
| 1–5 | ± | 2 |
| 6–10 | + | 3 |
| 11–20 | ++ | 4 |
| 21–50 | +++ | 5 |
| >51 | ++++ | 6 |

In practice no one actually counts the number of cells seen, but quickly learns with experience how to grade the activity of the anterior chamber consistently from a quick assessment of the appearance.

### *Using the slitlamp to check intraocular pressure*

Applanation tonometry is commonly done using a Goldmann tonometer. The end point is reached when the inner edges of the semicircles just touch, at the end of each cycle of oscillation which occurs with the pulse.

Too much tear or lid contact will give a falsely low reading, while pressing on the globe will induce an erroneously high reading.

### *Using the slitlamp to see the posterior segment of the eye*

The optics of the slitlamp allow only the anterior third of the vitreous to be seen. Use a narrow slit to examine the structure of the vitreous humour. Ask the patient to look up, then down quickly, and finally look straight ahead and keep the eyes still. The vitreous humour continues to move across the field of view and debris such as pigment cells and inflammatory cells are easier and more obvious to see.

To view the fundus, additional lenses have to be used which can either be contact or non-contact lenses. There is now a wide variety of non-contact lenses of high positive dioptre power on the market, but the principle of their use is the same. The slitlamp is focused on the cornea and then, holding the lens relatively close to the eye, the slitlamp is moved towards the eye until the retina comes into focus.

An alternative form of imaging is to use contact lenses that abolish refraction of the cornea. The eye is anaesthetised with a topical anaesthetic, and the contact lens placed on the eye, usually with a fluid interface between the cornea and the lens.

## Gonioscopy

The angle of the anterior chamber is not visible except through a gonio prism or mirror. The most commonly used lens for gonioscopy is the Goldmann single mirror contact lens. Gonioscopy is essential in evaluating the patient with high intraocular pressure.

### Structures in the angle

1 The most anterior structure is Schwalbe's line: an anterior opaque line which denotes the posterior limit of Descemet's membrane and the anterior limit of the trabecular meshwork.
2 Next the trabecular meshwork stretches from this line to the scleral spur. The anterior trabeculum is whitish but most have a greyish blue translucent appearance.
3 The next structure is the scleral spur; this is a narrow whitish band.
4 The most posterior structure is the ciliary body; it stands out behind the scleral spur as a dull brown band (Fig 1.11).

### The Schaffer grading system of the anterior chamber angle

The angle is recorded in four quadrants: superior, inferior, temporal, and nasal. The grading is as follows (Fig 1.12):

- Grade 4 is a wide open angle in which the ciliary body can be seen easily.
- Grade 3 is an open angle in which the scleral spur can be easily identified.
- Grade 2 is a moderately narrow angle in which only the trabeculum can be seen.
- Grade 1 is a very narrow angle in which perhaps only the top of the trabeculum can be seen.
- Grade 0 is a closed angle.

If the angle is apparently very narrow or closed, pressure can be put on the edge opposite the mirror to test if the angle is capable of opening.

## Using the direct ophthalmoscope

In the direct ophthalmoscope, revolving lenses from $+30$ to $-30$ D are mounted on discs, which allow compensation for any inherent refractive error in either the examiner or the patient.

# HISTORY TAKING AND EXAMINATION METHODS

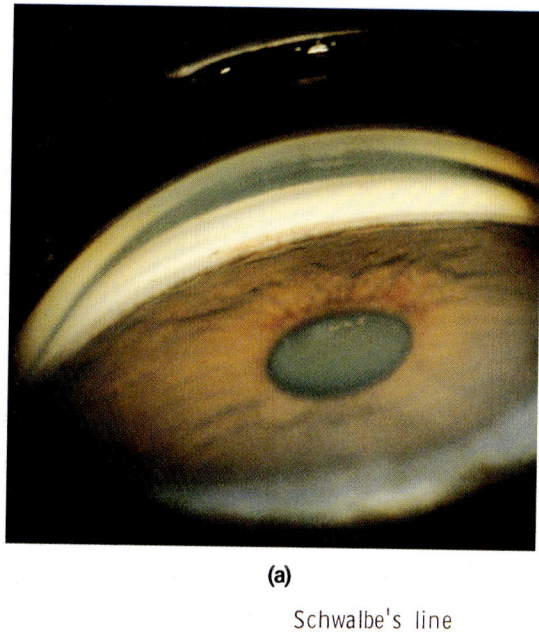

(a)

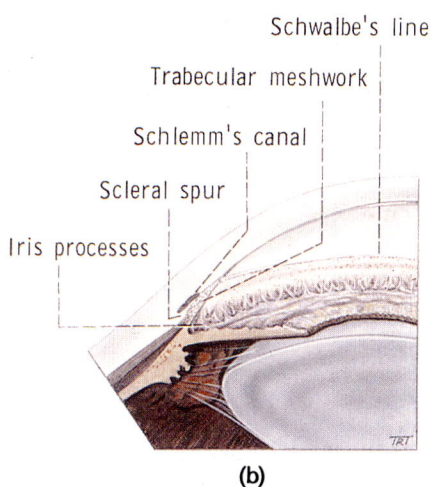

(b)

Figure 1.11 (a) Gonioscopic view of the anterior chamber; (b) diagrammatic view of the chamber angle which is also shown in cross section. (By kind permission of JJ Kanski.)

## *The red reflex*

The red reflex describes the reflected light from the retina seen through an ophthalmoscope or retinoscope. View the red reflex from about a foot away with a +1.0 D lens. Some books suggest

# EMERGENCY OPHTHALMOLOGY

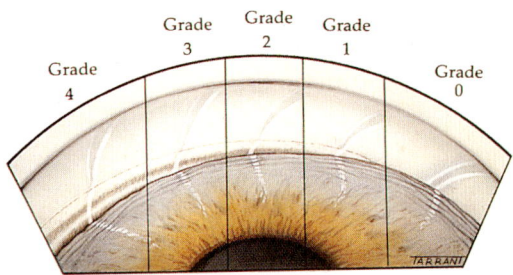

Figure 1.12   The Shaffer grading system of the chamber angle. (By kind permission of JJ Kanski.)

using a +10.0 D lens which will focus on the lens and will not show opacities in strong relief. Opacities in the lens and media show as dark silhouettes against the red reflex. In cases of severe infection, haemorrhage, or dense cataract, the red reflex will be lost.

After looking at the red reflex, with the patient fixing on a target, approach the eye adjusting the lenses in the lens wheel to focus on the retina. As the macula and disc lie on the same horizontal plane, the chance of finding the disc first time is increased if it is approached along this plane of fixation. Use the right eye when examining the patient's right eye, and the left eye when examining the patient's left eye. If the pupil is small, using a narrow beam avoids undue reflection and makes it easier to view the fundus. Without dilatation, it is not possible to examine the peripheral fundus thoroughly. The green or "red free" filter helps detail the nerve fibre layer and small vessels.

The magnification of the fundal image using direct ophthalmoscopy in an emmetrope is about 15 times larger, that is, three to four times larger than the image of indirect ophthalmoscopy.

## The binocular indirect ophthalmoscope

This gives a wide three dimensional view of the fundus and allows a more peripheral view. The pupil needs to be dilated.

The relatively high intensity of illumination and use of non-coaxial light mean that it is possible to overcome moderate media opacities such as cataract or a small vitreous haemorrhage to get a view of the fundus. In addition, by using scleral indentation, details can be brought into the path of the beam and there is a view out to the ora serrata. Indentation also adds a dynamic element to the examination in that, by rolling on the sclera, a tear

## HISTORY TAKING AND EXAMINATION METHODS

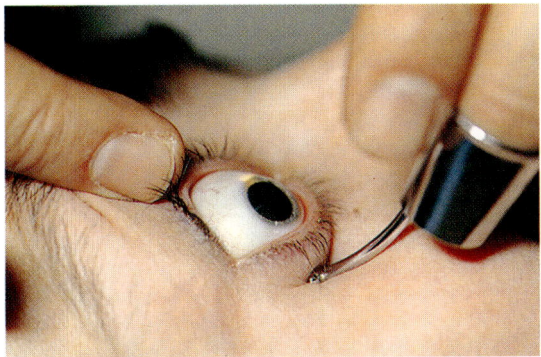

Figure 1.13  Indentation indirect ophthalmoscopy.

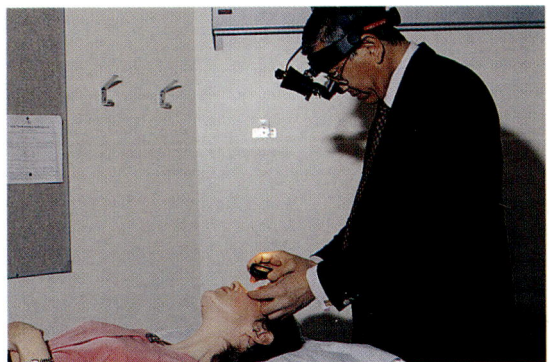

Figure 1.14  Indirect ophthalmoscopy.

can be opened on the apex of the indent, which may otherwise be difficult to see (Fig 1.13).

Expertise in the use of the indirect ophthalmoscope requires practice. To image the retina the lens needs to be kept at a certain distance from the eye of the patient and the examiner which is helped by resting a little finger on the face (Fig 1.14). By keeping the elbow against the body and moving the body and head as a unit, it increases the stability of the viewing system and helps to retain the image when trying to look at the rest of the fundus.

For the examination of eye movements, Chapter 7 will be of help; and for examination of the orbit, see Appendix C.

# 2 Visual loss

An appreciation of the anatomy of the visual pathway is of vital importance in understanding patients' symptoms. A brief description is found in Chapter 1.

Symptoms of visual "loss" vary greatly in meaning from patient to patient, ranging from blurring to complete blindness, and may affect one or both eyes. The different components of visual function, that is, acuity, field, colour, and brightness appreciation, may be affected jointly or separately, and a detailed history and examination are necessary to establish the extent and degree of involvement.

Anatomically, a lesion located anywhere between the cornea and the occipital cortex may cause visual loss but the topographical organisation of the visual pathway is such that a lesion at a particular site will give a characteristic visual defect (Table 2.1).

The first step in assessment is therefore to make an anatomical diagnosis, which is done by determining (1) the pattern of visual loss, followed by (2) the severity or degree of loss. After locating the lesion anatomically then proceed to find (3) the aetiology.

Diseases often have patterns, so knowledge of the anatomical diagnosis can eliminate a whole set of possibilities and frequently points to the true diagnosis.

Classification of visual loss by pattern and degree is shown in Fig 2.1.

## History

### Is the visual loss monocular or binocular?

Ocular or optic nerve pathology causes monocular visual loss, whereas a lesion at or posterior to the optic chiasma causes binocular loss. In the unusual event of simultaneous bilateral

Table 2.1 Characteristic visual defect by site

| Feature of defect | Location | | | | | | |
|---|---|---|---|---|---|---|---|
| | Cortex | Radiation | Tract | Chiasma | Nerve | Retina | Anterior segment |
| Pattern of field defect | Homonymous hemianopia | Homonymous hemianopia | Homonymous hemianopia | Bitemporal | Crosses midline | Depends on location | Diffuse |
| Steepness | Very | Very | No | No | No | No | No |
| Symmetry (congruity) | Yes 5+ | 3+–4+ | 2+–3+ | Not unless advanced 1+–4+ | No 0 | No 0 | No 0 |

Steepness describes the depth of loss; the steeper it is, the more absolute it is.
Symmetry describes the shape of the defect and the correspondence of the two sides (see Fig 1.4).

# EMERGENCY OPHTHALMOLOGY

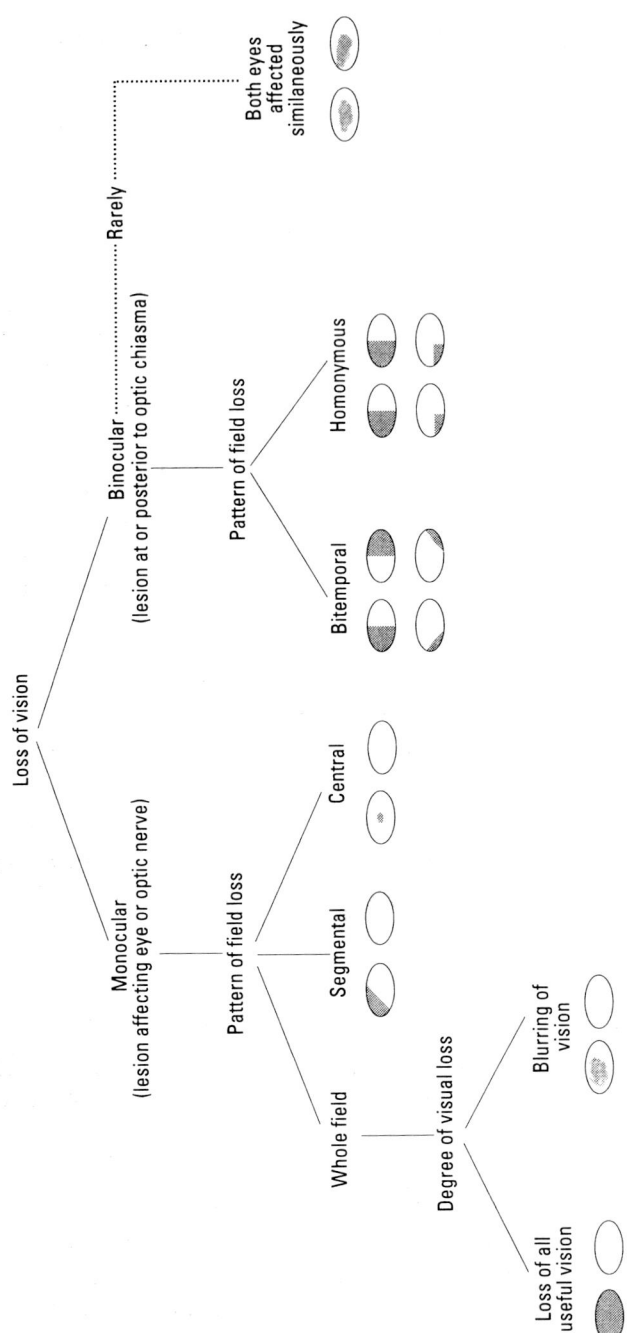

Figure 2.1 Classification of visual loss.

ocular or optic nerve disease, visual loss will involve both halves of the visual field of each eye and will not be limited by the vertical meridian.

Although differentiation between monocular and binocular visual loss is usually straightforward, the following should be borne in mind:

- Patients occasionally mistake a homonymous hemianopia for monocular loss.
- Retinal lesions cause "positive" scotomata in the visual field in that the patient is aware that part of the field is obstructed. By contrast, if the damage is posterior to the retina the patient does not "see" that a segment of the visual field is missing. Thus, for example, patients with a right homonymous hemianopia do not complain that there is something obstructing their right visual field, but they may have noticed that they keep bumping into objects on that side or that they are having difficulty reading because they cannot find the next word. Such "negative" scotomata are more difficult to describe and patients may complain of blurred vision instead.

### Does the monocular loss involve the whole or only part of the visual field?

Patients are usually able to distinguish between three patterns of visual field loss: whole, segmental, or central. Central loss caused by retinal disease is often associated with distortion of vision.

### How severely has monocular vision been affected?

It is useful to distinguish between eyes that have lost all useful vision and those that have blurred vision but are still able to see.

### Is binocular loss homonymous or bitemporal?

A lesion at the chiasma will cause bitemporal loss, often asymmetrical, whereas one located more posteriorly will cause a homonymous field defect. The more posterior the lesion, the more symmetrical and congruous the field defect.

## Examination

It is often possible to determine the pattern of visual loss (see Fig 2.1) from the history alone. Patients are not, however, always able to describe their visual loss accurately so it is important to perform a functional examination on both eyes of every patient.

### Acuity

For monocular visual loss, acuity is proportional to the degree of damage to either the central retina or the macular fibres in the optic nerve. By contrast, eyes with hemianopic field defects have a normal or only mildly reduced acuity (6/6 to 6/12) because the remaining half of the central field is intact. The field defect may, however, cause one half of the acuity chart to be ignored.

A relative afferent pupillary defect (RAPD) indicates either optic nerve disease or extensive damage to the retina. The following do not cause an RAPD:

- Opacification of the optical media—light is scattered but still reaches the retina.
- Focal lesions at the macula—although acuity may be greatly reduced, the small area of retinal damage does not cause a detectable change in pupil reactions.
- Lesions posterior to the optic nerves—because of the decussation of half of each optic nerve at the chiasma, and innervation of both Edinger–Westphal nuclei by each pretectal nucleus.
- Amblyopia—the pupil reflex arc is subcortical and intact.

### Colour perception

Colour perception is usually tested with isochromatic plates such as those designed by Ishihara. The following helps in interpretation of the results:

- About 8% of males and 0·5% of females are colour deficient; they are usually already aware of this.
- Colour perception is usually preserved in the remaining fields of patients with binocular hemianopias.
- Retinal lesions cause a parallel reduction in acuity and colour vision. Thus patients with an acuity of 6/36 or better will normally be able to read the Ishihara plates.

- Optic nerve diseases frequently cause a loss of colour vision that is disproportionate to the loss of acuity.

The rest of this chapter discusses in turn the differential diagnosis of each of the six patterns of visual loss outlined in Fig. 2.1.

## Profound loss of vision

This means that there is complete or greatly diminished vision affecting the whole field. Common conditions that frequently cause a profound loss of vision are listed in the box.

---

**Common causes of severe loss of vision**

Vascular
    Anterior ischaemic optic neuropathy
    Ischaemic central retinal vein occlusion
    Central reinal artery occlusion
    Vitreous haemorrhage
Inflammatory
    Optic neuritis
Infiltrative, compressive, inherited, nutritional
    Optic neuropathy
Mechanical
    Retinal detachment

---

### Differentiating features of the history
*Onset*

Sudden onset of visual loss indicates a vascular aetiology. Gradually enlarging field defect over hours to a few days indicates a retinal detachment. Progressive dimming of vision over hours to a few days indicates optic neuritis and optic neuropathy.

*Associated symptoms*

Optic neuritis is associated with ocular or retro-ocular pain which is exacerbated by eye movement. A retinal detachment is often preceded by flashes and floaters.

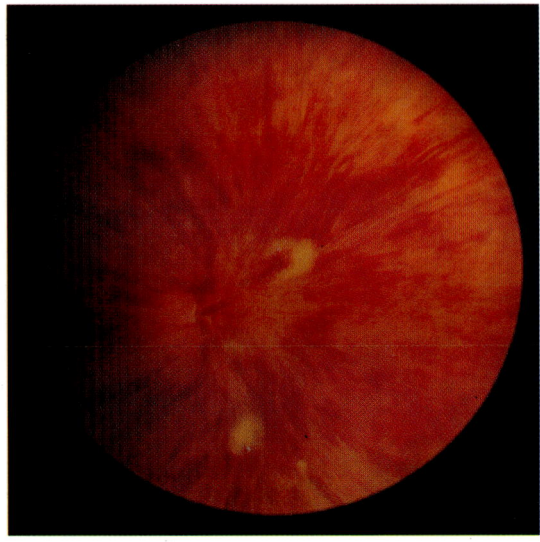

Figure 2.2 Central retinal vein occlusion (ischaemic) showing multiple retinal haemorrhages.

## Examination
### Abnormal retina

- No fundal view—vitreous haemorrhage
- Multiple retinal haemorrhages—ischaemic central retinal vein occlusion (Fig 2.2)
- Retinal pallor and arteriolar narrowing—central retinal artery occlusion (Fig 2.3)
- Elevated, mobile, grey looking retina—retinal detachment (Fig 2.4).

### Abnormal disc

Disc swelling indicates anteror ischaemic optic neuropathy (Fig 2.5); occasionally caused by optic neuritis or optic neuropathy.

### Normal disc and retina

There is optic neuritis and optic neuropathy.

## Anterior ischaemic optic neuropathy

Anterior ischaemic optic neuropathy (AION) is caused by occlusion of the posterior ciliary arteries supplying the preliminary optic nerve.

# VISUAL LOSS

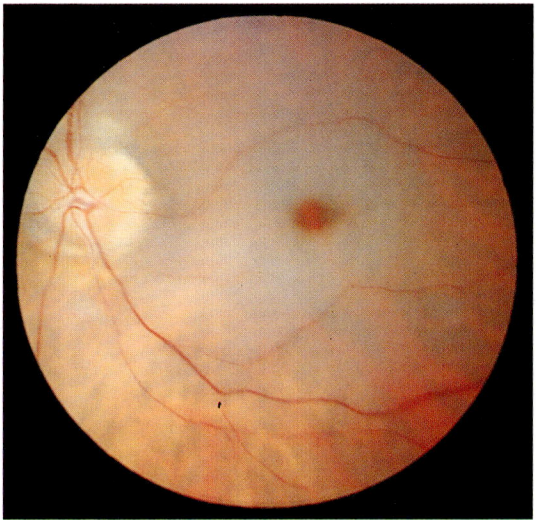

Figure 2.3 Central retinal artery occlusion showing cherry red spot, pale central retina, and narrowed arterioles.

**Symptoms and signs** There is sudden loss of vision and swelling of the optic disc. Two forms of AION are recognised: non-arteritic and arteritic AION.

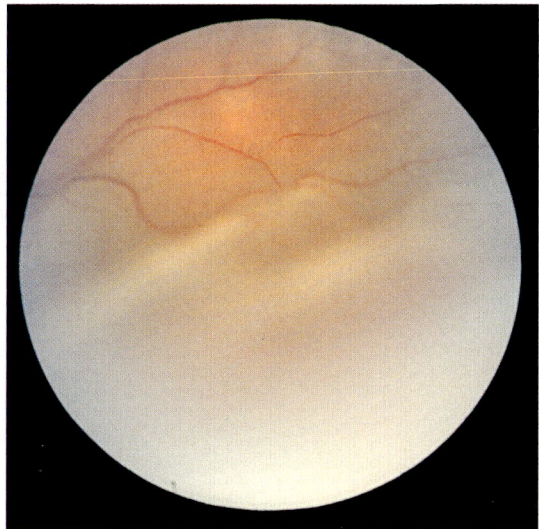

Figure 2.4 Retinal detachment showing grey undulating retina.

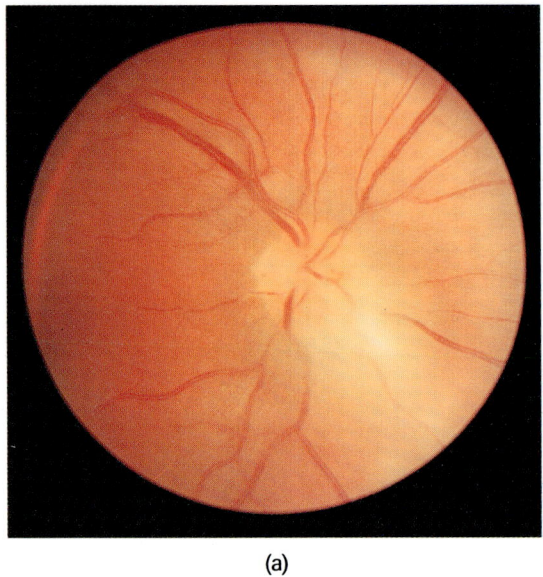

(a)

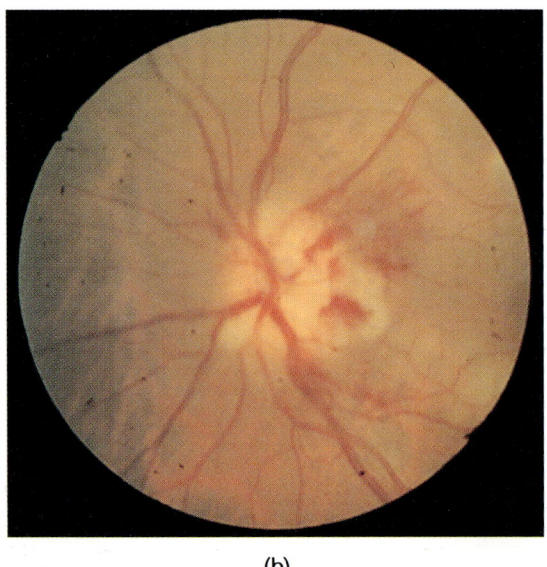

(b)

Figure 2.5 Anterior ischaemic optic neuropathy: (a) showing sectoral involvement; (b) a very pale disc with surface haemorrhages (some flame shaped).

# VISUAL LOSS

***Non-arteritic AION*** Peak incidence is in the 60–70 year age range but can occur in much younger patients. Field loss is usually altitudinal or arcuate, but may be total. Central vision is usually involved with resultant loss of acuity, but 40% of affeced eyes retain an acuity of 6/18 or better. Disc swelling may be subtle and limited to the sector corresponding to the field defect. Flame shaped disc haemorrhages are often seen (Fig 2.5).

***Arteritic AION*** This is most common beyond the age of 70 and very rare below 50. Patients usually present with profound loss of vision in one or both eyes, but partial field loss may occur. They may have experienced episodes of transient visual loss in the preceding few days. The disc is swollen and milky white in colour (Fig 2.6).

### Aetiology
- Non-arteritic AION: local arteriosclerosis (embolus is an extremely rare cause)
- Arteritic AION: giant cell arteritis (GCA).

### Immediate management
***Screen for GCA*** Systemic features include headache, pain, and tenderness of proximal muscle groups (polymyalgia rheumatica),

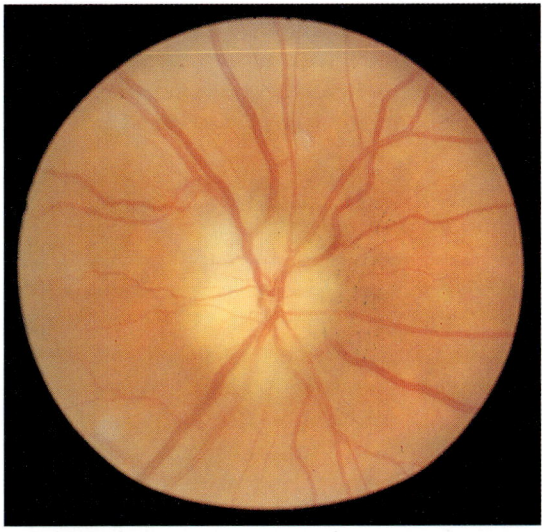

Figure 2.6   Arteritic AION waxy pallor and swollen disc in giant cell arteritis.

jaw claudication, fever, weight loss, scalp tenderness, and pulseless temporal arteries. On immediate erythrocyte sedimentation rate (ESR) measurement, most patients will have an elevated ESR, typically over 80 min/h. The age matched upper limit of normal is about half the patient's age in millimetres per hour.

*Treatment* This should be as though it were giant cell arteritis, the systemic features of which may be absent. Two per cent biopsy proven giant cell arteritis have a normal ESR. Giving immediate steroid treatment to a patient with giant cell arteritis may be sight saving, and a short course of steroids (until giant cell arteritis is definitely excluded) is unlikely to harm a patient with non-arteritic AION. Therefore, patients should be given hydrocortisone 200 mg intravenously, pending further investigation.

### Prognosis
*Non-arteritic AION* Simultaneous bilateral involvement is very rare but 40% of fellow eyes are affected within 10 years. It is very rare to have a further episode in the same eye. No treatment has proved effective in restoring vision to an affected eye, but low dose aspirin may reduce the incidence of second eye involvement.

*Arteritic AION* Untreated, 60% of patients who present with unilateral arteritic AION will develop second eye involvement within days. Treatment rarely improves vision in an affected eye but does greatly reduce the risk of visual loss in the fellow eye.

### Further management
*Temporal artery biopsy* A positive temporal artery biopsy establishes the diagnosis of giant cell arteritis. It is a low risk procedure which should be considered for all patients with AION who are over the age of 50, even if they have a normal ESR and no systemic features of giant cell arteritis. Even when the diagnosis of giant cell arteritis is obvious clinically, a biopsy should be performed before committing an elderly patient to a long course of steroid treatment with all its associated side effects.

Oral prednisone 1·5 mg/kg body weight per day, together with peptic ulcer prophylaxis, should be continued until the results of a temporal artery biopsy are known.

**Treatment of confirmed giant cell arteritis** High dose oral steroids are continued for several weeks and then gradually reduced. Treatment is monitored by serial ESR measurements and by the presence of systemic features of giant cell arteritis. Patients are likely to require treatment for several years.

**Treatment of non-arteritic AION** Patients should be prescribed aspirin 75 mg/day, and screened for hypertension and diabetes.

## Central retinal vein occlusion

**Symptoms and signs** Central retinal vein occlusion (CRVO) predominantly affects patients over 50 years old. Visual impairment varies from mild to severe. The key finding is retinal haemorrhages in all four quadrants.

Two forms of CRVO are recognised: non-ischaemic and ischaemic.

*Non-ischaemic CRVO* In about 70% of patients the occlusion is only partial, and causes a moderate reduction in visual acuity (typically 6/24 or better); there are no RAPDs, scattered retinal haemorrhages, few if any cotton wool spots, mild dilatation of the retinal veins, and mild disc swelling (Fig 2.7).

*Ischaemic CRVO* In the remaining 30% of patients the retina is rendered ischaemic. Visual acuity is severely reduced (6/60 or worse), an RADP is present, retinal haemorrhages and cotton wool spots are numerous, the retinal veins are markedly dilated and tortuous, and the optic disc is markedly swollen (see Fig 2.2). Fundus fluorescein angiography is useful in distinguishing between these two forms.

### Aetiology
- Ocular:
    raised intraocular pressure (IOP)
- Systemic:
    arteriosclerosis
    hyperviscosity syndromes
    systemic vasculitis.

### Investigations
- Full blood count
- Erythrocyte sedimentation rate

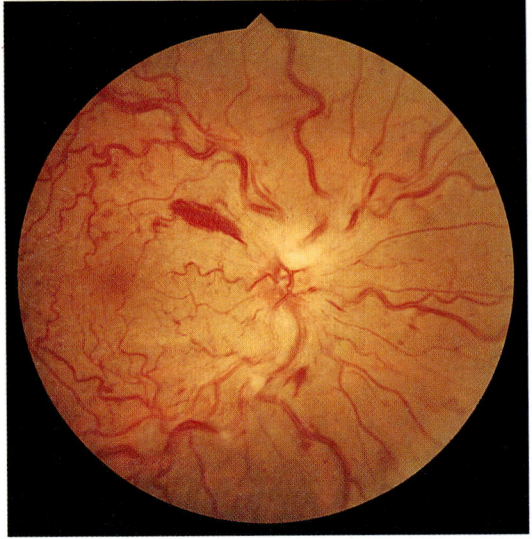

Figure 2.7 Non-ischaemic CRVO (or papillophlebitis): disc swelling, and tortuous and dilated veins with flame shaped haemorrhages in the nerve fibre layer.

- Plasma proteins and electrophoretic strip
- Glucose
- Lipid profile
- Antinuclear antibodies (ANAs)
- In young patients, clotting studies (for example, antithrombin III, proteins S and C deficiencies) should also be considered.

**Immediate management** Elevated intraocular pressure (IOP) in either eye should be treated.

**Prognosis**

*Non-ischaemic CRVO* Although there may be some spontaneous improvement, visual acuity is usually permanently reduced because of persistent macular oedema. Some affected eyes may go on to develop the ischaemic form of CRVO.

*Ischaemic CRVO* Visual acuity is permanently reduced as a result of macular ischaemia and oedema. Within six weeks to six months, 50% of these eyes will develop painful neovascular glaucoma in response to angiogenic factors released by the ischaemic retina.

# VISUAL LOSS

**Follow up and further treatment** Panretinal photocoagulation prevents rubeotic glaucoma following an ischaemic CRVO. Therefore patients should be reviewed in an ophthalmology clinic within two weeks, so that those with an ischaemic CRVO can be identified and retinal photocoagulation applied before the development of iris neovascularisation.

Persistent macular oedema is untreatable. Other possible treatments include:

- steroids for systemic vasculitis
- isovolaemic dilution
- oxyrutin.

These are not treatments that should be started in the A&E department and are for specialist clinics.

## Central retinal artery occlusion (CRAO)
### Symptoms and signs
- Most common in the seventh decade
- Visual acuity is usually down to counting fingers or less, but 11% of affected eyes retain some central vision because of a patent cilioretinal artery (Fig 2.8)
- Marked RAPD
- Pale fundus caused by infarction and swelling of the nerve fibre layer of the inner retina
- "Cherry-red spot" (see Fig 2.3) at the fovea where the retina is thin and the choroidal circulation is not masked
- Attenuated retinal arterioles
- An embolus is seen in 20% of affected eyes.

### Aetiology
- Embolus from the carotid arteries
- Cardiac embolus
- Locally formed thrombus
- Systemic vasculitis, particularly giant cell arteritis
- Coagulopathies
- Fat emboli after trauma (Purtscher's retinopathy).

### Investigations
- Urgent ESR
- Full blood count
- Glucose

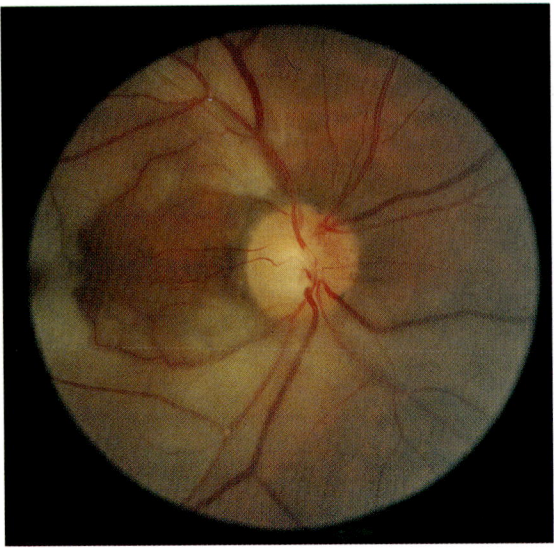

Figure 2.8 Retinal oedema with cilioretinal sparing: emboli at the first bifurcation of the temporal branch of the central retinal artery and more distally.

- Lipid profile
- Autoantibody screen: anti-DNA and anti-neutrophil cytoplasmic antibodies
- Carotid duplex ultrasonic scan
- Echocardiography.

**Immediate management** Measures to improve retinal perfusion by decreasing IOP:

- Intravenous acetazolamide 500 mg
- Ocular massage for 15/min by pressing on the eye for 10 seconds and then suddenly releasing
- Anterior chamber paracentesis: under topical anaesthesia about 0·2 ml of aqueous fluid is removed using a 25 gauge needle attached to a 1 ml syringe.

Giant cell arteritis must be considered for all patients over the age of 50. If any of the systemic features of this condition are present (headache, pain, and tenderness of proximal muscle groups, jaw claudication, fever, weight loss, scalp tenderness, or pulseless temporal arteries), or if the ESR is elevated, hydrocortisone 200 mg should be given intravenously and the patient investigated further (see page 32).

**Prognosis** Although treatment is occasionally beneficial if the patient presents within 24 hours, recovery of vision is rare. Patients have an increased risk of other cardiovascular disease, particularly myocardial infarction.

**Follow up and further treatment** If a paracentesis has been carried out the patient should be admitted and prophylactic antibiotic drops prescribed. All patients should be seen in an ophthalmology clinic within a few weeks for a review of the investigation results and management of identified risk factors.

Other forms of CRAO should be treated according to the aetiology.

## Optic neuritis and optic neuropathy

Although optic neuritis and optic neuropathy may present with severe loss of vision, they are more likely to cause loss of central field or blurring of vision, and are therefore discussed on page 54.

## Retinal detachment

Most retinal detachments present with partial rather than complete field loss so they are discussed on page 42.

## Vitreous haemorrhage

**Symptoms and signs** These can be from mild blurring with floaters to complete loss of vision depending on the amount of bleeding. Blood may accumulate within the substance of the vitreous or in the subhyaloid space between the vitreous and retina.

### Aetiology
- Retinal tears
- Ischaemic retinal neovascularisation:
    proliferative diabetic retinopathy
    BRVO (branch retinal vein occlusion)
    CRVO
    sickle cell retinopathy

- Abnormal retinal blood vessels:
    Angioma
    Macroaneurysm
- Intraocular tumours.

**Immediate management** First, establish the cause of the vitreous haemorrhage.

**History** Frequently the patient is known to have diabetes or sickle cell disease (SC or SThal are more likely to cause retinopathy than SS disease), or to have had a BRVO or CRVO. This does not exclude the possibility of a retinal tear.

**Examination** An RAPD indicates underlying retinal damage. The iris should be examined for rubeosis, indicating underlying retinal ischaemia. Both fundi should be examined because the fellow retina may provide clues to the underlying diagnosis. The indirect ophthalmoscope provides the best view through the haemorrhage.

**Ultrasonography** Unless ophthalmoscopy can confirm that the retina is not detached and that no tumour is present, the patient should have immediate ultrasonography to exclude these conditions.

**Follow up and treatment** Most vitreous haemorrhages are managed conservatively by waiting for several months for spontaneous reabsorption to occur, but immediate vitrectomy is required should a retinal detachment develop. Therefore funduscopy and ultrasound examinations should be repeated until the cause of the haemorrhage has been determined. Equally, if a retinal tear is strongly suspected vitrectomy should not be delayed. A suggested follow up plan is to review the patient at two days, one week, two weeks, one month, and thereafter at monthly intervals. (See also page 88 for management of vitreous haemorrhage.)

## Segmental loss of vision

The differential diagnosis of segmental visual field loss (box) is similar to that for loss of vision affecting the whole field (see Table 2.1). Within the affected field, vision may be mildly or severely reduced. Loss of acuity occurs if there is macular involvement.

# VISUAL LOSS

> **Causes of segmental visual field loss**
>
> **Vascular**
> Branch retinal artery occlusion
> "Branch" retinal vein occlusion
> Anterior ischaemic optic neuropathy
>
> **Mechanical**
> Retinal detachment

## *Differentiating features of the history*

### Onset
- Sudden onset visual loss—vascular aetiology
- Gradually enlarging field defect over hours to a few days—retinal detachment.

**Associated symptoms** A retinal detachment is often preceded by flashers and floaters.

## *Examination*

### Abnormal retina
- Multiple retinal haemorrhages mainly along a vein—branch retinal vein occlusion (Fig 2.9)
- Retinal pallor and arteriolar narrowing—branch retinal artery occlusion (BRAO) (Fig 2.10)
- Elevated, mobile retina—retinal detachment (see Fig 2.4).

### Abnormal disc
- Disc swelling—antrior ischaemic optic neuropathy (see Fig 2.5).

## Branch retinal vein occlusion (Fig 2.9)

### Symptoms and signs
- Sudden segmental loss of vision or ill defined blurring
- Loss of visual acuity occurs if the macula is affected
- Multiple haemorrhages in the area of retina drained by the occluded vein (Fig 2.9)
- Retinal oedema and cotton wool spots may also be present
- The occlusion may be seen to occur at the site of an arteriovenous crossing.

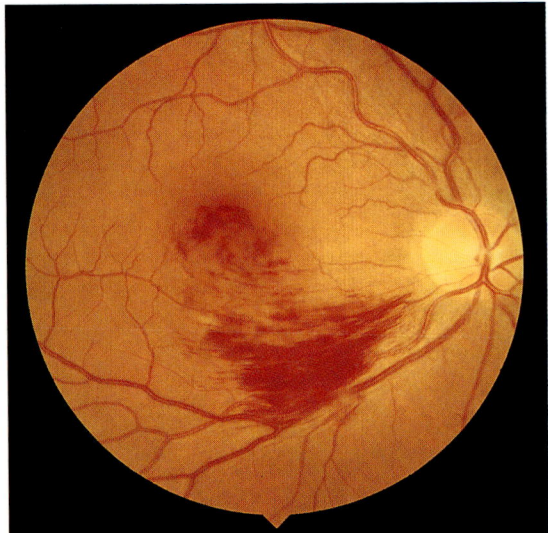

Figure 2.9 Branch retinal vein occlusion with involvement of the macula.

**Aetiology**
- Arteriosclerosis
- Systemic vasculitis.

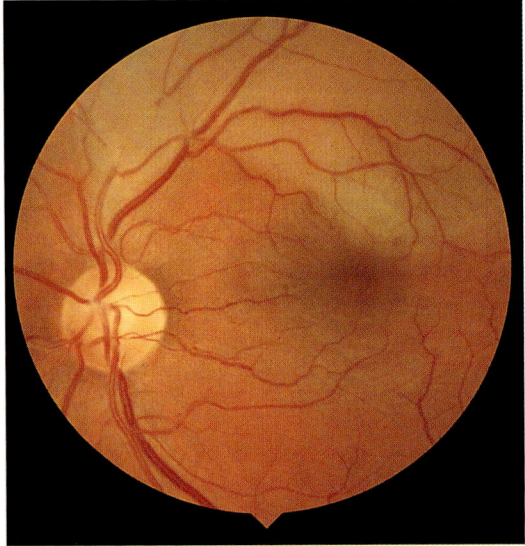

Figure 2.10 Branch retinal artery occlusion with resulting retinal oedema which has partially buried the retinal vessels.

## Investigations
- Full blood count
- ESR
- Glucose
- Lipid profile
- ANAs.

**Immediate management** BRVOs do not require immediate treatment.

**Prognosis** Visual acuity may be reduced by macular haemorrhage, oedema, or ischaemia. Over a period of several months spontaneous improvement occurs in one third to a half of affected eyes. Twenty per cent of BRVOs involving at least one retinal quadrant will develop neovascularisation and possibly vitreous haemorrhage. About 10% of patients will develop a BRVO in their other eye.

**Follow up and further treatment** Patients should be reviewed in an ophthalmology clinic initially every 2–3 months. At six months, if visual acuity has not spontaneously improved to better than 6/12, a fluorescein angiogram should be performed. If this shows that visual acuity is limited by oedema, laser photocoagulation to the oedematous macula (avoiding the fovea) may be beneficial. No treatment is available for macular ischaemia. If the angiogram shows large areas of peripheral ischaemia, the patient should be examined for neovascularisation every four months. If new vessels develop, laser photocoagulation should be applied to the ischaemic retina.

## Branch retinal artery occlusion (Fig 2.10)
### Symptoms and signs
- Sudden painless loss of visual field—90% involve the temporal retinal vessels
- Loss of visual acuity occurs if the fovea is affected
- The affected retina is pale (Fig 2.10)
- An embolus may be seen in the occluded arteriole.

**Aetiology and investigations** BRAOs and central retinal artery occlusions (CRAOs) are caused by the same range of systemic diseases (see section on CRAO for investigations).

**Immediate management** There is no treatment for a BRAO.

**Prognosis** About 80% of eyes retain or spontaneously regain an acuity of 6/12 or better.

**Follow up and further treatment** All patients should be seen in an ophthalmology clinic within a few weeks for a review of the results of the investigations and management of any identified risk factor.

### Anterior ischaemic optic neuropathy

Anterior ischaemic optic neuropathy (AION) may present with either complete or segmental visual loss. It is described on page 28.

### Retinal detachment

Separation of the retina from the retinal pigment epithelium (RPE) usually results from the development of a retinal tear.

#### Symptoms and signs
- Progressive loss of visual field
- Loss of visual acuity caused by macular involvement may occur within hours or may not occur for several months
- Patients frequently notice floaters and flashing lights (photopsia) before the onset of field loss
- A detached retina appears grey and slightly wrinkled
- Tears (frequently multiple) may be arrow shaped, circular, or long and irregular
- Brown RPE cells in the anterior vitreous indicate that a retinal hole is present.

#### Management
*Macula on* Immediate surgery, that is, the same day if possible, is necessary.

*Macula off* This should be managed as soon as possible and generally the sooner the better. However, where the macula has been off for some time a few days' wait will not affect the prognosis adversely. In case of delay admit the patient for rest in bed. There may be a call for rest and immobilisation of the eye by wearing slit spectacles until surgery is performed.

Depending on the configuration of the detachment, such surgery may include:

- Creating a chorioretinal scar around each break by laser or trans-scleral cryotherapy
- Using a silicone buckle (explant) to indent the sclera towards the breaks
- Draining subretinal fluid
- Injection of air or other gas into the vitreous cavity to press the retina against the retinal pigment epithelium
- Vitrectomy with intraocular repositioning of the retina.

**Prognosis** Well over 90% of retinas are successfully repositioned, but sometimes several operations may be required. Macula off detachments have a poorer visual prognosis than those in which the macula is still attached.

### Loss of central vision

Conditions that may cause a loss of central vision are listed in the box. Differentiating between them starts with determination of whether the disease process has affected the macula or the optic nerve.

---

**Common causes of loss of central vision**

*Degenerative*
  Age related macular degeneration
  Myopic macular degeneration
  Macular hole
*Vascular*
  Cilioretinal artery occlusion
*Inflammatory*
  Optic neuritis
*Infiltrative, compressive, inherited, nutritional*
  Optic neuropathy
*Idiopathic*
  Central serous retinopathy

## Macular versus optic nerve disease (Table 2.2)

### History

#### Effect on vision

- Positive scotoma is caused by macular disease—patients are constantly aware of an obstruction to the visual field.
- Negative scotoma is caused by optic nerve disease—patients are not constantly aware of an obstruction to the visual field, but only notice it when, for example, they try to read.
- Visual distorton (metamorphopsia), such as the apparent bending of straight lines, or a decrease (micropsia) or increase macropsia) in image size reflects a change in the relative position of the retinal photoreceptors and is characteristic of macular, rather than optic nerve, disease.
- Dimming of vision (reduced brightness perception) is a common symptom of optic nerve but not macular disease.

Table 2.2 Loss of central vision—differentiating features of macular and optic nerve causes

| Symptoms | Macular | Optic nerve |
| --- | --- | --- |
| Awareness | Positive scotoma | Negative scotoma |
| Metamorphopsia (distortion) | Usual | Absent |
| Micropsia or macropsia | Possible | Absent |
| Brightness perception | Not affected | Reduced |
| RAPD | Absent unless large lesion | Typical |
| Colour defect | Only if VA < 6/24 | Early |
| Maddox rod | Break | No break |
| Fundal appearance | Macula abnormal | Disc swelling or pallor |

VA, visual acuity.

### Examination

*Pupil reactions* Macular disorders do not cause an RAPD even if acuity is severely reduced, whereas an RAPD is characteristic of optic nerve disorders even if acuity is only mildly reduced.

*Colour vision* Loss of colour vision is an early sign of optic neuritis or neuropathy, but only occurs in macular disease when acuity is reduced to around 6/36.

### Differentiating between macular causes of loss of central vision

*Age* Central serous retinopathy typically occurs between the ages of 20 and 50. Mopic degeneration may also start in this age group, but the other macular conditions listed in the box typically affect older people.

# VISUAL LOSS

*Refraction* Eyes affected by myopic degeneration are usually at least −6·00 D myopic.

*Fundal appearance* Marked retinal pigment epithelial and choroidal degenerative changes indicate age related (Fig 2.11a, b) or myopic (see Fig 2.12) macular degeneration. The last usually also involves the peripapillary region. A central retinal hole with surrounding cuff of subretinal fluid indicates a macular hole (see Fig 2.13). A transparent blister of elevated retina indicates central serous retinopathy (see Fig 2.14). A pale macula associated with attenuated arteriole indicates cilioretinal artery occlusion (see Fig 2.15).

### Differentiating between optic neuritis and optic neuropathy

*Pain on eye movement* Optic neuritis typically causes periocular or retro-ocular pain which is exacerbated by eye movement. Although optic neuritis is (in retrospect) occasionally painless, patients should be investigated for causes of optic neuropathy.

### Age related macular degeneration (Fig 2.11)

Age related macular degeneration refers to a gradual degeneration of the macula involving the retina, pigment epithelium, Bruch's membrane, and choriocapillaris. It is the most common cause of visual loss in the over 75s and affects some 20% of individuals. Two patterns occur.

*Non-exudative ARMD*

For most patients with age related macular degeneration (ARMD), there is a gradual loss of receptors and pigment epithelium of the macula, presenting with patchy macular hyper- and hypopigmentation. Formation of drusen is also a feature. Eventually only large choroidal vessels may remain.

*Exudative ARMD* Less commonly, new vessels arising from the choroidal circulation grow through defects in Bruch's membrane to form a subretinal neovascular membrane (SRNVM). This may haemorrhage or cause a localised exudative retinal or RPE detachment. Subsequent fibrosis leads to the formation of a variable sized disciform scar.

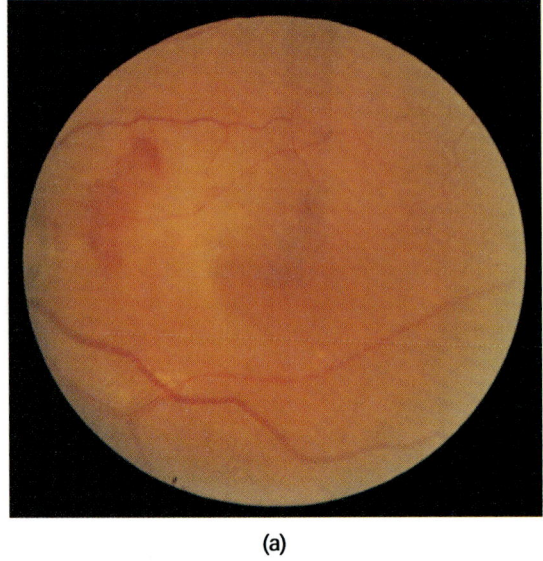

(a)

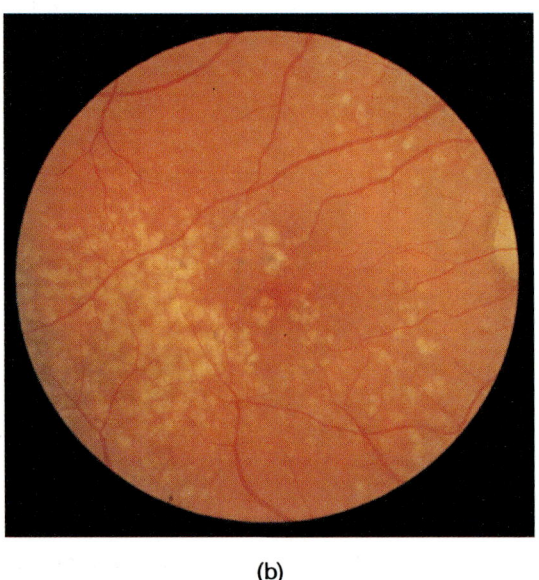

(b)

Figure 2.11 (a) Age related macular degeneration: subretinal neovascular membrane with haemorrhage; (b) non-exudative form with hard drusen.

### Symptoms and signs
***Non-exudative (see*** Fig 2.10)
- Gradual loss of central vision; patients often notice that they have to use a bright light to read and that the words tend to fade after a few minutes
- Small yellow–white spots: drusen
- Retinal pigment epithelial atrophy
- Pigment clumping.

***Exudative*** (see Fig 2.11)
- Sudden onset of central visual loss with distortion (or metamorphopsia)
- Drusen
- Retinal or subretinal haemorrhages
- Grey–yellow subretinal lesions: the SRNVM
- Focal elevation of the retina.

**Immediate management** Differentiating between non-exudative and exudative ARMD is important because, although there is no treatment for the non-exudative form, it runs a slow, albeit progressive course. The presence of an SRNVM may mean rapid progression and the membrane is treatable by laser in some instances, if it is not too near the fovea. If an SRNVM is suspected the patient should have an urgent fluorescein angiogram. Unfortunately, most membranes are not treatable because it is subfoveal, too extensive, or too ill defined. The limited scope of treatment should be made clear to the patient at the time of diagnosis in order not to raise false hopes.

**Prognosis** Both forms of ARMD are bilateral but often asymmetrical in onset. Although less common, exudative ARMD accounts for the majority of eyes with severe visual loss. The risk of developing SRNVM in the second eye is 10% per year. Non-exudative ARMD progresses gradually over a period of years. Peripheral, navigational vision is retained.

### Further management
- All patients with ARMD should be referred to an ophthalmology clinic to discuss their prognosis.
- As only early SRNVMs are treatable, patients should be provided with an Amsler chart and instructed in its use particularly if only one eye retains useful vision. They should

- be advised to return for review immediately if they detect any distortion or blurring in the fellow eye.
- Patients should also be referred to a low vision clinic where a variety of telescopes and magnifiers can be demonstrated.
- Eventually, blind or partial sight registration may be required to give social support.

Other causes of central SRNVM include presumed ocular histoplasmosis syndrome (POHS), idiopathic choroidal neovascularisation (CNV), and angioid streaks.

### Presumed ocular histoplasmosis syndrome
- Rare in the UK
- Endemic in the Ohio and Mississippi Valleys
- Age 25–50 years
- Otherwise, healthy people with no other symptoms.

**Associated signs** Punched out chorioretinal lesions in peripheral retina or peripapillary.

**Management** Laser treatment for extrafoveal membranes. Response to treatment and long term prognosis are better than for ARMD.

### Idiopathic CNV.

This is an arbitrary term used to describe the finding of an SRNVM wtihout an ARMD or associated condition.

### Angioid streaks
- SRNVM grows through the breaks in Bruch's membrane
- Cause of angioid streaks:
    pseudoxanthoma elasticum:
    Paget's disease of bone
    Ehler–Danlos syndrome
    sickle cell disease
    thalassaemia.

### Diagnosis and management
- Apart from the underlying disease, the diagnosis and management are the same as for SRNVM in ARMD
- Treatment is by laser if the membrane is not subfoveal
- Radiotherapy may be a possible treatment for subfoveal membrane which is undergoing clinical trials.

# VISUAL LOSS

**Myopic macular degeneration** (Fig 2.12)

Highly myopic eyes (> −8·00 D) frequently develop degenerative changes in the choroid and retina.

**Symptoms and signs** Central vision may be affected in two ways:

- It may gradually decline because of progressive macular chorioretinal atrophy.
- Cracks develop in Bruch's membrane through which choroidal vessels may grow. Haemorrhage from such vessels causes a sudden worsening of central vision giving rise to Fuchs' spot.

**Prognosis** With time severe bilateral central visual loss develops as a result of chorioretinal atrophy. Highly myopic individuals are also at risk of developing peripheral retinal holes which may progress to retinal detachment.

**Management** Although no treatment is available to arrest either the progressive enlargment of the globe or associated chorioretinal degenerative changes, patients should be referred to an ophthalmology clinic. This gives them another opportunity to

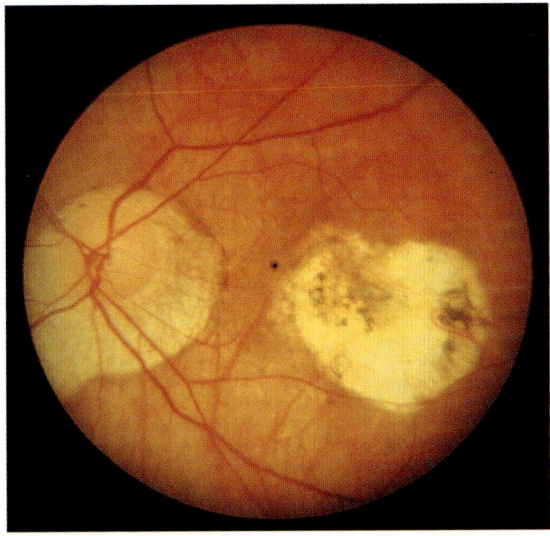

Figure 2.12  Myopic degeneration: peripapillary atrophy macular degeneration and thinning of the choroid and retina.

discuss their diagnosis and prognosis. They can also be examined for peripheral retinal holes. Patients should also be referred to a low vision clinic where a variety of telescopes and magnifiers can be demonstrated. Blind registration may eventually be required.

### Macular hole (Fig 2.13)

#### Symptoms and signs
- Gradual distortion of central vision or sudden discovery of poor vision
- Visual acuity is usually reduced to between 6/12 and 3/60
- Fundal examination reveals a central hole about one third of a disc diameter in size, which is surrounded by a cuff of subretinal fluid (see Fig. 2.13)
- Small yellow–white deposits may be seen at the base of the hole
- If a narrow slit beam is positioned across the hole, the patient may notice a gap in the light beam.

#### Aetiology
- Spontaneous—most common; probably caused by local vitreoretinal traction

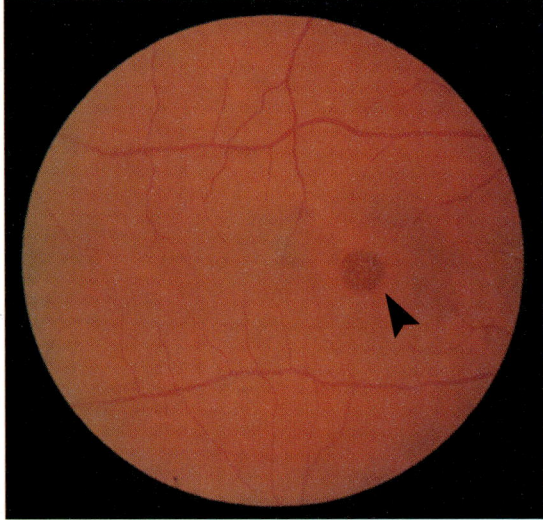

Figure 2.13  Macular hole: with cuff of detached retina and stippling at base of hole.

- High myopia
- Trauma.

**Prognosis** Vision usually remains between 6/36 and 3/60. Subsequent development of a retinal detachment is rare unless the eye is myopic. Macular holes will develop in about 10% of fellow eyes.

**Management** Patients, particularly those with early macular holes (acuity around 6/18), may benefit from surgery to relieve vitreoretinal traction. They should therefore be referred to a vitreoretinal surgeon.

### Central serous retinopathy (Fig 2.14)

Central serous retinopathy is a unilateral macular disorder of unknown aetiology which affects men nine times more commonly than women. As a result of focal damage to the retinal pigment epithelium, fluid accumulates beneath the retina forming a localised area of detachment.

#### Symptoms and signs
- Onset between the ages of 20 and 50
- Blurring of central vision
- Visual distortion (particularly micropsia)
- Visual acuity tends to be only mildly reduced but may range from 6/6 to 6/60
- Rare for acuity to be < 6/18
- Circular elevation of central retina is usually evident on ophthalmoscopy
- Transparent "blister" of elevated retina best seen on indirect ophthalmoscopy.

**Immediate management** If there is any doubt about the diagnosis a fluorescein angiogram should be performed. This will show characteristic fluorescein leakage through one or more defects in the retinal pigment epithelium (Fig 2.14b). No immediate treatment is required.

**Prognosis** Most episodes of central serous retinopathy heal spontaneously within three months. Up to 50% of patients will experience at least one recurrence.

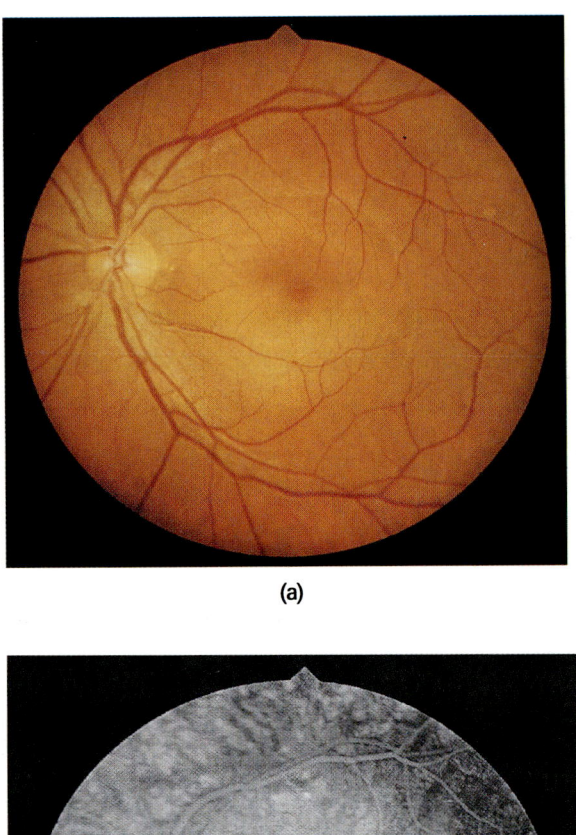

(a)

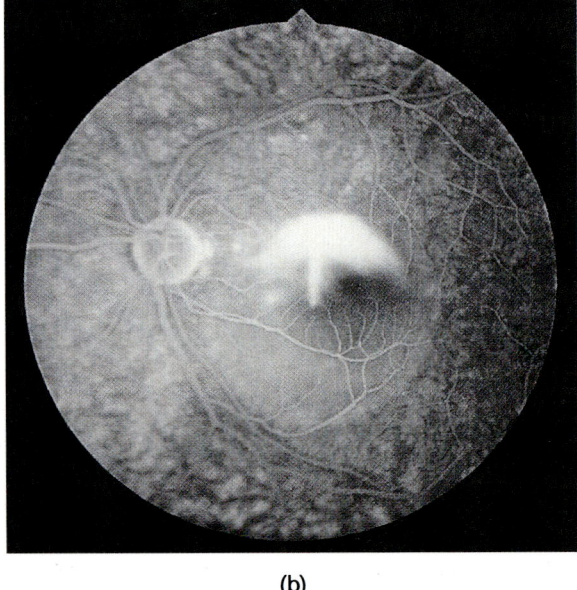

(b)

Figure 2.14  Central serous retinopathy: a bright reflex marks the edge of the elevated central retina with a fluorescein angiogram showing leakage through the pigment epithelium and the classic "smoke stack" sign.

# VISUAL LOSS

**Management** Patients should be reviewed in an ophthalmology clinic within a few weeks. In view of the high spontaneous resolution rate, treatment is not usually required. However, laser photocoagulation of the retinal pigment epithelium has been shown to promote resolution and decrease recurrence, and should be considered in persistent episodes.

## Cilioretinal artery occlusion (Fig 2.15)

Eleven per cent of eyes have a cilioretinal artery supplying a variable area of macula.

### Symptoms and signs
- Sudden loss of central vision
- Pallor of the retina adjacent to the artery.

**Aetiology and investigations** Predisposing factors are the same as for a CRAO (see page 35).

**Immediate management** No immediate treatment is required for a cilioretinal artery occlusion, but it is important to exclude giant cell arteritis as an underlying cause.

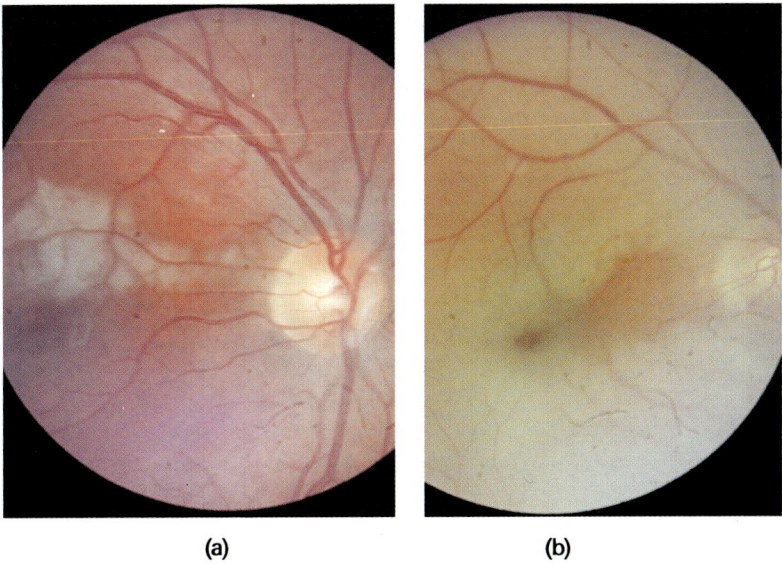

(a) (b)

Figure 2.15 (a) Cilioretinal artery occlusion showing retinal oedema of the papillomacular bundle; (b) cilioretinal sparing in central retinal artery occlusion.

**Prognosis** Most affected eyes will regain an acuity of at least 6/12 if there is no concurrent ischaemic optic neuropathy.

**Follow up and further treatment** All patients should be seen in an opthalmology clinic within a few weeks for a review of the investigation results and management of identified risk factors.

**Optic neuritis** Optic neuritis refers to inflammation of the optic nerve. Episodes are usually monocular, but may be bilateral particularly in children.

### Symptoms and signs
- Most common in adults between the ages of 20 and 40
- Progressive dimming of vision over a few days
- Periocular or retro-ocular pain which is exacerbated by eye movement
- Mild to severe loss of acuity
- Reduced colour perception
- An RAPD (or bilateral sluggish pupil responses to light if both nerves are affected)
- Visual field examination may show generalised contraction, a central scotoma, or an altitudinal defect
- The optic disc may be normal, but if the inflammation invoves the anterior part of the optic nerve it may cause disc swelling (Fig 2.16).

### Aetiology
- Demyelination: most adults with optic neuritis will develop multiple sclerosis; ask about previous or concurrent neurological dysfunction
- Viral infection
- Granulomatous inflammation (sarcoidosis, tuberculosis, syphilis)
- Adjacent sinusitis or meningitis
- Idiopathic.

**Prognosis** Within 2–3 weeks, vision starts to recover spontaneously, and over a period of several months only 13% fail to regain 6/12 acuity. In demyelination the optic neuritis treatment trial has demonstrated that oral steroids are ineffective at hastening visual recovery and predispose to further episodes. By contrast patients treated with intravenous methylprednisolone showed a modest reduction in the duration of visual loss, but no

VISUAL LOSS

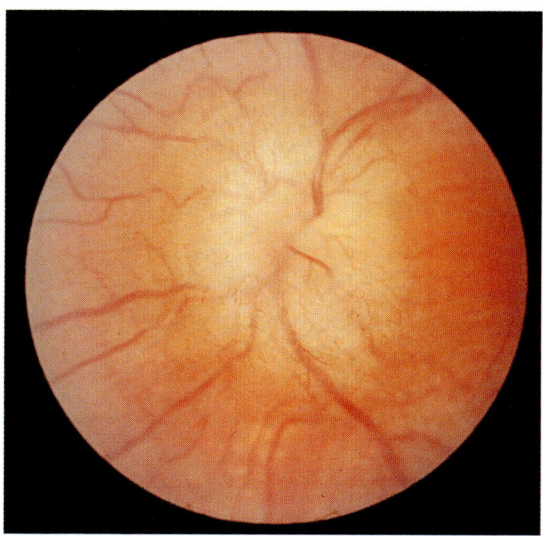

Figure 2.16  Optic neuritis showing disc oedema and dilated capillaries on surface of disc.

effect on final visual acuity. The same study also demonstrated that patients who had multiple periventricular white matter abnormalities on magnetic resonance imaging (MRI), who were treated with intravenous methylprednisolone, had a delayed onset of multiple sclerosis.

**Investigations** With a characteristic history and examination, investigations to establish the diagnosis are unnecessary. If there are any atypical features, however (for example, bilateral, painless, symptoms of a systemic disease or sinusitis), or if vision does not start to recover within three weeks of onset, the following investigations should be considered:

- Computed tomography or MRI for evidence of compressive or infiltrative lesions, sinusitis, or periventricular white matter abnormalities.
- Full blood count
- ESR
- VDRL/TPHA (Venereal Disease Research Laboratory/*Tregonema pallidum* haemagglutination) test
- ANAs
- Serum angiotensin-converting enzyme (sACE)
- Chest radiograph.

**Management** The association of optic neuritis with multiple sclerosis should not be discussed in the A&E department. Instead the patient should be referred to a neurologist or neuro-ophthalmologist for confirmation by further assessment and possible treatment.

### Optic neuropathy
#### Symptoms and signs
- Painless gradual or subacute visual loss
- Mild to severe loss of acuity
- Reduced colour perception
- An RAPD (or bilateral sluggish pupil responses to light if both nerves are affected)
- Visual field examination may show generalised contraction, a central scotoma, or an altitudinal defect
- The optic disc is pale or swollen but may be normal in early stages.

#### Aetiology
- Compression:
    orbital tumours—look for proptosis, limitation of ocular movement, and disc swelling
    intracranial tumours—look for a superotemporal field defect in the fellow eye
- Infiltrative:
    metastatic carcinoma
    lymphoma
    leukaemia
    sarcoidosis
- Inherited:
    autosomal dominant—bilateral mild to moderate visual loss in childhood
    autosomal recessive—bilateral severe visual loss in childhood
    mitochondrially inherited (Leber's optic neuropathy)—onset between the ages of 5 and 65, but usually in early adult life, with subacute visual loss and hyperaemic disc swelling; telangiectasis on or near the disc is characteristic
- Toxic:
    drugs commonly blamed: isoniazid, ethambutol, chloramphenicol, and chloroquine

- Nutritional:
  deficiencies of vitamins $B_1$, $B_2$, $B_6$, $B_{12}$, or folate "tobacco–alcohol amblyopia"
- Radiation:
  subacute unilateral or bilateral visual loss caused by vascular occlusion several months to years after radiation exposure; look for associated radiation retinopathy—haemorrhages, cotton wool spots, oedema, and neovascularisation.

**Immediate management** From the history it may be possible to identify the probable aetiology. The patient's past medical history, family history, medications, and systems enquiry are particularly important. Suspected medications should be withdrawn and the patient referred to a neuro-ophthalmologist or neurologist for investigation.

## Blurring of vision

In contrast to the other categories of visual loss, blurring of vision is not localised and may be caused by pathology anywhere from the cornea to the optic nerve. Therefore, it is essential to get an anatomical diagnosis first before considering the cause. Most patients will not be able to distinguish between general blurring and loss of central vision so the list of causes affecting central vision should also be considered (Tables 2.3 and 2.4).

### Differentiating features of the history
*Onset* Vitreous haemorrhage and occlusive vascular disease have a sudden onset. The other diagnoses listed in Table 2.3 develop more gradually.

### Differentiating features of the examination
*Pinhole acuity* If vision is improved by looking through a pinhole, then the blurring results at least partly from a refractive error. In retinal lesions (especially macular), visual acuity is reduced.

*Pupil reactions* Clouding or distortion of the optical media and focal retinal pathology do not cause an RAPD, but optic neuropathy and optic neuritis do.

Table 2.3  Anatomical causes

| | | | |
|---|---|---|---|
| 1 | Cornea and lens | Refractive change | |
| | | Loss of transparency | |
| 2 | AC and vitreous | Clouding | |
| 3 | Retinal disease | Macular | Inner retina, for example, cotton wool spots |
| | | Peripheral retinal involving macula | Outer retina, for example, choroiditis |
| 4 | Optic nerve | Swollen | |
| | | Pallor or atrophy | |
| | | Normal appearance | |
| | | Intra-disc changes | |

***Media opacities*** Opacification: cataract; these can be identified by slitlamp examination.

### *Abnormal retina*
- Hazy fundal view—vitreous haemorrhage or cataract
- Multiple retinal haemorrhages, especially if limited to distribution of veins—non-ischaemic CRVO (see Fig 2.7)
- Microaneurysms, haemorrhages, exudates, and oedema—diabetic retinopathy.

### *Abnormal disc*
- Disc swelling—occasionally caused by optic neuritis or optic neuropathy.

### *No ocular abnormality seen*
- Optic neuritis and optic neuropathy (but RAPD if unilateral).

**Refractive error**

Unlikely to present acutely but patient may self refer because of anxiety.

### Symptoms and signs
- Monocular or binocular blurring of vision without distortion
- Visual acuity improves with the use of a pinhole.

### Management
***Pinhole acuity 6/9 or better*** Exclude ocular diseases that may present with a refractive error, particularly:

- Keratoconus—look for corneal distortion or central thinning
- Early cataract or acquired myopia from undiagnosed diabetes mellitus

Table 2.4 Common causes of blurring of vision that are likely to present acutely

| Causes | Anatomical site | | | | | |
|---|---|---|---|---|---|---|
| | Cornea | Anterior chamber | Lens | Vitreous | Retina/choroid | Optic nerve |
| Refraction | | | Undiagnosed Diabetes mellitus | | | |
| Loss of transparency | Surface disease Keratopathy Corneal decompensation Scarring | Debris from iritis or blood | Cataract | Cells from inflammation or blood | | |
| Inflammation | Keratouveitis | Cells from debris | | Cells from: intermediate uveitis choroidoretinitis | Choroidoretinitis Retinitis | Neuritis |
| Vascular | | | | Blood | Occlusive disease Bleeding disease Diabetic retinopathy Abnormal permeability, e.g. CSR | |
| Infiltrative/compressive | | | | | Choroidal metastases | |
| Nutritional/inherited | | | | | | Optic neuropathy |
| Degeneration | | | | | ARMD | |

- Central serous retinopathy—the mild exudative macular detachment will make the eye hypermetropic by effectively shortening the eye's axial length, so a fundal examination is required.

After excluding any ocular pathology, those patients whose vision improves to at least 6/9 with a pinhole should be refracted. Follow up is only required if spectacles do not restore normal vision.

### Pinhole acuity 6/12 or worse
This indicates that the refractive error is not the only cause of reduced vision, so a full ocular assessment is required. Even if no other diagnosis is apparent, patients should be referred to an ophthalmology clinic for review.

## Cataract
Cataract is the most common non-refractive cause of visual impairment.

### Symptoms and signs
- Misting or blurring of vision
- Glare caused by scattering of light
- Change in refraction: commonly a progressive myopia which causes previously emmetropic patients difficulty with distance vision, but enables them to read once again without spectacles
- Reduction or distortion of the red reflex
- Focal or diffuse opacification of the lens.

### Aetiology
- Age related—increasingly common after the age of 50
- Congenital
- Familial
- Metabolic—particularly diabetes mellitus
- Traumatic.

**Immediate management** The high prevalence of mild lens opacities in the elderly population makes it necessary to exclude other causes of visual loss. Thus, for example, a history of sudden visual loss or an RAPD is not compatible with a diagnosis of cataract. If retinal examination is prevented by lens opacification, ultrasonography of the eye should be performed.

**Further management** Patients should be referred to an ophthalmology clinic for assessment. If vision improves significantly with a pinhole the patient should be refracted and new spectacles prescribed. When vision is no longer adequate (this varies from person to person) surgery is required.

### Vitreous haemorrhage
See pages 86–8.

### Diabetic retinopathy

Diabetic retinopathy is a microvascular complication of diabetes mellitus resulting in capillary closure and abnormal permeability. It is still the most common cause of blind registration for patients between the ages of 20 and 65. Its major risk factors are duration and control of diabetes. Vision may be impaired because of oedema in maculopathy or proliferative disease causing vitreous haemorrhage or macular traction. Diabetic maculopathy is more common and affects predominantly patients with type II or non-insulin dependent diabetes. In spite of public awareness and screening programmes, diabetic maculopathy is still a fairly frequent presentation of diabetes in the elderly population.

#### Symptoms and signs
- Blurring of vision—gradual onset in maculopathy
- Sudden drop in vision if haemorrhage from proliferative retinopathy
- Background lesions are retinal microaneurysms and haemorrhages (dots and blots), exudates, and cotton wool spots
- Proliferative retinopathy comprises new vessels of fibrous tissue and these may arise from vessels of the disc or the peripheral retina
- Maculopathy will have background lesions plus macular oedema, best observed with slitlamp either with a 90 D lens or contact lens but suggested by the absence of a foveal reflex on direct ophthalmoscopy.

**Prognosis** Untreated, diabetic maculopathy will eventually cause severe visual loss. Focal laser treatment is effective at halting or reversing progression, particularly when vision is only mildly affected.

**Management** Known diabetic individuals with maculopathy should be referred to an ophthalmology clinic within a few weeks. Patients with a vitreous haemorrhage should be referred urgently for fuller assessment or treatment. When typical features of diabetic maculopathy are found in someone who is not known to be diabetic, a random blood glucose should be measured (BM Stix and venous sample) and the patient's general practitioner informed of the result.

### Non-ischaemic central retinal vein occlusion

See page 33.

### Optic neuritis and optic neuropathy

See page 54.

## Homonymous hemianopia

A homonymous hemianopic field defect indicates damage to optic tract (rare), lateral geniculate body (very rare), optic radiation (common), or occipital cortex (common) on the side opposite to that of the field loss. The possible causes of such a field defect are shown in the box.

Although a homonymous hemianopia is usually obvious on confrontation testing, accurate plotting of the visual fields with a perimeter may help to localise the site of the lesion. If the hemianopia is incomplete, the following patterns of field loss may be observed:

---

### Causes of a homonymous hemianopia

*Vascular lesions*
   Thrombosis
   Embolus
   Haemorrhage
   Vasospasm
   Hypotension
*Tumours*
   Primary
   Metastatic
*Inflammatory lesions*

- Temporal lobe lesions cause predominantly upper field loss
- Parietal lobe lesions cause predominantly lower field loss
- The blood supply to the tip of the occipital lobe is derived either from the middle cerebral artery or from a more distal branch of the posterior cerebral artery to that which supplies its medial surface. Thus the macular field may be selectively spared or involved after a vascular event in this area.

**Symptoms and signs** Patients may complain that they are unaware of things approaching from the side of the field defect. They may also report difficulty with reading because either they cannot follow a line of text or they cannot find the next line. Speed of onset and history of cardiovascular or malignant disease may help to identify the aetiology.

Visual acuity is usually only mildly reduced in both eyes because at least half of the cortical representation of each macula is intact. While reading the Snellen chart, however, a patient may not see the letters on the side of the chart corresponding to the patient's field defect. Colour vision is unaffected and an RAPD will not be present.

**Management** Patients should be referred to a neurologist for further investigation.

## Bitemporal hemianopia

Bitemporal field loss usually indicates chiasmal pathology or bilateral retinal disease. Most chiasmal lesions result from compression by tumours arising from adjacent structures (see box). Such tumours usually cause a gradual deterioration of the visual fields but a sudden worsening can occur if they rapidly increase in size as a result of internal haemorrhage.

It is important to be aware of the variety of field defects that can be caused by a tumour in the region of the optic chiasma:

- Posterior chiasmal compression causes predominantly inferotemporal loss
- Anterior chiasmal compression causes principally superotemporal loss
- The field defects are usually asymmetrical and may be confined to macular fibres

> **Causes of chiasmal compression**
>
> Pituitary adenoma
> Meningioma
> Craniopharyngioma
> Aneurysm

- Compression of an adjacent optic nerve may cause a central field defect in one eye and a temporal field defect the other.

**Symptoms and signs** Patients may complain of blurring of the temporal fields, difficulty with driving, or that objects immediately beyond fixation are not seen. For example, cutting fingernails may be difficult because, while looking at the scissors, the patient cannot see the fingers. Vertical steps in the binocular visual field may occur with severe temporal field loss because each occipital lobe is receiving information from only one eye. Reduced acuity or colour perception, and a relative afferent pupil defect in one eye, suggest concurrent optic nerve involvement.

Fundal examination may reveal mild bilateral optic disc pallor resulting from loss of optic nerve fibres. Frequently, however, the fundi appear normal.

Tumours around the chiasma may also cause pituitary dysfunction and oculomotor cranial nerve palsies. The patient should therefore be asked about diplopia and symptoms suggestive of a pituitary endocrine abnormality, and ocular movements should be examined.

**Management** Patients should be referred to a neurologist for further investigation.

# 3 Transient visual loss

Transient visual loss refers to temporary visual impairment of variable duration lasting from seconds to hours. Typically, episodes have an abrupt onset, progressing over a few seconds to involve the whole or part of one or both visual fields. Within the affected area vision may be dimmed or completely lost. Sight usually returns within seconds or minutes but, exceptionally, attacks may last several hours. The range of possible aetiologies is large and is listed in the box. As many of the conditions are treatable, transient visual loss requires immediate investigation and prompt action to prevent irreversible loss of function.

---

**Causes of transient visual loss**

*Vascular*
Thromboembolic: carotid artery disease, cardiac, vertebrobasilar
Carotid occlusion: slow flow retinopathy
Vasculitis: giant cell arteritis, systemic lupus erythematosus, pararteritis nodosa, rheumatoid arthritis

*Neurological*
Papilloedema
Migraine: ocular, classic

*Ocular*
Angle closure glaucoma
Hyphaema
Optic disc anomalies: drusen, coloboma
Retrobulbar tumour

*Haematological*
Hyperviscosity: polycythaemia, thrombocythaemia, multiple myeloma
Coagulopathies
Anaemia

## Initial diagnosis

Thromboembolic disease is the most common cause of transient visual loss and, if an alternative diagnosis cannot be made, the patient should undergo cardiovascular investigation. At presentation there are four important causes:

- Giant cell arteritis
- Intermittent angle closure glaucoma
- Slow flow retinopathy
- Papilloedema.

These can be either diagnosed or excluded (Table 3.1).

Table 3.1 Key features of common or important causes of transient visual loss

| Diagnosis | Key findings |
| --- | --- |
| Giant cell arteritis | Age > 50, ± systemic symptoms, ± raised ESR, ± disc swelling |
| Intermittent angle closure glaucoma | Shallow angles, ± aching pain |
| Slow flow retinopathy | Peripheral haemorrhages, narrow arterioles, central retinal arteriole pulsation with minimal pressure on the globe |
| Papilloedema | Swollen discs |
| Thromboembolic disease | Normal fundus ± peripheral embolus |

## History

A complete ocular and systemic history is essential in the assessment of transient visual loss because ocular examination is often normal. The following are of particular importance.

### Is the visual loss in one or both eyes?

Observant patients will have noticed this but, more often, patients may not be sufficiently aware to be certain.

Beware of the error of confusing homonymous hemianopia with monocular loss. Retinal embolisation from carotid artery disease typically produces monocular transient visual loss ("amaurosis fugax"). The loss is often described as a shutter being lowered or raised.

## Duration of each attack

This may vary but typical patterns are as follows:

- Embolic disease—seconds to minutes
- Migraine—minutes
- Papilloedema—seconds and related to posture
- Glaucoma—minutes to hours.

   Often the causes are variable but usually last over 30 seconds.

## Precipitating factors

- Posture—standing up for papilloedema and systemic hypotension
- Turning the head for carotid artery disease
- Eye movements in some tumours of the orbit
- Eating chocolate as trigger factor for migraine.

## Associated symptoms

   Current or previous symptoms include:

- Other neurological deficit in thromboembolic disease
- Headache in papilloedema and giant cell arteritis
- Visual aura and other symptoms in migraine
- Haloes around lights in congestive glaucoma.

## Risk factors for cardiovascular disease

- Smoking
- Raised BP
- Diabetes mellitus and hyperlipidaemia.

# Examination

   Full ocular and cardiovascular examinations are required.

## Visual function assessment

   This should include:

- visual acuity
- visual field
- pupil reactions.

Most cases will have negative findings but a number of cases of transient visual loss may leave permanent visual loss of which the patient is unaware. For example, papilloedema causes enlarged blind spots.

### Anterior segment

- Depth of anterior chamber (AC) for narrow angle glaucoma—use a gonioscope if in doubt
- Measure intraocular pressure (IOP)
- Look for causes of transient obstruction of the visual axis, for example, soft lens matter occluding pupil after cataract surgery
- Or sources of spontaneous hyphaema—for example, iris clip lens or AC intraocular lens.

### Posterior segment

- Retinal vessels for patterning and signs of old embolism
- Disc for swelling, atrophy, or drusen
- Retina for peripheral haemorrhages:
    midperipheral haemorrhage in slow flow retinopathy
    scattered punctate haemorrhage in preretinal vein occlusion
- Retinal tear with shifting fluid in posterior pole (rare).

### Cardiovascular system

- Pulse and rhythm
- BP
- Carotid auscultation
- Cardiac auscultation
- Peripheral pulse when indicated.

## Investigations

The erythrocyte sedimentation rate (ESR) should be measured immediately for all patients. A high ESR in patients over the age of 50 strongly suggests giant cell arteritis, whereas in younger patients it may be associated with other vasculitic causes of transient visual loss.

Doppler studies are needed for carotid stenosis. Angiography is carried out only if carotid surgery is being considered.

## Management of specific conditions
### Giant cell arteritis
#### General features
- Malaise, weight loss, fever
- Headaches and scalp tenderness; classically painful to put head on pillow
- Pain on chewing in severe cases and jaw claudication
- Aches and pains from polymyalgia.

#### Ocular features—non-pulsatile temporal late stage arteritis
- Ischaemic optic neuropathy
- Central retinal artery occlusion on moving eyes
- Diplopia from nerve palsy
- No signs in early stage.

#### Diagnosis
- ESR typically >80
- Temporal artery biopsy to demonstrate focal arteritis with giant cells.

#### Management
- Immediate intravenous injection of hydrocortisone 200 mg
- Oral steroids to be started at the same time
- Admission for biopsy and control of arteritis.

See also section on ischaemic optic neuropathy (page 28).

### Intermittent angle closure glaucoma
**Symptoms** Symptoms of transient visual loss caused by intermittent angle closure glaucoma are usually accompanied by the following:

- Eye ache and headache
- Haloes and lights
- Intermittent blurring of vision.

#### Signs
- Shallow anterior chamber (Fig 3.1)
- Positive van Herrick's sign where the peripheral cornea is in contact with the iris
- Raised intraocular pressure (IOP) is not always present except during an attack.

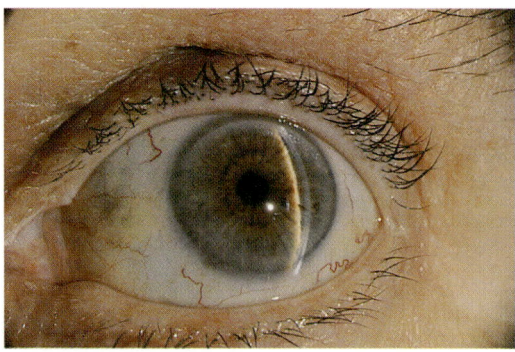

Figure 3.1 Shallow anterior chamber: note that the already shallow anterior chamber tapers at the limbus where the cornea and the iris appear to touch.

**Diagnosis** Demonstrate narrow or closed angle by gonioscopy. (See Chapter 5 for full account.)

### Management
- Medical therapy to lower pressures or as adjunct:
  acetazolamide (Diamox)
  miotics—pilocarpine
  β blockers
  osmotic agents (see Chapter 5)
- Laser—urgent iridotomies to relieve acute attack.

### Slow flow retinopathy (Fig 3.2)

Slow flow retinopathy is caused by severe stenosis of the carotid circulation. It may be monocular or binocular.

### Symptoms and signs
- Intermittent blurring or loss of vision; residual blurred vision may occur because of retinal ischaemia
- Photopsia
- Midperipheral retinal haemorrhage
- Cotton wool spots
- Marked arterial attenuation and mild venous dilatation
- Occasionally new vessels on disc and vitreous haemorrhage (Fig 3.2)
- Low perfusion pressure in artery results in closure of artery with minimally applied pressure.

# TRANSIENT VISUAL LOSS

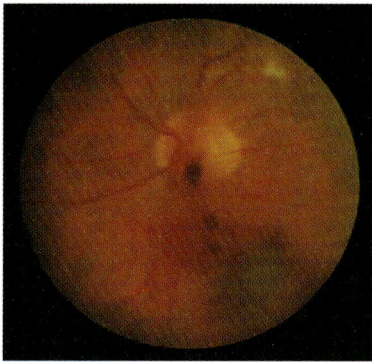

Figure 3.2   Slow flow retinopathy: showing cotton wool spot haemorrhage from disc vessel in a patient with almost complete obstruction of both carotids. Peripheral paravenous haemorrhages are not shown.

**Management** This is similar to that for transient visual loss caused by thromboembolic disease (see below).

### Papilloedema (Fig 3.3)

Transient visual loss associated with papilloedema characteristically lasts for a few seconds and usually affects one eye at a

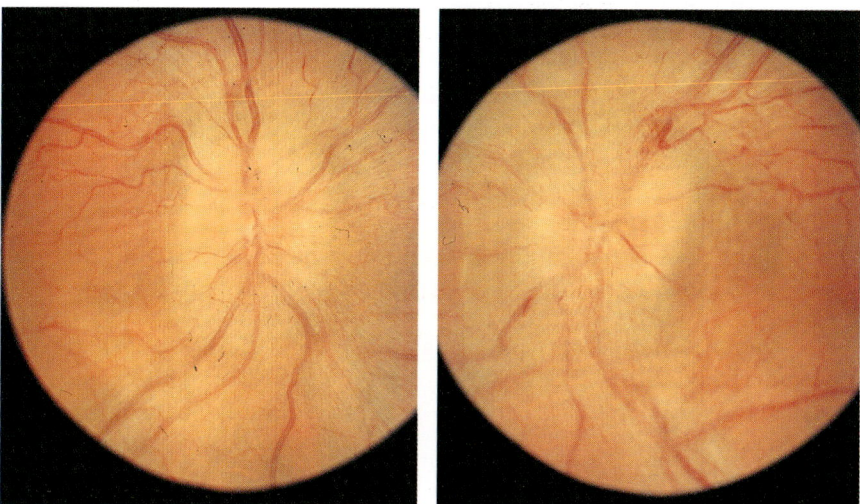

Figure 3.3   Papilloedema in raised intracranial pressure: the disc margins are blurred, the vessels emerging from the disc are partly buried, and the capillaries on the nerve head are congested.

time. Recurrences and repeated episodes are the rule. Visual loss may be precipitated by alterations of posture and can often be reproduced by gentle pressure on the globe. Other features of raised intracranial pressure may be elicited, including headache, which is typically worse in the morning and exacerbated by coughing or changes in posture, nausea, or vomiting, and horizontal diplopia caused by cranial nerve VI palsies.

### Signs
- Swollen and hyperaemic discs
- Overlying capillaries and dilated peripapillary flame shaped haemorrhages
- Engorged retinal veins—no spontaneous venous pulsation.

### Differential diagnosis
*Bilateral drusen of optic nerve head*
- Nodule on surface
- Spontaneous venous pulsation
- No venous engorgement
- Autofluorescence
- Typical appearance on computed tomography or ultrasonography.

*Other causes of disc swelling*
- Papillitis or optic neuritis—visual acuity usually decreased
- Malignant hypertension—BP increased
- Central retinal vein occlusion (CRVO)—rarely bilateral—peripheral retinal haemorrhage
- Infiltrations of optic nerve head:
    granuloma, for example, sarcoid
    neoplasia, for example, leukaemia
- Uveitis—signs of inflammation—commonly affects only one eye. No congestion of vessels and seldom bilateral.

**Management** Urgent investigation is needed to establish the underlying cause. Blood pressure must be measured to exclude malignant hypertension, and the patient referred for neurological assessment.

Treatment is that of the cause, although if cause is pseudotumour cerebri, then treatment may include the following:

- Acetazolamide and /or frusemide
- Repeated lumbar punctures

# TRANSIENT VISUAL LOSS

- Fenestration of optic nerve
- Peritoneal shunts.

## Thromboembolic disease

Transient thrombosis or embolism associated with atheromatous disease of the internal carotid or ophthalmic arteries accounts for most cases of monocular transient visual loss. Such cases were previously said to have "amaurosis fugax" or "fleeting blindness". Less commonly, they may be caused by emboli originating from the heart or proximal vessels. The risk of subsequent stroke, at 3–5% per annum, is five times greater than in an age matched population and 30% of patients will have a myocardial infarction within five years.

Concurrent neurological symptoms are rare but there may be a history of previous transient or permanent neurological deficits within the distribution of the carotid arteries. Retinal emboli, when present, are diagnostic.

Episodes of transient visual loss resulting from ischaemia in the vertebrobasilar circulation are binocular and usually less than a minute in duration. They may be associated with other features of brainstem ischaemia such as drop attacks, dysarthria, and vertigo.

### Symptoms
- Transient loss of vision usually lasts seconds to minutes; impairment lasts a little longer, up to 20 min
- Loss of vision may begin as if a curtain was drawn up or down the field of vision and recovery has the reverse effect.

### Signs
- Old emboli in peripheral arterial tree
- No signs if the cause is platelet emboli which pass through the circulation.

**Management** The investigation and treatment of transient visual loss resulting from a thromboembolism are ideally coordinated by someone (possibly a neurologist, cardiologist, ophthalmologist, or vascular surgeon) who has an interest in this field. The aims of treatment are to reduce the risks of subsequent stroke and myocardial infarction. The approach to treatment can be summarised as follows.

Carotid endarterectomy improves survival for patients with

severe carotid stenosis (70–99% reduction in diameter). Therefore patients experiencing monocular transient visual loss, and who are fit for surgery, should be screened for such a lesion. Contraindications include recent myocardial infarction and unstable angina, but age alone should not necessarily be considered a limiting factor. The initial screening investigation is likely to be carotid duplex ultrasonography, which may be followed by angiography. There is no equivalent surgical procedure for vertebrobasilar stenosis so angiography is not required for binocular transient visual loss.

Aspirin 300 mg per day has been shown to reduce the risk of non-fatal stroke by 30% after transient visual loss caused by thromboembolism. There is no definite evidence that anticoagulation with either warfarin or heparin is of benefit.

All patients require a cardiac assessment looking for ischaemia and sources of emboli. Investigations will include an ECG and echocardiograpy.

Cardiovascular risk factors such as smoking, hypertension, diabetes, and hyperlipidaemia should be reviewed.

Therefore, while in the A&E department, the following baseline investigations should be arranged: full blood count, urgent ESR, plasma glucose and lipids, and ECG. Carotid duplex ultrasonography and echocardiography can later be requested by the specialist. Patients should be advised to stop smoking and started on aspirin (unless they have a history of allergy or peptic ulceration).

## Other causes of transient visual loss

- Transient visual loss is an unusual presentation for a *retrobulbar tumour* but it should be considered if episodes are precipitated by eye movement.
- Patients with a spontaneous hyphaema should be referred to an ophthalmology clinic for investigation.
- Optic disc drusen and colobomas may be coincidental findings, so other causes of transient visual loss must be ruled out (Fig 3.4).
- Vasculitis other than giant cell arteritis may occasionally cause transient visual loss. If there are any suggestive symptoms or signs, such as arthritis, skin rashes, and Raynaud's phenomenon, the antinuclear antibody titre and rheumatoid factor should be measured.

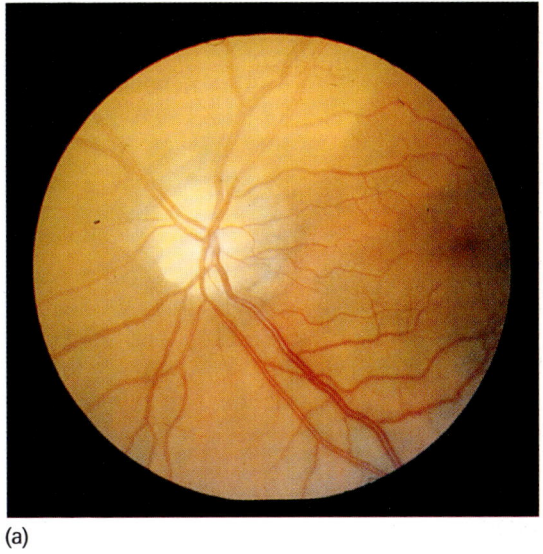

(a)

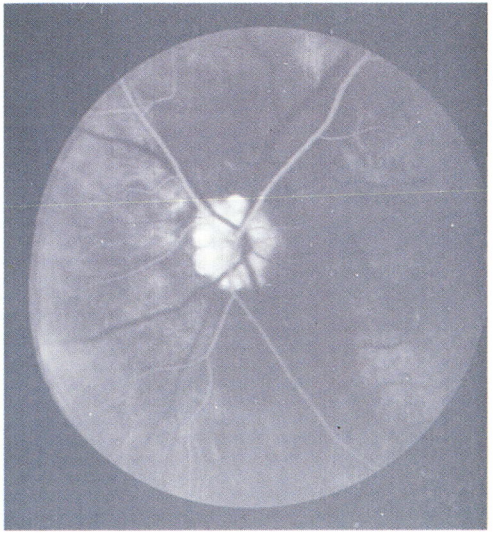

(b)

Figure 3.4  Disc drusen: (a) glistening grape like nodules best seen on nasal side; (b) autofluorescence (same eye) in blue light.

- Coagulopathies are an uncommon cause of transient visual loss, but should be considered in young patients and those with known malignancy. Screening for the lupus anticoagulant and coagulation factor abnormalities may be indicated.
- Hyperviscosity syndromes and anaemia will be detected by a full blood count and ESR.
- Migraine: there are no distinguishing features of monocular transient visual loss resulting from ocular migraine. In particular, headache does not always occur with this type of migraine and occasionally accompanies transient visual loss caused by thromboembolic disease. The diagnosis of ocular migraine must therefore be one of exclusion. When the transient visual loss is binocular and associated with headache, migrating scintillations, and a family history of migraine, the diagnosis of classic migraine is almost certain. If there are any atypical features other causes of occipital ischaemia should be considered.

# 4 Flashes and floaters

## Floaters

Patients may complain of "spots", "flies", or a "cobweb" in front of the eye.

### Causes of floaters

*Mechanical*
 Posterior vitreous detachment (PVD)
 Retinal tear

*Vascular*
 Vitreous haemorrhage

*Inflammation*
 Intermediate and posterior uveitis

*Neoplastic*
 Infiltrates, leukaemia (rare)

*Idiopathic*
 Muscae volitantes

Both retinal tear and PVD are common and both may present in the same way. In the absence of obvious alternatives it is important to exclude a retinal tear.

## History

The following are important points to establish:

- Establish that spots are floaters by asking if the spots have a motion independent of eye movement. Vitreous opacities will move with the eye but will continue to move from inertia when the eye stops.
- Ascertain the shape and size of the spots:

large spots are usually blood clots
  small spots are cells which may be white blood cells (WBCs), red blood cells (RBCs), or pigment epithelial cells
  filaments, "cobwebs", or ill defined shapes are usually elements on the posterior vitreous face or in the gel.
- Onset:
  sudden onset in a matter of minutes or seconds usually means a PVD, retinal tear, or haemorrhage
  if floaters appear after flashing lights a retinal tear must be excluded
  inflammatory cells are built up slowly.
- Duration: myopic patients will have had similar floaters for a long time.
- Ask about current systemic disease, for example, diabetes and systemic hypertension are strongly associated with vitreous haemorrhage and sarcoid with ocular inflammation.
- Other known ocular conditions may explain the symptoms, for example, myopia for "muscae volitantes", vein occlusion for neovascularisation, and toxoplasmosis for choroiditis.

## Examination

The aim is to determine the following:

- Whether there are abnormal vitreous opacities
- What the nature of the opacities or "floaters" is
- The source of origin.

Key manoeuvres in the examination are shown in the box.

See Fig 4.3 for the scheme of steps in management.

## Diagnosis and management of specific conditions
### *Posterior vitreous detachment*

The type of patient is aged 50 and over, although could be younger if myopic.

### Symptoms
- Flashing lights on rising or in the dark
- Usually unilateral but may be bilateral
- Seen as "arcs" or crescents and could be in any field; the position of the flashing has no localising value

# FLASHES AND FLOATERS

## Key manoeuvres in examination

- Check visual function (which should have been done at the beginning) and cross check by doing relative afferent pupil response, especially if the media are little cloudy and vision is reduced
- Look at the red reflex with a direct ophthalmoscope; opacities stand out in silhouette
- Slitlamp biomicroscopy:
  Look at the anterior vitreous for cells
    RBC and pigment cells are often difficult to differentiate although pigment cells tend to be bigger and look like "tobacco dust"
    RBCs seldom occur without a trace of frank blood in the retina or vitreous especially inferiorly
  Look for the presence of a PVD
  Look at the posterior vitreous face with a 90 D (or equivalent) lens and look for a Weiss ring which confirms a PVD (Figs 4.1 and 4.2)
- Examine the peripheral fundus with a binocular indirect ophthalmoscope for complete inspection of the periphery—with indentation if necessary
- Inspect any suspicious areas with the three mirror lens, which gives better magnification but does not go as far to the periphery
- Look at the fellow eye for bilateral disease
- Use ultrasonography if visualisation is poor

---

- Often difficult to describe but dramatic and alarming to patient
- Less dramatic forms tend to be recurrent (if vitreous detachment was incomplete)
- Floaters described as spots or a spider.

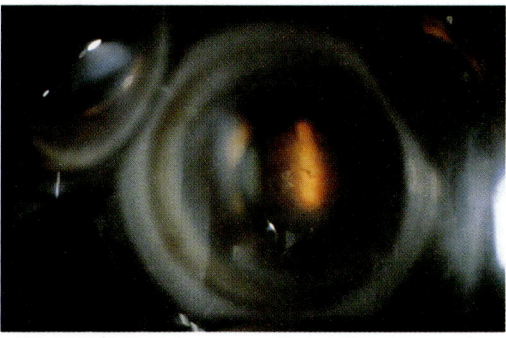

Figure 4.1  Posterior vitreous face and a Weiss ring in PVD, photographed through a three mirror contact lens.

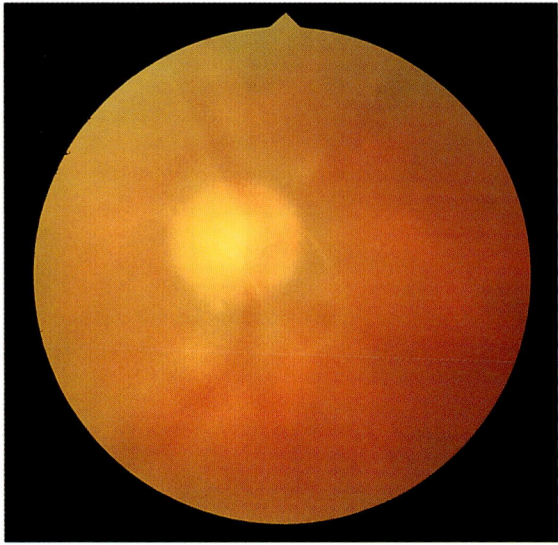

Figure 4.2  Weiss ring photographed by a fundus camera focused anteriorly (hence retinal details out of focus).

### Associations
- Myopia
- Blunt trauma.

### Differential diagnosis
- Retinal tear with or without retinal detachment
- Other retinal pathology, for example, degeneration
- Migraine—typical history and negative examination
- Retinal neovascularisation with small haemorrhages
- Vitritis—history of uveitis and non-pigmented cells.

### Management
- Exclude retinal pathology
- PVD may be on going: see again if symptoms worse or if there is loss of vision or field
- Treat retinal pathology accordingly:
    flat holes by laser if located posterior or cryotherapy if near the ora serrata
    detachment by surgery
    degenerative retina by watching or ablation.

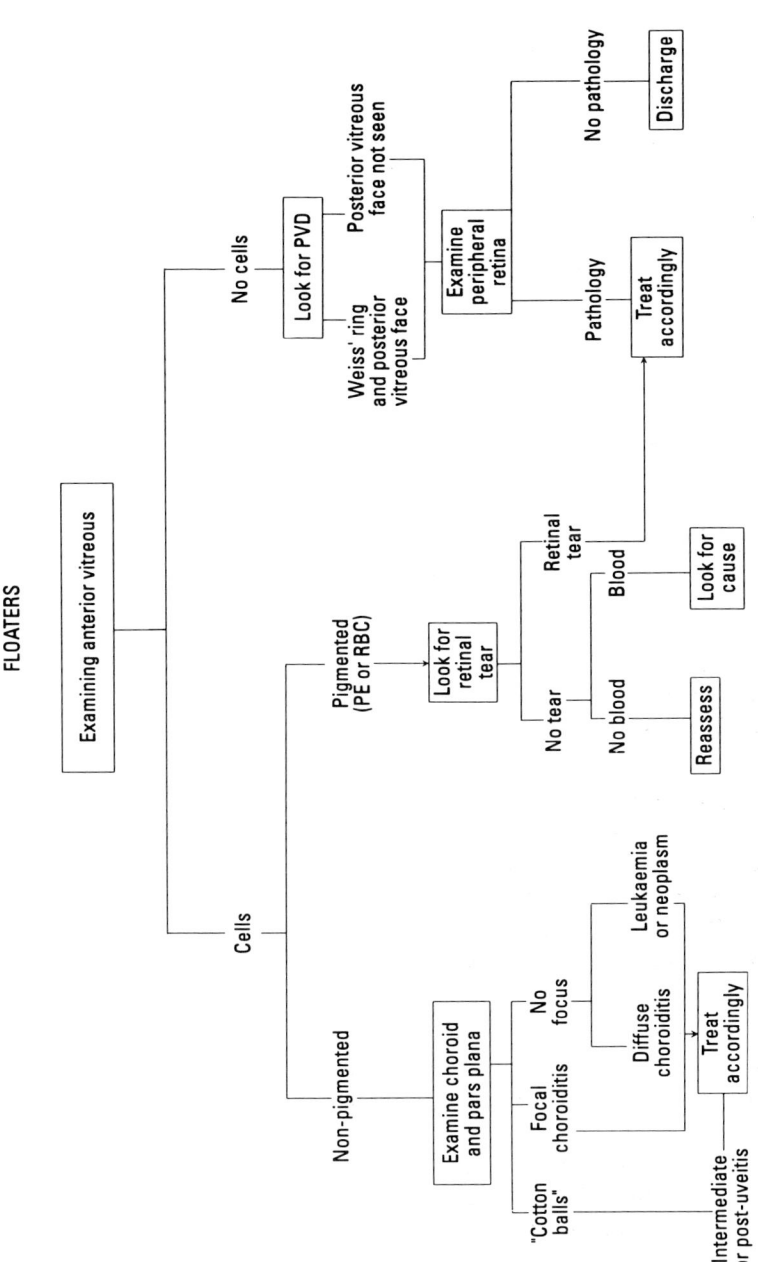

Figure 4.3 Steps in management of floaters. PE, pigment epithalium.

## Retinal tear

### Symptoms
- May be indistinguishable from those of PVD
- Floaters often more pronounced if there is a lot of blood
- Often, flashes cease when floaters appear.

### Signs
- Pigment cells in vitreous (or anterior vitreous)
- Blood in inferior vitreous or inferior part of fundus
- Haemorrhage at the edge of the tear
- Visible tear often "U" or tongue shaped (Fig 4.4).

### Associated features
- Myopia
- Previous tear or detachment in fellow eye
- Previous retinal scarring.

### Management
- Without retinal detachment:
    laser: if tear is accessible
    cryotherapy: if anterior edge of the tear is too peripheral to be reached by laser (unless indirect delivery is available)

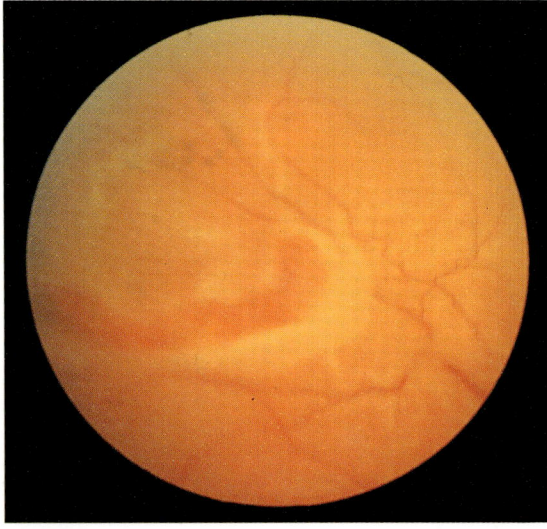

Figure 4.4  A large "U" tear of the retina with surrounding detachment—note wrinkling of vessels in the detached retina posterior to the tear.

- With associated retinal detachment:
  buckling procedure and cryotherapy
  other detachment procedure
- Macula on—immediate admission and surgery
- Macula off—planned surgery when possible.

## Other causes of floaters

### Vitreous opacities: muscae volitantes

This is a common complaint in patients with moderate or high myopia. Symptoms usually start at an early age and may worsen with time.

**Symptoms** Moving spots, best seen against a light background. Symptoms usually in excess of findings which are frequently negative apart from a mobile vitreous. This is the result of ability of myopic individuals to form images of small opacities within the eye.

**Signs** Fluid vitreous or syneresis which is liquefaction of the vitreous followed by cavitation. This is not an easy sign to pick up and requires dark adaptation and experience on the part of the examiner. May give the false impression of PVD but the Weiss ring is absent.

### Inflammatory cells

#### Cause
- Intermediate uveitis (or pars planitis)
- Posterior uveitis or choroiditis.

#### Symptoms and signs (common to both)
- Non-specific reduction in vision by varying amounts
- Floaters of insidious onset
- Occasional discomfort
- May have associated anterior uveitis.

#### Symptoms and signs of intermediate uveitis
- Clumps of fluffy material or "snowball" deposits on inferior retina or pars plana; also "snowbanking"
- Peripheral vascular sheathing or periphlebitis
- Cystoid macular oedema.

### Symptoms and signs of posterior uveitis
- Focal scars in localised choroiditis; away from the macula inflammation may be dense and recurrent but vision may not be greatly reduced
- Diffuse inflammation may leave no visible scar
- Disc oedema in long standing cases.

**Anterior uveitis** tends not to present with floaters as the predominant symptom. An intermediate uveitis or panuveitis may have anterior chamber signs.

**Investigations for intermediate and posterior uveitis** First line tests should include:

- Full blood count
- ESR
- Serum calcium
- Angiotension converting enzyme
- Toxoplasmosis titre
- Antinuclear factor (ANF)
- RPR + fluorescence treponema antibody absorption (FTA-Abs)
- Chest radiograph.

Tests should then be used to identify the common causes of intermediate or posterior uveitis: sarcoidosis, toxoplasmosis, TB, syphilis, systemic lupus erythematosus.

More esoteric tests can be used later to identify less common causes which include Behçet's disease, multifocal choroiditis, Lyme disease, toxocariasis, fungal infection, Whipple's disease, and the Vogt–Koyanagi–Harada syndrome.

### Common inflammatory disorders presenting with floaters
*Sarcoidosis*

#### Symptoms and signs
- Vision decreased by varying amounts
- Floaters
- Symptoms of anterior uveitis: pain, photophobia, redness
- Signs of granulomatous uveitis: mutton fat keratic precipitates, vitritis, yellow deposits ("candle-wax drippings"), and retinal vasculitis

- Less specific features:
    granuloma of conjunctiva, iris, and optic disc
    retinal neovascularisation, disc oedema, retinal haemorrhage, and cystoid macular oedema
- Extraocular involvement affects many systems including hilar lymphadenopathy, salivary glands, facial nerve, CNS, erythema nodosum, hepatosplenomegaly, and bone "cyst".

**Diagnosis** Differentiate from TB and other forms of uveitis. Critical tests include:

- Chest radiograph for hilar lymphadenopathy
- Angiotension converting factor in serum
- Calcium levels in serum (raised in bone involvement)
- Purified protein derivative for anergy (in 50% of cases of sarcoid)
- Conjunctival or lymph node biopsy.

### Management
- Treat anterior uveitis with topical steroids and mydriatics
- Posterior uveitis is treated according to the level of vision and progression of disease; treatment is by systemic steroids or by orbital floor injection (short term)
- As with all patients receiving steroids, warning should be given of side effects.

## Toxoplasmosis

This is primarily a retinitis but the choroid is invariably involved. The age group is chiefly young adults.

### Symptoms and signs
- Floaters and varying degrees of diminished vision
- If macula is involved, vision may be profoundly affected
- Active lesions look yellow–white and have a fluffy edge; they may be adjacent to an old scar or arise *de novo*
- Inflammatory cells in the vitreous
- Anterior chamber cells and flare occasional.

**Diagnosis** Differentiate from other forms of posterior uveitis, for example, TB, sarcoidosis.
Tests include:
- Serum anti-toxoplasma antibody titres
- Serum IgM antibody levels—positive in current infection
- Dye test if confirmation needed.

### Management
- Small peripheral lesions—no treatment but serial observation
- Anterior uveitis—treat with topical steroid and mydriatic
- Lesions within one disc diameter of the macula, lesions causing massive exudation, or those threatening vision may all need treatment.

**Treatment** Treatment consists of using pyrimethamine + folinic acid + sulphadiazine ± clindamycin.

There are several regimens:

- Pyrimethamine, loading dose of 75–100 mg, then 25–50 mg once daily for 3–4 weeks (bone marrow toxicity: avoid in AIDS patients)
- Folinic acid 10 mg/day reduces the side effects of thrombocytopenia
- Sulphadiazine, loading dose of 2 g then 1 g four times daily for 3 weeks
- Clindamycin 300 mg four times daily for 3 weeks (risk of *pseudomembranous colitis*; patient should be warned)
- Prednisolone by mouth may be added after starting antibiotics
- Co-trimoxazole 960 mg twice daily is an alternative substitute for sulphadiazine.

## *Neoplastic cells giving rise to floaters*

This is rare but important; it should be considered in cases where there is (1) an absence of inflammatory signs, and (2) no response to treatment.

## *Vitreous haemorrhage*

### Symptoms and signs
- Black worm like floaters or showers of spots
- May be preceded by flashing lights
- Varying degrees of reduced vision depending on the density of the haemorrhage
- Blood in the vitreous varies according to severity, ranging from a few cells in the anterior vitreous to a blood filled cavity with no fundus view; in general:
    mild cases give a hazy view
        moderate amounts produce clumps seen as black silhouettes on retroillumination or as sheets lying inferiorly

# FLASHES AND FLOATERS

severe cases will lose the red reflex and RBCs seen in the slitlamp.

## Causes
- Retinal tear (rarely PVD without tear)
- retinal new vessels, for example, proliferative diabetic retinopathy, old branch retinal vein occlusion (BRVO), sickle cell disease, and Eales' disease
- Subretinal neovascular membrane in age related macular degeneration (ARMD) where blood has broken through the retina
- Intraocular tumours
- Systemic hypertension
- Bleeding diseases
- Subarachnoid haemorrhage (Terson's syndrome).

**Management** This depends on the cause:

- Slitlamp examination for rubeosis
- Look for clues from the other eye (dilate both pupils for funduscopy)
- Simple baseline investigations to include BP, BM Stix on urine, full blood count
- Stop aspirin ingestion and do international normalised ratio if on warfarin
- B scan if no fundal view
- Bed rest with slit spectacles for 24–48 hours if laser may be possible in vasoproliferative cases (Fig 4.5).

## Treatment
- Retinal break—laser coagulation or cryotherapy
- Retinal detachment—surgical repair
- Proliferative retinopathy—laser when view permits
- Tumour—enucleation, radiotherapy, or excision
- ARMD (usually not treatable)—counselling, registration
- No view of fundus—follow with B scan
- Vitrectomy—indications:
    persistent haemorrhage > 6 months
    haemorrhage plus tear or detachment
    haemorrhage plus rubeosis
    haemorrhage with known proliferative retinopathy where haemorrhage is not clearing after 3–4 weeks.

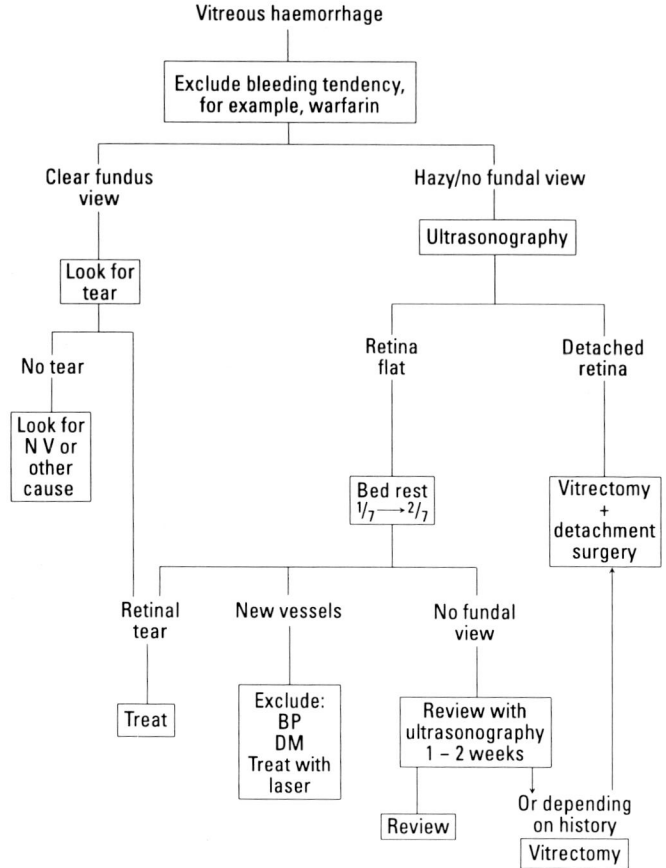

Figure 4.5   Management of vitreous haemorrhage.

## Flashing lights

Flashing lights as a term is used by patients to describe a variety of experiences, ranging from linear lightning like flashes to well formed colour patterns which do not flash in an on/off manner.

### Causes
- Mechanical stimulation of the retinal neurons by direct traction or pressure
- Ischaemia of the retina as in incipient vascular occlusion
- Cerebral phenomenon as in migraine.

### Important points in history taking
- Get the patient to describe more exactly what the symptoms are:
    central or peripheral?—central flashing is never caused by a retinal tear
    linear or patterned?—patterned is likely to be migraine
    episodic or rhythmic?—migraine may be rhythmic; retinal traction may be spasmodic but not rhythmic
    diffuse or focal?—retinal traction typically relates to movement; ischaemia does not
- Are there any floaters? A tear may be associated with floaters and often the flashing ceases when floaters appear
- Duration—recent or long standing?
    Migraine—long standing
    PVD—recent
- Associated with other symptoms—migraine will have a set of related symptoms
- Family history is typically present in migraine—doubtful if one should diagnose migraine without it (probably not in the over 50s without neuroimaging)
- Other illnesses or conditions:
    arteriopathic patient more likely to have vein occlusion
    vasculitis may predispose to retinal ischaemia

### Examination
Important points to look for:

- Any retinal vascular abnormality centrally or peripherally
- Peripheral retinal pathology, for example
    retinal tear
    degenerate areas
    pigmented areas where there might be retinal adherence and traction during PVD
- Signs of temporal arteritis
- Listen for carotid bruit
- Check intraocular pressure (IOP) for raised pressure (may be lowered in retinal detachment or ocular ischaemia).

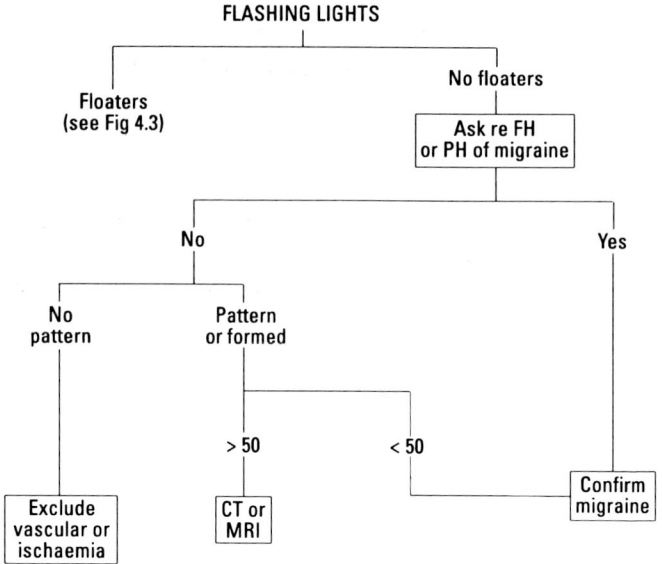

Figure 4.6 Management of flashing lights. FH, ???; PH, ???; CT, computed tomography; MRI, magnetic resonance imaging

## Important causes of flashing lights
*Migraine* (see Chapter 8)

**Symptoms** These are very variable:

- Flashing lights may be part of an aura
- Lights have a specific configuration—typically like fortification spectra
- Other visual symptoms include paracentral scotoma, hemifield flashing lights, distortion of vision, or shimmering effects often described as "jazzy"
- Ensuing headache is often one sided but may be bilateral
- Frequently, patients want to lie down in a darkened room
- Nearly always a positive family history.

Signs are negative and the diagnosis is based entirely on history.

**Management** (Fig 4.6) (See Chapter 8).

### *PVD with or without a retinal tear* (see pages 78–83)

- Flashing is typically peripheral and often confined to one sector of the visual field
- Associated with eye movement
- Floaters common and their appearance may coincide with cessation of flashes
- Examination to exclude a retinal tear is of prime importance.

### *Vascular events*

Three common conditions need to be ruled out:

- Retinal vein occlusion or threatened occlusion
- Temporal arteritis
- Transient ischaemic attacks.

(See Chapter 3.)

### *Intracranial causes*

Rarely, tumours or occipital arteriovenous malformation can cause flashing lights but patients will have other symptoms and signs such as field defects, headache, and progressive neurological deficits.

# 5 Red eye

A red eye is a presenting feature for a large number of ophthalmic conditions and accounts for a large volume of referrals to the A&E department. Quite often the red eye will have some accompanying symptoms such as pain, soreness, reduced vision, or some features worrying to the patient.

There are numerous causes of "a red eye", but essentially the redness is caused by dilatation of the vessels of the conjunctiva, episclera, and sclera, or by extravasated blood. The stimulus is either the products of inflammation, ischaemia, or reflex dilatation, or a combination of these factors.

The conditions giving rise to redness can be broadly classified anatomically into those in Table 5.1.

Table 5.1 Conditions

| Diseases of | Examples |
| --- | --- |
| The ocular surface | Conjunctivitis |
|  | Keratitis |
| The intermediate coat | Episcleritis |
|  | Scleritis |
|  | Uveitis |
| The inner eye or global | Endophthalmitis |
|  | Congestive glaucoma |
| The lids and orbit | Blepharitis |
|  | Orbital congestion |

Orbital conditions will be dealt with in Chapter 10 and contact lens related problems in Chapter 11.

## History taking

The key symptoms that need to be noted are those in the box.

> **Key symptoms**
> - Pain
> - Visual loss or reduced vision
> - Any photophobia?
> - Stickiness or watering of eye

Is the eye painful? This question starts to subdivide red eyes into basic symptomatic groups (Table 5.2).

Table 5.2 Symptomatic classification of the red eye

| Chief secondary symptom | Condition |
|---|---|
| **Painful red eye** | |
| Loss of vision or markedly diminished | Severe inflammation |
| |   severe acute anterior uveitis |
| |   infective endophthalmitis |
| | Acute congestive glaucoma |
| | Central corneal lesion with loss of axial transparency, for example, abscess |
| No loss of vision or small reduction of vision | Peripheral corneal lesion |
| | Early anterior uveitis |
| | Anterior scleritis |
| | Keratitis or corneal abrasion |
| Herpes zoster | |
| **Non-painful red eye (or minor discomfort)** | |
| Purulent discharge | Infective conjunctivitis |
| |   bacterial |
| |   viral |
| |   chlamydial |
| Itchy ± sticky, watery | Allergic conjunctivitis |
| |   hay fever |
| |   acute allergy |
| |   vernal conjunctivitis (atopy) |
| Photophobia ± lacrimation | Keratitis |
| | Abrasion |
| General irritation/grittiness (foreign body sensation) | Blepharitis |
| |   blepharoconjunctivitis |
| | Sicca syndrome |
| Sectoral redness | Marginal ulcers/keratitis |
| | Episcleritis |
| | Pterygium |
| | Pinguecula |
| | Subconjunctival haemorrhage |
| | Rosacea keratitis |

## Visual loss or reduced vision

Is the vision affected? Any disease process causing loss of transparency of the media or that affects the central retina will reduce vision.

Severe reduction in vision with a red eye indicates a potentially serious problem such as acute glaucoma, severe iritis, or endophthalmitis.

## Is there any photophobia?

Disturbance of the corneal epithelium and inflammation of the anterior uvea (anterior uveitis) cause excessive sensitivity to light.

## Is the eye sticky or watering?

**Discharge** Eyes sticky from a mucopurulent discharge may be caused by a discharge that is secondary to conjunctival irritation. This can be infective, allergic, or toxic.

**Watering** Watering can be secondary to corneal epithelial disturbance of any aetiology. When acute, it is usually accompanied by photophobia. Watering will also occur with tear duct drainage problems such as blocked nasolacrimal duct or everted punta.

## Other clinical features
### Duration of symptoms

This can indicate whether it is an acute or chronic condition.

### Previous history

This is important because the present complaint may be a sequel or recurrence, for example, iritis, episcleritis, anterior scleritis, recurrent corneal erosions, herpes simplex, and marginal ulcers are all potentially recurrent problems.

### Extraocular symptoms

Are there any symptoms outside the eye? Ocular pathology can be one of the manifestations of a systemic disease, for example, anterior scleritis in rheumatoid arthritis. Conversely, the severity of the ocular condition may cause systemic upsets such as nausea and vomiting as a result of high pressures in acute glaucoma.

## Steps in the examination of the red eye

### Check distance visual acuity (VA) with correcting spectacles or pinhole

If VA is reduced:

- look for media opacities
- test RAPD
- examine fundus through dilated pupil
- check for compatibility of diagnosis with the degree of loss of VA.

### Assess general appearance before detailed examination

Look for:

- ocular asymmetry
- size of interpalpebral aperture—lid retraction or ptosis
- proptosis or enophthalmos
- exposure if any.

### Assess pattern of redness

Examples:

- maximal redness in fornices—conjunctivitis
- segmental—episcleritis
- segmental, maximal near limbus—focal keratitis
- limbal and circumferential (that is, ciliary)—iritis, glaucoma
- brawny red—scleritis (mostly segmental)
- interpalpebral—dry eyes
- deep crimson red and confluent—subconjunctival haemorrhage.

### Assess the lid margin and eye lids as a prelude to detailed examination

Look for:

- position of the lid margin in relation to the globe, for example, entropion, ectropion
- position and state of the lashes—trichiasis
- contour of lid margin, for example, irregular and rounded in chronic blepharitis.

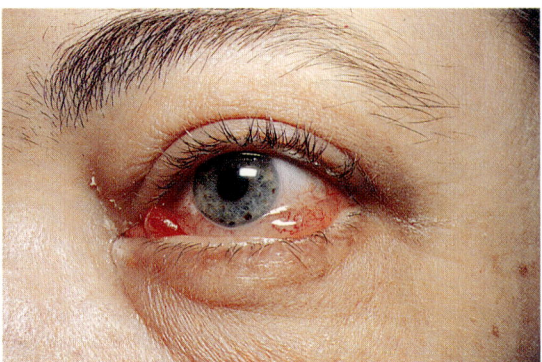

Figure 5.1   Chemosis: swelling and redness of lower bulbar conjunctiva.

## Examine the conjunctiva

The conjunctiva should be examined for:

- surface changes—ulceration
- oedema (chemosis (Fig 5.1))
- membrane or pseudomembrane formation indicating underlying ulceration (Fig. 5.2)
- focal abnormalities, for example, pingecula or nodules.

## Examine the cornea
### *Macroscopic*

Check brightness or sheen of the two eyes—epithelial oedema shows as loss of sheen at an early stage.

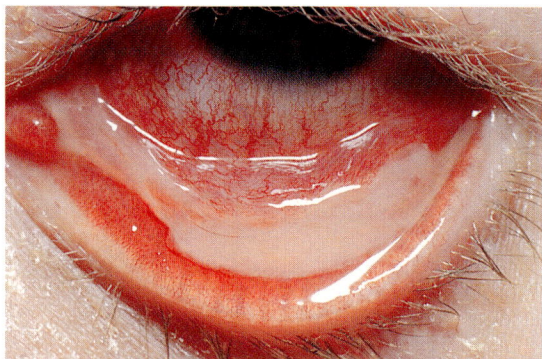

Figure 5.2   Pseudomembrane in ulcerative conjunctivitis.

## *Microscopic (slitlamp)*

See history taking: use of ophthalmic instruments.
Examination with slitlamp should include looking for:

- surface changes
- loss of transparency
- vascularisation
- limbal disease.

## *Use topical dyes* (see Appendix A)

- Fluorescein for epithelial defects
- Rose bengal for inflammation, dead or damaged cells.

## Evert lids for subtarsal changes

Look for:

- subtarsal foreign body
- follicles—which are collections of lymphocytes—prominent in chlamydial (Fig 5.3) and viral infection
- papillae—conjunctival elevation with a vessel in the centre; prominent in allergic reactions (Fig 5.4).

## Examine the anterior chamber

The anterior chamber should be examined for:

- depth—expecially especially the periphery for iridocorneal contact

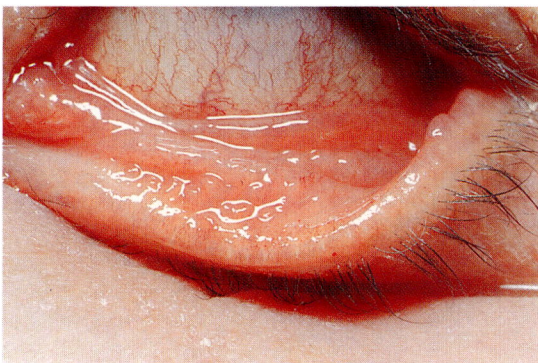

Figure 5.3 Follicles in the lower fornix: smooth, round elevations with avascular centre—a case of chlamydial infection.

# EMERGENCY OPHTHALMOLOGY

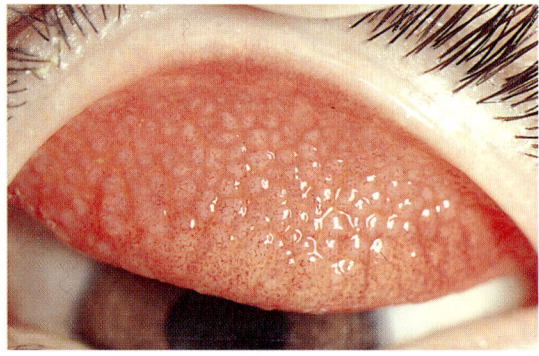

Figure 5.4 Papillae under the upper tarsus, typified by the vascular tufts in the centre.

- keratic precipitates (KPs) in iritis—clumps of cells on corneal endothelium
- flare and cells—light scatter by protein and particles in inflammation
- fluid levels of deposits.

(See Appendix B for more details on techniques of examination.)

## Assess pupil

The pupil should be assessed for:

- size, shape, and regularity of margin
- reaction to light.

## Dilate pupil and examine fundus.

This should be done where fundal pathology is suspected and where the loss of vision is not compatible with the amount of aterior segment disease.

# Painful red eyes with loss of vision

> ### Causes of painful red eye with loss of vision
> Acute congestive glaucoma
>     Angle closure attacks
> Severe inflammation
>     Severe acute anterior uveitis
>     Endophthalmitis
> Central corneal lesions
>     Keratitis
>     Corneal abscess

## Diagnosis and management of specific conditions
### Acute glaucoma

In the present context the term refers to any acute rise in pressure sufficient to cause pain, redness, and reduced vision. Most cases are caused by angle closure but some are rubeotic or secondary (Fig 5.5).

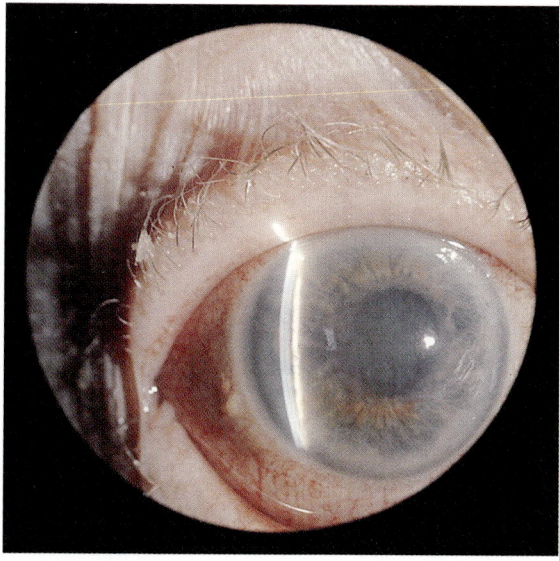

Figure 5.5 Acute angle closure glaucoma: note the hazy cornea, shallow anterior chamber, torsion of iris, and mid-dilated pupil.

### Symptoms and signs
- Usually asymmetrical and presents unilaterally; occasionally bilateral
- Headache, nausea, and vomiting
- Haloes around bright lights
- Visual acuity usually reduced
- Cornea oedematous and cloudy
- Eye feels hard to digital palpation.

In angle closure glaucoma, the anterior chamber looks shallow and the pupil is oval, fixed, and mid-dilated in an attack.

In rubeotic glaucoma the pupil also tends to be mid-dilated and there are blood vessels visible on the surface of the iris or in the drainage angle on gonioscopy.

In phacolytic and uveitic glaucoma the pupil may be miosed but reacting to light.

### Associated factors
- Angle closure is more common in hypermetropic individuals and elderly women.
- Rubeotic glaucoma occurs with ocular ischaemia, for example, diabetes or previous vein occlusion
- Phacolytic and phacomorphic (that is, related to enlargement of the lens) glaucomas are associated with cataract.

**Management of acute angle closure glaucoma** Acute angle closure glaucoma is related to decreased anterior chamber depth, pupil block, and obstruction to aqueous outflow. It produces the typical picture shown in Fig 5.5. Untreated, acute angle closure glaucoma causes severe visual loss and eventual blindness. Gonioscopy of both the presenting and fellow eye should be carried out to confirm the diagnosis.

Admit the patient for control of the nausea and vomiting, and effective monitoring of the response to treatment.

Immediate treatment is medical with intravenous acetazolamide 500 mg.

Topical pilocarpine 4% breaks the pupil block by inducing miosis. Intensive pilocarpine is ineffective when the intraocular pressure is over 40 mm Hg because of pupillary muscle ischaemia. Pilocarpine toxicity can occur from systemic absorption of intensive pilocarpine drops. Instil one drop and wait 15 minutes. If no response (miosis) repeat up to four applications.

Put pilocarpine 2% into the fellow eye as prophylaxis against angle closure.

Check the response of the intraocular pressure to treatment after 1–2 hours. If there is no response at all use hyperosmotic agents, for example, oral glycerol in a 50% solution, 1–2 g/kg body weight or intravenous mannitol in a 20% solution 1–2 g/kg body weight. The general health of an elderly patient must be taken into consideration because of potential side effects.

If medical treatment fails to control the pressure within 12–24 hours, then YAG (yttrium–aluminium–garnet) laser iridotomy or surgical iridectomy may be necessary to relieve the pupil block.

Usually YAG laser iridotomy, surgical iridectomy, and drainage operations are performed after successful medical treatment to prevent recurrence. Do not forget prophylactic laser or surgery to the fellow eye.

**Management of rubeotic glaucoma** Rubeotic glaucoma is evident from the neovascularisation on the iris and in the drainage angle. It occurs in ocular ischaemia, most commonly in diabetes and after central retinal vein occlusion. In an early case, treatment is with urgent laser panretinal photocoagulation or retinal cryotherapy, which could bring about regression of vessels. For advanced cases, treatment is for symptomatic relief. Ablation of the ciliary body may help.

**Management of other acute glaucomas** Glaucoma can occur secondary to mature or dense cataracts either from leakage of lens proteins or from the bulk of the lens precipitating angle closure. Extraction of the lens is usually necessary.

### *Acute anterior uveitis (iritis)* (Fig 5.6)

**Symptoms and signs**
- Usually unilateral, pain, photophobia, and tearing
- Redness maximal at limbus (ciliary flush)
- Visual acuity affected to varing degrees
- Pupil irregular and miosed
- Keratic precipitates on the lower corneal endothelium
- There may be a hypopyon in severe inflammation.

**Associated factors** Most cases of uveitis are idiopathic.

There are many systemic associations. The more common are linked to infective conditions such as: herpes zoster and other viral infections; HLA types (notably HLA-B27); inflammatory

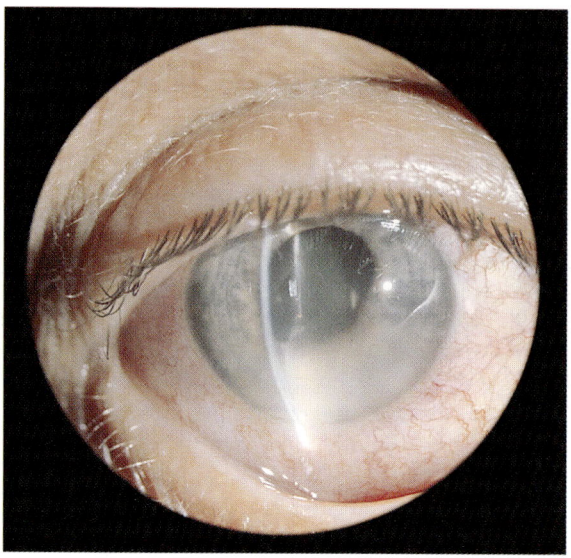

Figure 5.6 Acute anterior uveitis (iritis): note ciliary injection, plasmoid aqueous (cellular deposit) in lower part of the anterior chamber and over the lens, and a small hypopyon. The irregular pupil is atypically dilated.

bowel disease; and ankylosing spondylitis, sarcoidosis, syphilis, and tuberculosis. Ocular associations with iritis include intraocular tumours, rhegmatogenous retinal detachment, corneal inflammation, and intraocular foreign body.

**Investigations** If a patient presents with iritis for the first time, both fundi should be checked for evidence of chorioretinitis, vitritis, and retinal detachment.

Appropriate history taking may indicate whether there is any ocular or systemic cause. There is a potential for doing countless investigations but the most useful are: full blood count, ESR and C-reactive protein, chest radiograph for sarcoidosis (abnormal in 90% of patients with sarcoidosis and uveitis), and tuberculosis; a rheumatological opinion; VDRL for syphilis; and measurement of antinuclear antibody and angiotensin converting enzyme.

**Relief of symptoms** The inflammation of the iris causes a painful miosis. Mydriatics such as cyclopentolate or atropine relieve pain and prevent the formation of synechiae in a miosed pupil, that is, the iris adhering to the lens. Dilate the pupil in the A&E department using both tropicamide and phenylephrine if not medically contraindicated. The use of steam in hot spoon bathing may help break stubborn synechiae.

When synechiae form around the entire pupil margin, normal aqueous flow is prevented, the iris will bulge forward, forming an iris bombé. When the chamber angle is occluded, the intraocular pressure will rise. In this situation, if medical measures fail to break the synechiae, YAG laser iridotomy will relieve the obstruction to aqueous flow.

Suppress inflammation with frequent topical steroids, hourly or two hourly for the first week and then tailed off gradually over a month or two. Once treatment has been started the patient should be reviewed in a week, on the understanding that he or she should return earlier if there is no improvement or the symptoms worsen.

If the iritis has been neglected and the patient presents late in the course of the disease, subconjunctival injections of steroids (for example, betamethasone 4 mg) and mydriatic agents (for example, Mydricaine [I or II]) may be necessary. Ensure that patient is well anaesthetised before the injection with topical anaesthetics, including cocaine drops if necessary (also helpful because of its mydriatic effect).

If the patient cannot or will not put in the drops, consider admission to hospital and systemic treatment.

Management of posterior uveitis is detailed in Chapter 4.

### *Infective corneal ulcers and abscesses* (Fig 5.7)

Infective bacterial and fungal corneal lesions with suppuration cause significant pain and loss of visual function. In endophthalmitis, the whole eye is involved (see Postoperative complications).

### Symptoms and signs
- Pain, photophobia, and tearing
- Usually a mucopurulent discharge with generalised conjunctival injection
- Visual acuity affected, especially if visual axis is involved
- Anterior chamber inflammation or hypopyon
- Dense white or grey opacities in corneal stroma
- Satellite lesions surrounding the main lesion may suggest fungal infection.

Stromal melt can occur: a descemetocele (Descemet's membrane bulging forward) forms and perforation is then possible.

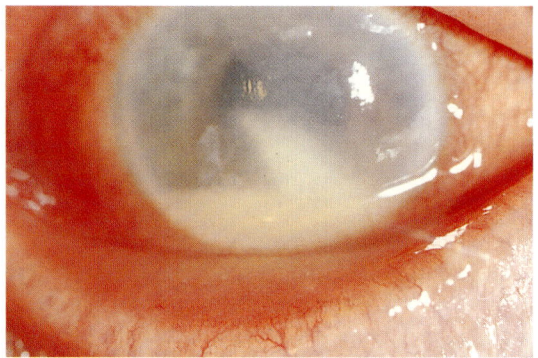

Figure 5.7   Infective corneal abscess with hypopyon.

### Associated factors
- Contact lens wear, especially soft and extended wear lens
- Recent history of corneal trauma
- Topical steroid drops for other eye problems
- History of exposure to vegetable matter in suspected fungal ulcers.

**Management**   Infective corneal lesions need to be scraped for a Gram stain and cultures. Using a sterile needle or spatula, place the samples directly onto agar plates, glass microscope slide, and into broth for prolonged culture (see Chapter 11). In contact lens wearers, microbiology of the contact lens cases is invaluable.

If there is a dense infiltrate or anterior chamber activity, admit the patient and start intensive topical drops half hourly, 24 hours a day, while waiting for Gram stain or culture results.

In addition, subconjunctival injections of antibiotic can be used, although similar anterior chamber concentrations can be achieved with half hourly drops alone.

Antibiotics commonly used before culture sensitivities are known include those in the box.

For severe infections, topical antibiotics can be given in fortified preparations, for example, 1·5% gentamicin versus the normal 0·3% strength.

Recognised treatment regimens for an unknown organism include the following:

- Cefuroxime 5% and gentamicin forte alternately on the half hour

> ### Antibiotics used before culture results received
>
> Ciprofloxacin: active against many Gram-positive and Gram-negative bacteria including the ocular pathogens *Pseudomonas aeruginosa* and *Staphylococcus aureus*. It has limited activity against streptococci (including *Streptococcus faecalis*), however, and non-aeruginosa pseudomonads.
>
> Ofloxacin: active against many Gram-positive and Gram-negative bacteria, including *Pseudomonas aeruginosa*, staphylococci, and moderate activity against most streptococcal organisms.
>
> Gentamicin: broad spectrum antibiotic; effective against *Pseudomonas aeruginosa* and *Staphylococcus* sp.
>
> Cefuroxime: active against a wide range of Gram-positive and Gram-negative bacteria including *Staphylococcus aureus*, many steptococci, but not *Streptococcus faecalis*. It is ineffective against *Pseudomonas* species. Cefuroxime combined with gentamicin has been shown not only to have an additive effect, but is occasionally synergistic in the elimination of bacteria.

- A topical quinolone and gentamicin forte alternately on the half hour
- A topical quinolone (ciprofloxacin or ofloxacin) half hourly.

## Painful red eye with little or no loss of vision

> ### Causes of painful red eye with little or no loss of vision
>
> Peripheral corneal lesions, keratitis, or corneal abrasion:
>     marginal ulcers, viral keratitis, recurrent erosions, keratoconjunctivitis sicca, abrasions from trichiasis, dellen, entropion
> Early acute anterior uveitis
> Anterior scleritis

**Diagnosis and management of specific conditions**
*Marginal ulcers* (Fig 5.8)

### Symptoms and signs
- Pain, photophobia, and watering
- Tend to be recurrent
- Peripheral, discrete infiltrate, and ulcer
- Associated eyelid margin disease (blepharitis).

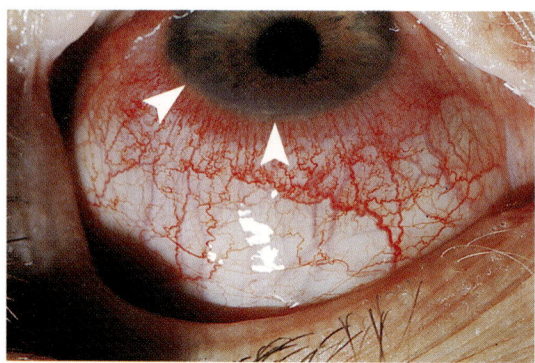

Figure 5.8   Marginal ulcers in staphylococcal sensitivity reaction: note microabscesses at 6 and 8.30 o'clock and the intense redness at the corneal margin.

**Management**  Marginal ulcers are a hypersensitivity reaction to staphylococcal eyelid disease. They respond rapidly to a combination of topical antibiotic and steroid. Regular eyelid hygiene (see Blepharitis) will help reduce the number of recurrences. Occasionally herpes simplex can mimic marginal ulcers, but decreased corneal sensation and the pattern of epithelial loss help differentiate the two.

***Viral conjunctivitis and herpetic keratitis***  Although viral and herpetic problems can cause a patient significant pain, they are more likely to result in discomfort and feelings of grittiness and therefore more details are included later (see Non-painful eye).

### *Recurrent abrasions (recurrent corneal erosion syndrome)*

#### Symptoms and signs
- Generalised injection with pain, photophobia, and watering
- Typically symptoms occur on waking first thing in the morning
- Visual acuity can be affected if the pupillary axis is involved
- Fluorescein staining will show areas of epithelial loss.

Examination of the cornea with the slitlamp may show features of microcystic corneal dystrophy, such as epithelial microcysts, fingerprint, or map and dot changes, or there may be a history of previous corneal trauma, for example, fingernail in eye.

**Management** This consists of topical antibiotics while the lesion is healing. Cycloplegia, for example, with atropine or cyclopentolate, helps decrease discomfort from reactive miosis. There is controversy regarding corneal padding. A poorly applied loose pad, under which the patient's eye can open, prolongs symptoms by abrading the cornea. A firmly applied pad can, however, increase comfort and assist healing. The patient should not drive with one eye occluded because this may invalidate a car insurance policy.

After the erosion has healed, a simple lubricating ointment last thing at night for a few months prevents disturbance of the epithelium first thing in the morning on opening the eye. Taping the eyelid shut at night encourages the patient to open the eye gently in the morning and ensures protection of the cornea during sleep.

If symptoms continue to recur despite ocular lubrication, refer the patient to a clinic where débridement, microcyst puncture, or therapeutic contact lenses can be tried.

## *Dellen*

These result from localised drying of the cornea adjacent to a raised limbal lesion, for example, trabeculectomy bleb.

### Symptoms and signs
- Discomfort, photophobia, and watering
- Corneal thinning and epithelial staining with fluorescein.

**Management** Topical lubricants keep the epithelium hydrated and reduce symptoms.

## *Entropion* (Fig 5.9)

### Symptoms and signs
- Irritation, pain, and watering
- Inferior corneal abrasions
- Eyelid rolled in.

### Associated factors
- Increasing age
- Conjunctival scarring
- Ocular irritation causing a blepharospasm.

# EMERGENCY OPHTHALMOLOGY

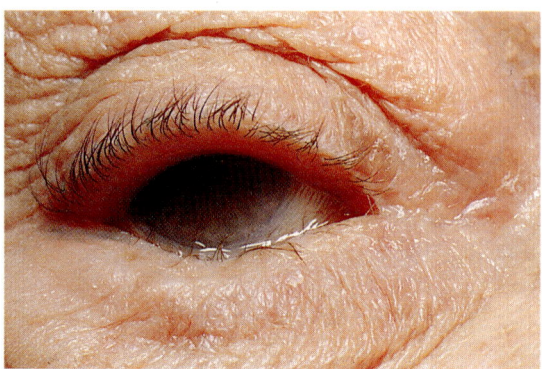

Figure 5.9 Entropion showing lid margin rolled inwards with lashes rubbing against cornea.

**Management** Exclude corneal disease and foreign bodies and treat any concurrent infection. Taping from the lower lid to the cheek will minimise patient discomfort by pulling the lashes away from the eye. Alternatively use temporary eyelid everting sutures.

A minor operation is needed to correct the entropion to prevent corneal scarring and visual loss.

## *Trichiasis*

This is caused by misdirected eyelashes rubbing on the cornea.

### Symptoms and signs
- Irritation, pain, and watering.

### Associated factors
- Blepharitis
- Previous lid trauma, surgery, or trachoma.

**Management** Immediate relief can be gained by epilating the affected lashes, although regrowth in six weeks is common. For a more permanent cure use electrolysis and cryotherapy.

## *Dry eyes*

Although dry eyes can be distressing and painful in severe cases, most patients experience predominantly gritty symptoms and therefore more details are included in the section Non-painful red eyes.

# RED EYE

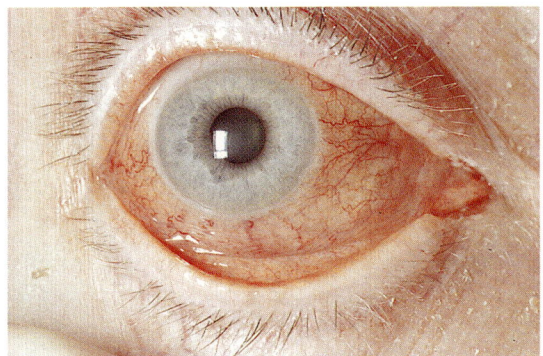

Figure 5.10   Scleritis showing a brawny redness.

### *Anterior scleritis—painful, brawny red eye* (Fig 5.10)

**Symptoms and signs**
- Severe pain, typically waking patient at night
- Intense brawny red colour
- Can be nodular or diffuse
- Visual acuity usually normal unless posterior scleritis or uveitis is present.

**Associated factors**
- Rheumatoid arthritis, systemic lupus erythematosus, polyarteritis nodosa, Wegener's granulomatosus, sarcoidosis, tuberculosis
- Herpes zoster.

**Management**   There are two main categories: necrotising and non-necrotising scleritis. In necrotising scleritis, there is vascular occlusion often associated with a widespread systemic vasculitis. There are areas of non-perfused sclera, peripheral corneal opacity, uveitis, and glaucoma. Look for a systemic vasculitis using tests for rheumatoid factor, antinuclear factor, and antineutrophil cytoplasm antibody (ANCA).

Untreated, visual prognosis is poor. Treatment is with high dose systemic steroids and other immunosuppressant drugs. The patient may need to be admitted for a general medical work up.

In non-necrotising scleritis, destructive tissue necrosis is absent and the condition will usually respond to systemic non-steroidal anti-inflammatory drugs administered as an outpatient.

## Painful red eye with ophthalmic herpes zoster (Fig 5.11)

About half of the patients with ophthalmic herpes zoster develop a variety of ocular problems. This section summarises the problems that an A&E officer should be aware of.

### Symptoms and signs
- Pain and tingling occur in the region of skin supplied by the ophthalmic division of the trigeminal nerve a few days before the appearance of the rash
- Not all branches of the nerve are affected
- Malaise and fever
- The rash is initially papulomacular, then becomes pustular; it may be limited to one or two spots
- A mucopurulent conjunctivitis, uveitis, glaucoma, episcleritis, scleritis, keratitis, and retinitis can all occur
- Neurological complications include cranial nerve palsies and optic neuritis.

### Associated factors
- Increasing age
- Immune deficiency
- Stress.

**Management** Most patients can be managed as outpatients. The effectiveness of systemic acyclovir 800 mg, five times a day for a week, depends on early administration, preferably within 48 hours of the appearance of the rash.

In patients with ophthalmic herpes zoster affecting the first division of nerve V there is a 40% chance of ocular complications. The nasociliary nerve is involved if the skin rash involves the tip of nose, and in these patients the eye is nearly always affected.

The ocular complications are treated as they arise with appropriate medication.

Uveitis is usually treated with topical steroids and cycloplegics, although some authorities argue that topical acyclovir alone is sufficient.

Ophthalmic zoster is associated with a rise in IOP, even with minimal anterior chamber activity probably as a result of inflammation of the trabecular meshwork. Treatment with topical glaucoma medication (e.g. β blockers) is usually sufficient, combined with a topical steroid four times a day.

# RED EYE

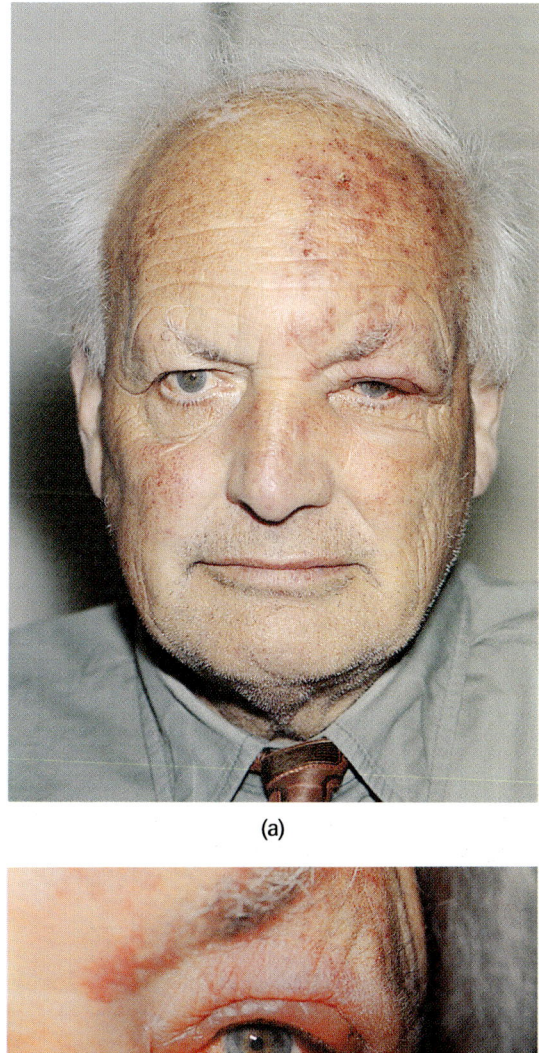

(a)

(b)

Figure 5.11 Ophthalmic shingles (herpes zoster ophthalmicus): involvement of left nerve VI and nasociliary branch.

Using steroids to treat zoster uveitis is associated with a relatively high rate of relapse on withdrawal of the treatment, so these patients need to be followed for some time in the outpatient department while the drops are slowly tailed off.

## Non-painful red eyes

This group is large and it is helpful to subdivide them according to the chief secondary symptoms as in Table 5.3.

Table 5.3  Subdivisions of non-painful red eyes

| Chief secondary symptoms | Condition |
| --- | --- |
| Purulent discharge | Infective conjunctivitis<br>    bacterial<br>    viral<br>    chlamydial |
| Itchy ± sticky, watery | Allergic<br>    acute allergic<br>    hay fever<br>    chronic conjunctivitis<br>    vernal conjunctivitis/atopy |
| Photophobia ± epiphoria | Keratitis<br>Iritis |
| General irritation/grittiness | Keratoconjunctivitis sicca<br>Blepharitis |
| Sectoral redness | Marginal ulcers/keratitis<br>Episcleritis<br>Pterygium<br>Pinguecula<br>Subconjunctival haemorrhage<br>Rosacea keratitis |

### Gritty non-painful red eyes with purulent discharge
***Acute bacterial conjunctivitis*** (Fig 5.12)

**Symptoms and signs**
- Gritty
- Mucopurulent discharge, eyelids stuck together on waking
- Redness—maximal in fornices.

**Management**  This is usually a self limiting disease resolving in 10–14 days if untreated. Staphylococci are the most common infecting organism followed by *Streptococcus pneumoniae* and *Haemophilus* spp.; treatment with antibiotics that are usually

# RED EYE

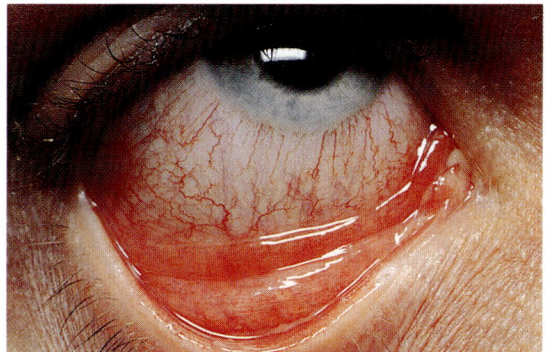

Figure 5.12 Acute bacterial conjunctivitis showing redness maximal towards inferior fornix.

effective against staphylococci should reduce symptoms within three days, for example, chloramphenicol or fusidic acid. Microbiology and culture are only necessary in very severe cases, if the diagnosis is uncertain, or if there is no resolution on treatment; they are mandatory in neonates. (For actual details of taking conjunctival culture, see Appendix G.)

## Chlamydial (adult inclusion) conjunctivitis

### Symptoms and signs
- Usually bilateral
- Gritty with mucopurulent discharge
- Maximal redness in the fornices
- Conjunctival chemosis may be a feature
- Pronounced *follicular reaction* on the tarsal conjunctiva
- Epithelial keratitis particularly affecting the superior cornea.

### Associated factors
- Preauricular lymphadenopathy
- Infection is usually through sexual contact; the eye lesions present about one week after sexual exposure and may be associated with a non-specific urethritis or cervicitis.

### Diagnosis
- ELISA (enzyme linked immunosorbent assay) test
- Scrapings for inclusion bodies (stains with Giemsa)
- Culture in special medium (special transport medium available).

**Management** Chlamydial conjunctivitis is treated for several weeks with topical tetracycline, usually in combination with an equivalent oral antibiotic, for example, erythromycin or doxycycline. Any patient with proven chlamydial infection should be referred to the family doctor or the sexually transmitted disease clinic for genital swabs (and, ideally, treatment of the sexual partner).

### Ophthalmia neonatorum

Conjunctivitis occurring in the first month of life is termed "ophthalmia neonatorum". It is a *notifiable* disease. It can either be chemical, gonococcal, bacterial, herpetic, or chlamydial.

#### Symptoms, signs, and associated factors

***Chemical conjunctivitis*** This is secondary to the silver nitrate or antibiotics used routinely in some countries as prophylaxis against gonorrhoea. It appears as a transient mild hyperaemia resolving in 24 hours.

***Chlamydia*** This is probably the most common cause of ophthalmia neonatorum in Europe. There is a mild mucopurulent conjunctivitis, lid oedema, chemosis, and conjunctival injection. Pneumonitis is a potential systemic complication.

***Gonococcal conjunctivitis*** In this, there is purulent exudate, chemosis, membranes, and pseudomembranes. Corneal ulceration can lead to rapid perforation unless treatment is started. Systemic involvement is common, and may involve the central nervous system.

***Bacterial conjunctivitis*** This may occur secondary to mild ocular trauma allowing access for bacteria. Lid oedema, chemosis, and discharge are common. Systemic involvement is possible with virulent bacteria such as *Pseudomonas* spp.

***Herpetic conjunctivitis*** This occurs in the context of a viraemia, acquired by the infant during birth. Central nervous system involvement and chorioretinitis are common. The viraemia can be fatal. Vesicles may be present on the eyelids and other parts of the body.

***Congenital nasolacrimal duct obstruction*** In this, the child has a recurrent conjunctivitis and a watering eye from the first few weeks of birth. Pressure over the lacrimal sac may express mucoid material out through the lacrimal puncta.

The following are distinguishing features from all the above causes:

- Usually unilateral
- The onset is seldom in the first week
- The sac is usually distended
- The discharge is often more than the redness.

### Management
***Evaluate the general well being of the infant*** If the baby is systemically unwell, admit and refer to paediatricians.

Paediatricians should be involved in all cases of chlamydial, gonococcal, herpetic, or generalised infection.

***Swabs*** Take conjunctival swabs for Gram stain and bacterial, chlamydial, and viral culture. Giesma staining can be used to identify the intracytoplasmic inclusion bodies of chlamydial conjunctivitis present in 60–80% of infections.

***General management*** With all forms of neonatal conjunctivitis, keep the eyes clean with physiological saline.

### Specific treatments
- Gonococcal: treat gonococcal conjunctivitis with systemic third generation cephalosporins in areas where there is resistance to penicillin.
- Bacterial: with mild and moderate bacterial conjunctivitis, ocular hygiene may be sufficient treatment alone, but with severe conjunctivitis start treatment with a broad spectrum topical antibiotic until culture results are known.
- Chlamydia: a 14 day course of oral erythromycin (50 mg/kg per day in four divided doses) with or without topical tetracycline or erythromycin. Remember to refer the parents for evaluation for sexually transmitted diseases.
- Herpes simplex: treat herpetic conjunctivitis with systemic acyclovir.

# EMERGENCY OPHTHALMOLOGY

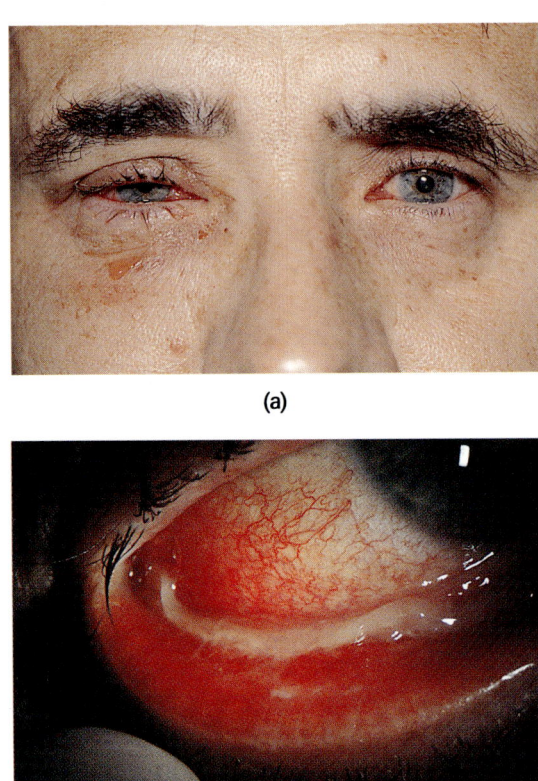

Figure 5.13 Acute adenovirus infection.

**Management of nasolacrimal duct obstruction** Treat the acute conjunctivitis with topical antibiotics and massage the lacrimal sac. The stenosis at the inferior end of the nasolacrimal duct resolves spontaneously in most cases by one year. If the problem persists beyond a year, the tear duct is probed to release the block. Dacryocystis may occur secondary to the block and is treated conservatively with systemic antibiotics. Arrange probing of the nasolacrimal system if problems persist when the infection settles down (see Chapter 10).

*Viral conjunctivitis* (Fig 5.13)

Most viral conjunctivitis is caused by an adenovirus. Primary herpetic infection can present with a similar picture to that of an adenovirus described below, except that it is unilateral, may have vesicles on the eyelids, and is predominantly found in children under six years of age.

### Symptoms and signs of adenovirus
- Two thirds of patients have bilateral disease; usually one eye is affected first, and when the second eye is involved the symptoms are less severe
- Gritty, predominantly watery, although can be sticky in the mornings
- Severe infection is associated with subconjunctival haemorrhages, chemosis, and pseudomembranes
- Tarsal conjunctival follicular reaction
- Visual acuity may be affected by the focal white subepithelial infiltrates of viral keratitis
- These infiltrates may persist for many months as anterior stromal opacities.

**Associated factors** There are two recognised syndromes of adenoviral infection, one associated with preceding fever and sore throat, the other mainly causing a viral keratitis. Both types are associated with preauricular lymphadenopathy and are highly infectious. (Primary herpes simplex is also associated with a preauricular lymphadenopathy.)

**Management** Treatment of adenovirus is reserved for cases of secondary infection or severe inflammation. Topical steroids are used only for severe symptoms or if vision is compromised, because it can be difficult to wean the patients off the drops.

(Treatment of primary herpes simplex is with an antiviral agent for 21 days—see below.)

The patient has to be warned that viral conjunctivitis (particularly adenoviral) is highly infectious, and not to share towels, face flannels, and pillowcases. Equally the examiner must make sure that, after the examination, hands and equipment are cleaned.

### Red eyes with itching as predominant symptom

Itching is usually a symptom of allergy. There are several different presentations depending on the type of allergic response involved.

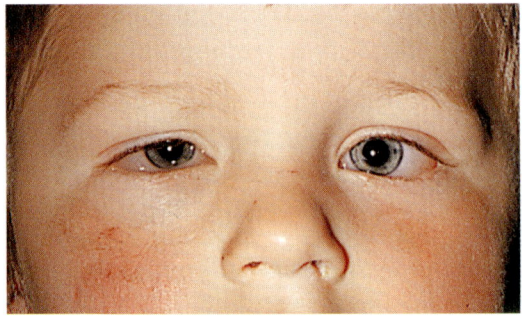

Figure 5.14 Acute allergic chemosis showing greater swelling of the right side.

## *Allergy*

There are various types of conjunctivitis caused by allergies:

- Acute allergic conjunctivitis
- Hayfever conjunctivitis
- Chronic allergic conjunctivitis
- Vernal conjunctivitis.

### *Acute allergic conjunctivitis* (Fig 5.14)

Acute allergic reactions usually occur during the early months of summer.

#### Symptoms and signs
- Acute unilateral or bilateral chemosis with a pale, jelly like appearance
- Recent exposure to an allergen such as grass pollen, cats, or horses
- The patient is otherwise well, and visual function is normal.

**Management** This is a type 1 allergic response and mild cases will resolve spontaneously over 24 hours with no treatment. Otrivine (Antistin) drops may help.

In severe cases, a mild steroid, for example, fluorometholone three times daily for one week will help.

## Hayfever conjunctivitis

This seasonal conjunctivitis is very common. There may be an associated history of eczema or asthma, or a family history of allergic tendencies.

### Symptoms and signs
- Bilateral, itching, and watering red eyes
- Stringy white discharge
- Mild chemosis
- Conjunctival papillary reaction.

### Management
- Difficult to abolish symptoms completely.
- Topical sodium cromoglycate preparations with topical steroids in severe cases. The sodium cromoglycate should be used continuously throughout the hayfever season with a short course of topical steroids in acute exacerbations
- Systemic and topical antihistamines.

## Chronic allergic conjunctivitis (Fig 5.15)

Chronic allergic conjunctivitis covers a variety of conditions resulting from hypersensitivity to various allergens including drops and preservatives.

### Symptoms and signs
- Chronic itching, red eyes
- Conjunctival papillary or follicular reactions

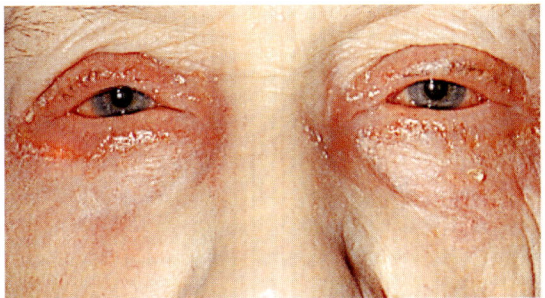

Figure 5.15 Allergic dermatitis and conjunctivitis.

- Cornea may show punctate epithelial changes
- Patient may be a contact lens wearer
- The lids may show evidence of contact dermatitis.

### Management
- Remove allergen if identified
- Have a break from contact lens wear for at least a couple of weeks and change to low allergy cleaning systems
- Topical sodium cromoglycate or equivalent preparations
- If there is severe dermatitis of the lids, a weak topical steroid cream, such as hydrocortisone 0·5%, relieves symptoms. Do not use a prolonged course of a steroid, because of the risk of chronic glaucoma or lens changes.

## *Vernal keratoconjunctivitis/atopy*

### Symptoms and signs
- Intense itching, photophobia, lacrimation, and mucus discharge
- Large subtarsal papillae (see Fig 11.6 in Chapter 11)
- Limbal inflammation
- Superficial corneal ulceration and plaque formation.

### Associated factors
- Uncommon, usually affecting children with a history of atopy
- More prevalent in the spring.

### Management
- Continuous treatment with topical sodium cromoglycate
- Topical steroids during acute exacerbations.

## *Toxic conjunctivitis*

### Symptoms and signs
- Gritty, sometimes painful eyes
- Associated with topical ocular treatment and any drops can be implicated
- A conjunctival follicular or diffuse papillary reaction
- Speckling of the inferior cornea with fluorescein
- Mucus discharge.

**Management** Often just stopping the drops is sufficient, but occasionally a short course of a topical steroid will hasten resolution.

## Photophobia and watering as chief symptoms

Any keratitis may cause the symptoms of photophobia and watering, for example, trauma, viral infection, and exposure, but most will have some leading history or other signs such as pain.

### Herpetic keratitis

After primary infection with herpes simplex, recurrent infection can occur in the presence of host antibody, the most common complaints being dendritic ulcers (Fig 15.16) and disciform keratitis.

#### Symptoms and signs
- Varying irritation, pain, and photophobia
- Generalised conjunctival injection.

Herpetic ulcers have a branching shape (dendritic) which can be outlined with fluorescein or rose bengal staining (Fig 5.16).

In disciform keratitis (probably a hypersensitivity reaction to the herpes virus), there is a coin shaped area of stromal oedema which can reduce vision (Fig 5.17).

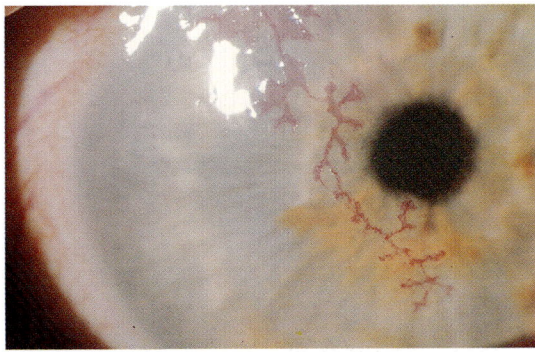

Figure 5.16   Dendritic ulcer stained with rose bengal.

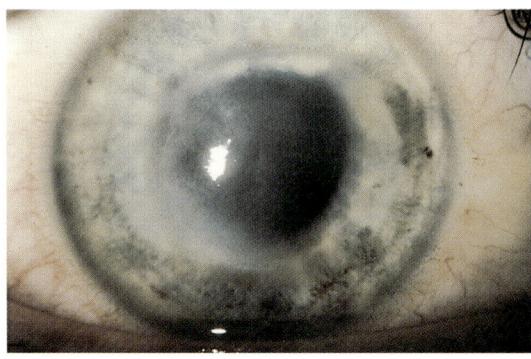

Figure 5.17 Disciform keratitis showing central corneal opacity caused by stromal oedema.

## Management

***Dendritic ulcers*** Topical acyclovir ointment five times a day, for 1–2 weeks or until the epithelium has been healed for three days. Acyclovir is less toxic to the epithelium than other available antivirals (idoxuridine (ID4), vidarabine (Vira-A), and trifluorothymidine ($F_3T$)). All antivirals, including acyclovir, can delay healing with prolonged usage. Review at one week and, if there is no sign of healing, consider resistance to the antiviral or toxicity.

*Do not* treat a dendritic ulcer with topical steroids becase this may promote the development of an amoeboid ulcer (Fig 5.18) or even corneal perforation.

***Disciform keratitis*** If there are no active epithelial ulcers, disciforms away from the pupillary axis can be treated with mydriatics alone. Otherwise, treatment is with mydriasis and weak steroid drops (for example, 0·1–0·025% prednisolone drops) three to four times a day with antiviral cover at the start of treatment. The steroids have to be tailed off slowly to avoid recurrence.

Scarring of the cornea (Fig 5.19) can occur with repeated attacks of inflammation.

### *Iritis*

This has been described under painful red eye but, if mild, there may be no visual loss. Photophobia and pain or discomfort

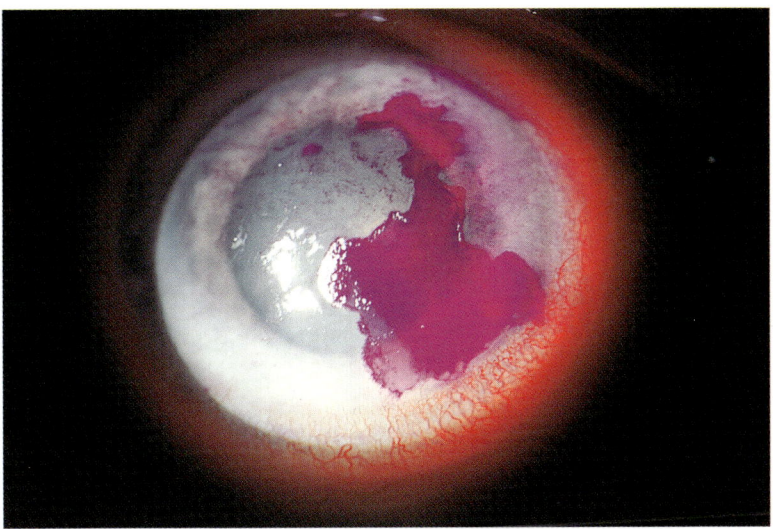

Figure 5.18  Herpetic amoeboid ulcer stained by rose bengal

may be the presenting symptoms with ciliary injection. Diagnosis is based on the following:

- Cells and flare in the anterior chamber
- Miosis
- Typical limbal or ciliary injection.

See also page 101.

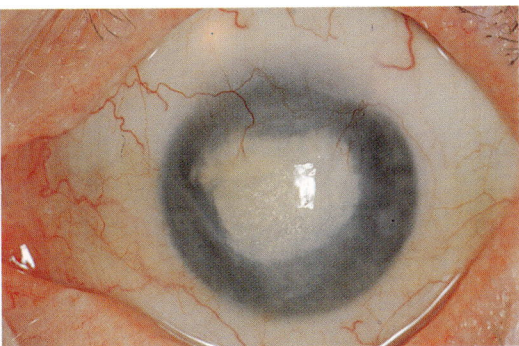

Figure 5.19  Dense vascularised corneal scar from repeated attacks of herpes simplex keratitis.

## General irritation and grittiness

### Blepharitis (Fig 5.20)

Chronic eyelid disease (blepharitis) is very common, and causes more symptoms than would be expected from the clinical signs. Blepharitis is poorly understood but is probably a combination of staphylococcal infection, malproduction of lipids, and tear film instability.

#### Symptoms and signs
- Gritty sore eyes
- Red rimmed eyelids with mild to severe crusting along the lash line
- Recurrent styes or infected meibomian glands
- Loss of sharp edge to lid margin, uneven contour, and marginal corneal ulcers
- Misdirected and inverted lashes (trichiasis)
- Reduced eyelashes (madarosis).

#### Associated factors
- Dry eyes
- Atopic eczema
- Rosacea.

**Management** It is a chronic condition and treatment rationale is aimed at relief rather than cure with regular lid hygiene. The lid

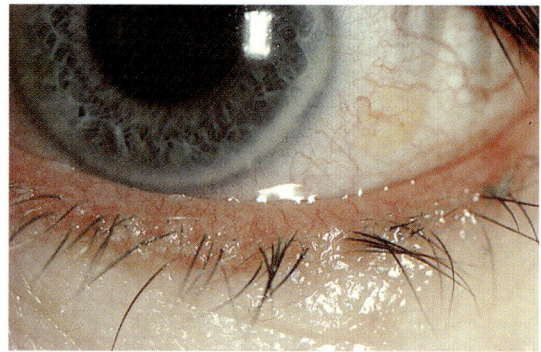

Figure 5.20   Blepharitis showing telangiectasis of eyelid margin, crusting on the base of the lashes, some of which are matted and misdirected.

margins are "scrubbed" daily using a pledget of cotton wool soaked in dilute sodium bicarbonate lotion or cotton wool buds dipped in mild shampoo (for example, Johnson's Baby Shampoo), to remove crust and debris.

During exacerbations, antibiotic ointment is rubbed into the inflamed margins after lid toilet twice a day. In addition, use a topical steroid three to four times a day for a few weeks if itching is pronounced.

Systemic tetracycline over several months is especially useful in rosacea.

Styes and meibomian gland inflammation (Fig 5.21) are treated with topical antibiotics and hot compresses. If there is surrounding cellulitis, oral systemic antibiotics, for example, flucloxacillin or co-amoxiclav, may be necessary. Treatment of chronic chalazia is by incision and curettage.

## Dry eyes (Fig 5.22)

### Symptoms and signs
- Gritty, burning, tired, and dry
- Chronic, interpalpebral redness
- May complain of watering, but does not have to wipe tears from cheek; frequently has tried a large number of drops with no relief
- Conjunctival and cornea stains with rose bengal and fluorescein, especially in the interpapebral area
- Confirm diagnostic Schirmer's test and check tear break up time (BUT) (see Appendix B).

### Associated factors
- Increasing age
- Blepharitis
- Autoimmune conditions and infiltration of the gland, for example, Sjögren's syndrome, thyroid eye disease, sarcoidosis.

**Management** Use tear substitutes, of which there are a number on the market. Some patients find certain brands provide more relief than others, so it is worth trying several (e.g. hypromellose and polyvinyl alcohol—Hypotears, Liquidfilm Tears). Viscotears (Carbomer 940) is more viscous and may be more effective in severe cases or where the tear BUT is very short.

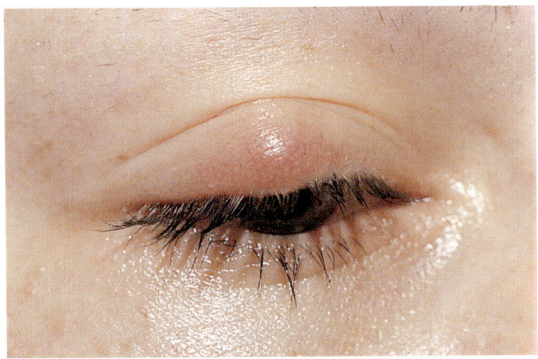

Figure 5.21  Inflamed meibomian cyst.

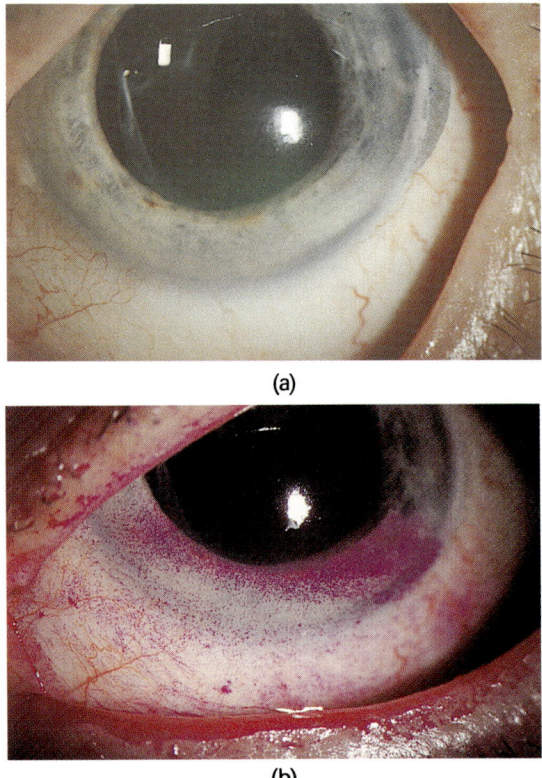

(a)

(b)

Figure 5.22  Dry eye: (a) no stain, (b) stained with rose bengal. Note the dense, almost confluent, punctate stain in the interpalpebral area, which is invisible without the dye.

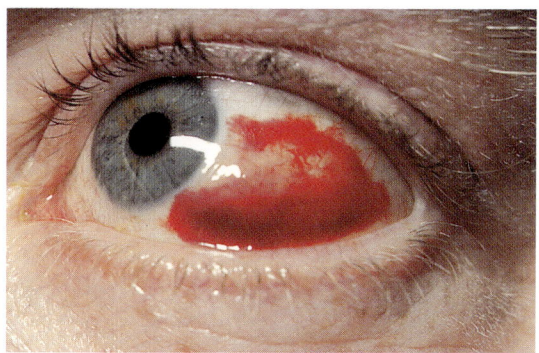

Figure 5.23 Subconjunctival haemorrhage consists here of bright red confluent blood.

If abnormal mucus or filaments are present, use acetylcysteine, for example, Ilube drops.

At the start of treatment put the drops in frequently, up to every hour for very dry eyes. If preservatives cause problems with toxicity, use preservative free preparations (for example, Minims Artificial Tears—hydroxyethyl cellulose).

If these simple measures fail, consider (1) punctal occlusion, (2) wearing humidification goggles, or (3) soft contact lens (highly selective), some of which may help.

## Non-painful conditions with sectoral redness

### *Spontaneous subconjunctival haemorrhage* (Fig 5.23)

#### Symptoms and signs
- Usually no symptoms; pointed out by an observer
- Painless, occasionally mild discomfort
- Blood red patch on eye
- Spontanous or associated with coughing, sneezing, and straining
- Rarely hypertension and bleeding diatheses.

Small subconjunctival haemorrhages can occur in infective conditions, particularly with picornavirus, adenovirus, pneumococci, and *Haemophilus* spp.

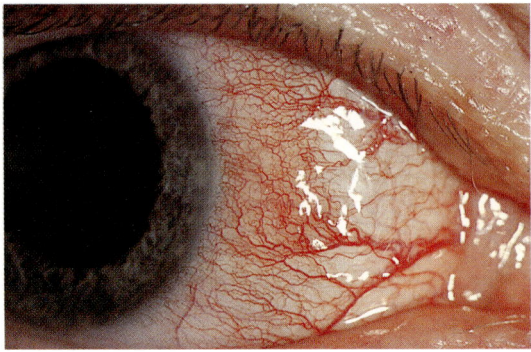

Figure 5.24   Episcleritis showing sectoral injection of episcleral vessels.

### Management
- Eliminate trauma
- Check blood pressure
- Ask about medication such as aspirin or warfarin
- Reassure the patient that it will take about two weeks to resolve
- For recurrent cases check blood count.

## *Episcleritis*
### Symptoms and signs
- Segmental redness wich may rarely be nodular
- Mildly uncomfortable
- May be tender to the touch.

### Associated factors
- Tends to be recurrent
- Typically affects young adults
- Seldom associated with a systemic disorder but may be associated with rheumatoid disease.

**Management.** Inflammation of the episclera is common, non-specific, and resolves spontaneously after three weeks or so. No treatment is necessary unless there is significant discomfort, and then topical steroids or non-steroidal drugs, three to four times a day for five days, should help.

## *Phlyctenulosis*

Phlyctenules are small pinkish white nodules of lymphoctes usually located near the limbus which may stain with fluorescein.

### Symptoms and signs
- Photophobia and watering.

### Associated factors
- Typically children aged 6–10 years
- Tuberculosis used to be the main cause, but nowadays it is hypersensitivity to staphylococci.

## *Exposure keratitits*

### Symptoms and signs
- Gritty sore eye
- Inadequate eye closure (for example, Bell's palsy, proptosis, thyroid eye disease), or poor blink rate:
    may be associated photophobia and watering
    fluorescein shows speckling of cornea
    there may be conjunctival chemosis.

### Associated factors
- Loose, lax lids
- Tendency to sleep with eyes partly open.

### Management
- Topical lubricants (for example, Lacri-Lube ointment at night)
- Taping eyelid shut at night.

Refer to clinic for further managment, for example, tarsorraphy or botulinum toxin injection, if exposure is likely to be a long term problem.

## *Ectropion* (Fig 5.25)

### Symptoms and signs
- Gritty eyes with soreness of exposed conjunctiva
- Watering if puntum is everted
- Tendency to recurrent conjunctivitis.

### Associated factors
- Increasing age
- Scarring from facial injury

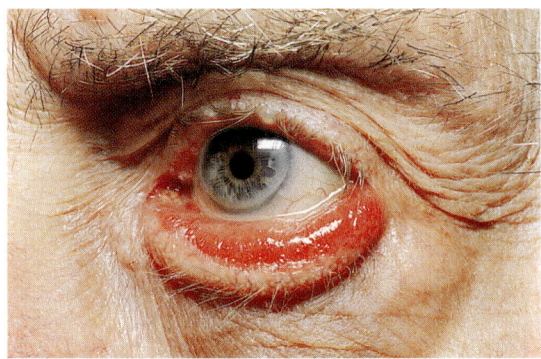

Figure 5.25   Ectropion in which the redness is limited to the lid.

- Palsies of nerve VII
- Blocked tear duct may give rise to secondary ectropion from patient repeatedly wiping lid downwards.

**Management**
- Use ocular lubrication and antibiotics for associated conjunctivitis
- Surgical correction.

## *Pingueculum* (Fig 5.26)

A common raised yellow–white degenerative change in the bulbar conjunctiva, next to the nasal or temporal limbus.

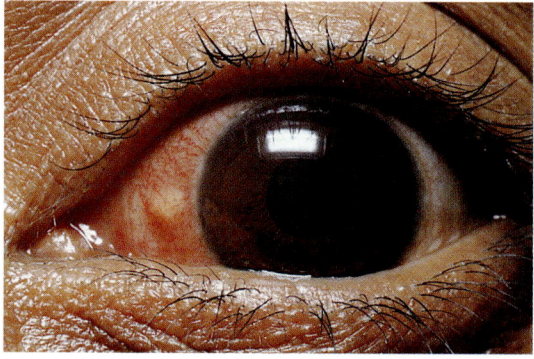

Figure 5.26   Inflamed pingueculum in which the redness surrounding the nodule is again sectoral.

# RED EYE

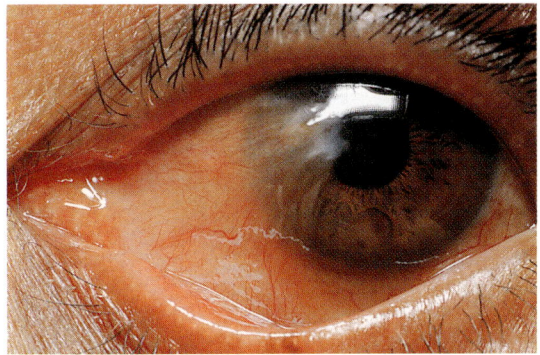

Figure 5.27 Pterygium: redness is limited to the overgrowth of conjunctiva.

### Symptoms and signs
- May be asymptomatic; patient aware only after being pointed out by an observer
- Sore uncomfortable eye
- Injection if inflamed
- Staining with fluorescein in cases of dry eye.

### Management
- Topical lubrication in dry eyes
- If the patient is very uncomfortable, topical anti-inflammatory agents three to four times a day for about a week.

## *Pterygium* (Fig 5.27)

A triangular fold of conjunctiva with subconjunctival fibrovascular tissue encroaches on to the surface of the cornea. In advanced cases the apex encroaches on to the visual axis.

### Symptoms and signs
- A sore gritty eye
- Inflammation and injection around the pterygium.

**Management** Usually topical treatment with lubricants is sufficient, but topical steroids or other anti-inflammatory agents can be used if there is significant discomfort. Excision is carried out for cosmetic reasons or if the growth of the pterygium is threatening the visual axis.

# 6 Trauma

Ocular trauma is a major cause of visual impairment accounting for between 4% and 11% of cases of blindness. Unilateral visual loss that is trauma related is 10 times more common. Children and young adults are at particular risk and males are affected four times more commonly than females.

The aim of this chapter is to provide: (1) a classification of the major types of trauma; (2) methods of diagnosis; and (3) management appropriate to the A&E setting.

It is not our intention to give detailed accounts of the definitive treatment that takes place after admission of the patient to hospital or referral to the follow up clinic. The emphasis is on immediate management so that the correct diagnosis and categorisation of the case can be made and steps initiated to achieve an optimum outcome.

## Classification

---

**Classification**

*Non-penetrating injuries*
  Blunt trauma (contusion)
  Surface injuries

*Penetrating injuries*
  No intraocular foreign body (IOFB)
  Retained IOFB

*Burns*
  Chemical
  Thermal
  Radiation

---

## Preliminary assessment of ocular trauma

In adults a history of the incident provides a good guide to the nature of the trauma and the probable injuries sustained.

In general, for physical injuries, the damage depends on the magnitude and direction of force; for chemical burns, this depends on the nature of the chemical and delay in having it washed out.

In the case of penetrating injuries, the sharper the object, the more the damage is limited to the direct path of entry, whereas the blunter the object, the more damage results from secondary effects.

For intraocular foreign bodies, the outcome depends on intraocular damage remote from the site of entry which is often small and insignificant.

In children the history cannot be relied on unless there is an eye witness account from an adult. In young children and infants, non-accidental injury must be borne in mind.

## Documentation

Complete and accurate records are essential both for patient management and as a reference for future medicolegal reports. Guide to the documentation of ocular trauma is shown in the box.

---

### Documentation of ocular trauma

*Identification*
  Name, address, and date of birth
  Date and time of arrival
  Names of accompanying relatives of injured children

*History*
  When, where, and how the injury occurred
  Ocular symptoms caused by the injury
  First aid treatment given
  Previous ocular disorders and their effect on vision
  Whether spectacles, contact lenses, or protective eye wear was worn
  Tetanus status

*Examination*
  Examination of both eyes

*Management*
  Investigations
  Treatment
  Follow up arrangements

## Advice to patients

Patients with major ocular trauma should be told that it is impossible to predict the final visual outcome at presentation. Occasionally, a severely damaged eye which is a non-penetrating injury at presentation regains some useful vision. On the other hand, complications such as infection or scarring may seriously limit the final outcome for eyes that had good acuity initially. Patients should also understand that visual rehabilitation may sometimes require many operations over months or years.

## Blunt trauma

Blunt trauma causes injury by distorting the globe and abrading tissues. Although partially protected by the orbital bones, the eye is vulnerable anteriorly and laterally to blunt trauma. A blow to the cornea causes anteroposterior compression of the globe and a corresponding stretching of ocular and orbital tissues in the coronal plane. Obliquely directed forces may also cause rotation of the globe. The degree of tissue damage depends on the amount of energy dissipated.

### Symptoms and signs of blunt ocular trauma
*Injury to the ocular surface*

- Pain and watering if cornea involved
- Varying degrees of reduced vision if the central cornea is abraded
- Subconjunctival haemorrhage if conjunctiva is damaged.

*Internal ocular injury*

- Symptoms include transient loss of vision, varying amounts of persistent visual loss depending on the tissues damaged
- Aching pain resulting from traumatic iritis or hyphaema
- Anterior segment signs may include:
    cells and flare—traumatic iritis
    hyphaema (Fig 6.1)—bleeding from peripheral iris
    iridodialysis (Fig 6.2)—separation of iris from ciliary body
    traumatic mydriasis—damage to sphincter muscle
    angle recession—stretching of the drainage angle
    lens subluxation or dislocation (Fig 6.3) following zonular rupture

# TRAUMA

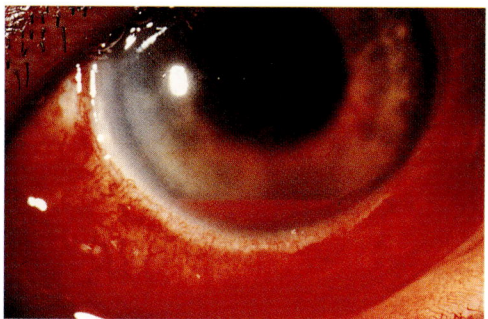

Figure 6.1  Traumatic hyphaema with large subconjunctival haemorrhage.

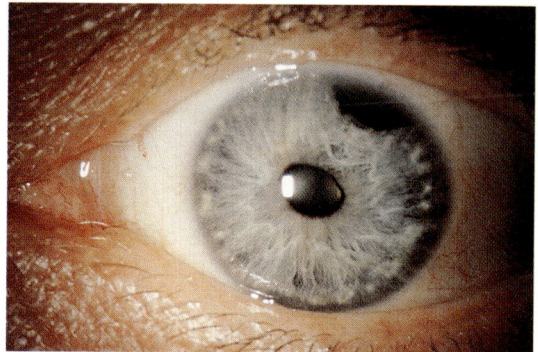

Figure 6.2  Iridodialysis at 2 o'clock; note the distorted pupil.

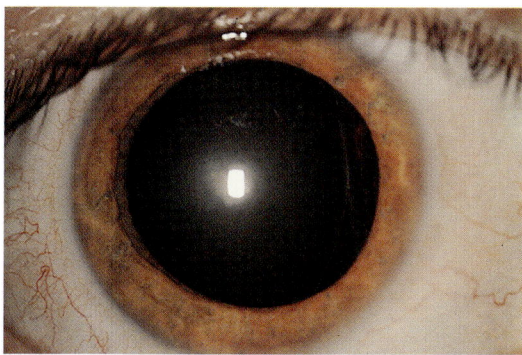

Figure 6.3  Subluxed lens: the edge of the lens is showing, abutting against a thin wedge of vitreous (right edge of pupil).

cataract
- Posterior segment signs may include:
    detachment of the vitreous base
    retinal dialysis—separation of the retina from the ora serrata
    retinal tear or detachment
    vitreous haemorrhage
    commotio retinae (Fig 6.4)—retinal haemorrhages and oedema
    macular hole (Fig 6.4)
    choroidal rupture (Fig 6.4)
    optic nerve contusion.

### *Scleral rupture*

Scleral rupture usually occurs just behind the insertion of the rectus muscles or at the limbus. It is a severe injury that is associated with extensive intraocular damage.

Signs suggestive of a scleral rupture include severe loss of visual acuity, an RAPD, conjunctival chemosis, subconjunctival pigmentation from exposed choroidal tissue, a deep anterior chamber, low IOP, and vitreous haemorrhage.

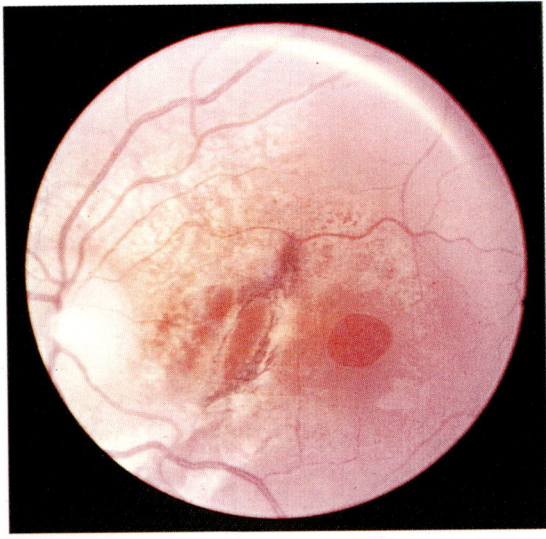

Figure 6.4  Commotio retinae: with macular hole and choroidal rupture.

# TRAUMA

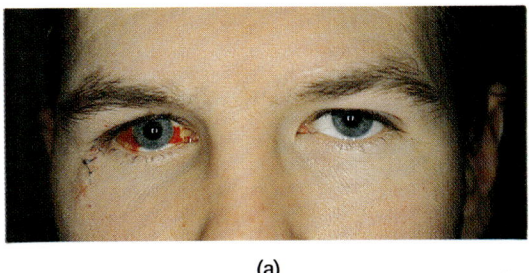

(a)

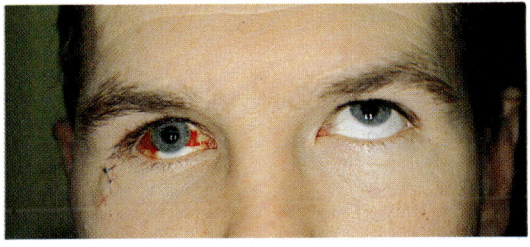

(b)

Figure 6.5  Blowout fracture: (a) eyes in primary position; (b) eyes looking up. Note the subconjunctival haemorrhage which has no posterior edge.

## Blowout fracture of the orbital wall

- The medial wall and floor are commonly affected
- Pain in direction of action of the muscle, bruised, or entrapped
- Diplopia with limitation of eye movement (Fig 6.5)
- Numbness over the lower lid (floor fractures) and the gum over the anterior and middle alveolar processes
- Crepitus in acute stage
- Enophthalmos.

Where there is a hyphaema the force of injury may be sufficient to cause a fracture of the floor or medial wall of the orbit. A blowout fracture may cause prolapse of muscle or more commonly of the surrounding fibrous septa which tethers the inferior or medial rectus, causing diplopia and limitation of ocular movement both along and away from the direction of action of the affected muscle. Fractures of the floor of the orbit may also damage the infraorbital nerve causing loss of sensation over the cheek and upper gum (out to premolar). Enophthalmos is usual from prolapse of orbital contents but, acutely, orbital bruising

137

may cause proptosis. Later, the loss of orbital volume associated with large orbital floor fractures causes enophthalmos.

## Surface injuries

### Subtarsal foreign body

Unless severe pain prevents examination of the eye, it is advantageous not to instil a topical anaesthetic because the patient can confirm, by the relief from pain, that the foreign body has been removed. The upper lid should be everted and the foreign body removed, preferably under direct vision provided by a slitlamp, with a cotton tipped applicator. The corneal abrasion may require treatment (see page 141).

### Conjunctival laceration

- Exclusion of any underlying scleral perforation is a first priority. If necessary, the conjunctiva can be moved with a cotton tipped applicator after instilling a topical anaesthetic. If there is any uncertainty, further exploration should be performed in the operating room.
- Small conjunctival lacerations (up to 5 mm) heal rapidly without suturing.
- Larger defects, over 5 mm, should be repaired with 6/0 or 8/0 Vicryl. This can often be done under topical anaesthesia but children will require a general anaesthetic. In children therefore defects may be left if no globe perforation is suspected unless the tear is very large.

### Corneal foreign body

A foreign body should be removed using the slitlamp. During the procedure the patient's forehead should be firmly pressed against the headrest. Several drops of topical anaesthetic are instilled and, with the doctor's hand resting on the patient's cheek to minimise relative movement, the foreign body is removed using the edge of a 21 gauge needle held tangential to the globe. Residual rust staining will delay epithelial healing and should be removed. Once the foreign body has been removed, the remaining corneal abrasion should be treated (see page 141).

## Corneal laceration
### Partial thickness lacerations

These rarely require suturing, but shelving wounds may need to be stabilised with a bandage contact lens. Dirty wounds should be irrigated with balanced salt solution. Prophylactic antibiotic drops should be prescribed and the patient reviewed daily until the epithelium has healed and the eye is comfortable. Increasing pain, redness, and the development of a stromal infiltrate suggest an infective keratitis. Mixed organisms, including fungi, are likely to be present. The patient should be admitted for treatment.

### Full thickness lacerations

Patients with full thickness lacerations should be admitted in case of infection or instability. Small self sealing wounds can be treated with a bandage contact lens and prophylactic antibiotics. Larger full thickness lacerations require suturing.

## Eyelid lacerations
### Types of laceration

Eyelid lacerations may be partial or full thickness, and involve the lid margins, canthal tendons, or canaliculi (Fig 6.6).

### General principles of management

Lacerations should be cleaned with saline and all foreign material removed. The vascular supply to the eyelids is so good that all attached tissue is usually viable and should not be excised. Wounds are then covered with a moist dressing until repaired. Prophylactic antibiotics should be prescribed for bite injuries. If necessary, surgery can be deferred for up to 48 hours without affecting outcome. It can be performed under a local block unless there is an associated ocular injury when it should be performed under general anaesthesia.

Bear in mind that where there is a full thick laceration there is always a possibility of globe penetration.

### Special features

Lacerations involving the lid margin must be accurately apposed and repaired to prevent notching of the margin,

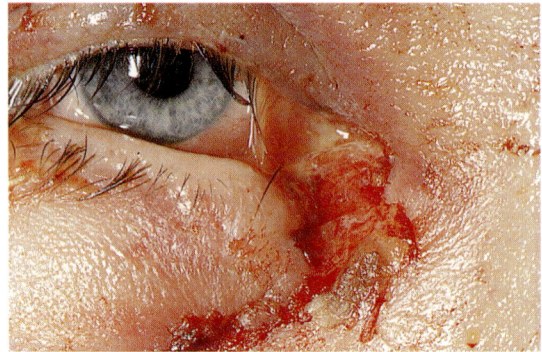

Figure 6.6  Laceration of lower lid: the lower canaliculus is torn.

ectropion, entropion, or damage to the nasolacrimal system. Partial thickness lacerations are closed with 6/0 silk or synthetic sutures. Full thickness vertical lacerations are repaired in layers. The cut ends of the tarsal plates are joined with absorbable sutures such as 6/0 Vicryl. Accurate alignment is essential. Silk sutures are then used to unite the lid margin and skin.

### Torn canaliculus

The management of canalicular injuries is debatable. Most would attempt to repair a combined upper and lower canalicular laceration, but not isolated upper canalicular lacerations for fear or damaging the more important lower canaliculus during the attempt. It is debatable whether repair of the lower canaliculus is worth while if the upper one is intact because repair of the lower one takes 40% of the tear drainage. There is a theoretical risk to the remaining canaliculus and the common duct. Audit of results has not been conclusive.

## Management of specific ocular injuries

### Subconjunctival haemorrhage

Anterior subconjunctival haemorrhages with a definable posterior border are usually caused by damage to superficial vessels—no need for special treatment but check for fracture of orbit.

Subconjunctival haemorrhages without a posterior border may be caused by blood tracking anteriorly from a basal skull fracture.

Therefore, following a significant head injury the absence of a posterior limit to the haemorrhage is an indication for imaging by computed tomography of the skull.

A subconjunctival haemorrhage resolves spontaneously over a few weeks. Occasionally, extensive conjunctival swelling may interfere with the tear film, causing discomfort resulting from localised drying and thinning of the cornea (a dellen). Lubricating ointment should be used until the swelling has resolved.

## Corneal abrasion
### Débridement

Corneal abrasions usually heal within a few days from spread of adjacent cells. Loose epithelium impedes this process and, if present, should be removed under topical anaesthesia at the slitlamp using a cotton tipped applicator. The size of the abrasion should be measured with the variable height beam of the slitlamp so that the response to treatment can be monitored.

### Padding

Although there is some debate as to the effectiveness of padding, it is probable that healing is promoted by keeping the eyelids closed. Two eye pads should be used, the first folded in half and the second taped firmly over it.

### Medication

Before covering the eye, use a cycloplegic (for example, cyclopentolate drops 1%) to relieve pain caused by ciliary spasm, and an antibiotic ointment for prophylaxis and lubrication. The patient should be aware that the aim of treatment is to prevent eyelid opening. Oral analgesia is often required. Topical anaesthetic drops must never be prescribed because their repeated use will delay healing. Patients should be reviewed daily and treatment repeated until the epithelial defect has healed.

## Hyphaema

**Problems** Blood may block the trabecular meshwork and cause a rise in intraocular pressure (IOP). A sustained rise in IOP will lead to corneal blood staining and, for patients with sickle cell disease or its trait, even a modest rise in IOP may be sufficient to cause optic nerve infarction. A force that is large enough to produce a hyphaema also frequently causes other serious ocular injuries, including angle recession, lens subluxation, and peripheral retinal tears.

**Management** The aims of management are to decrease risk of future bleeding, reduce complications, and screen for other ocular injuries.

### *Decrease the risk of further bleeding* (Fig 6.7)

Most hyphaemas are spontaneously reabsorbed within a week. During this period there is a risk of further bleeding from the

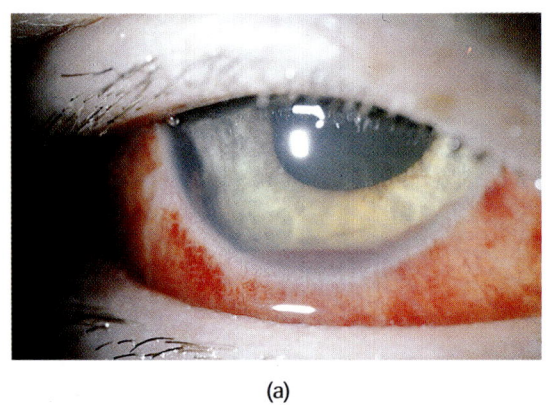

(a)

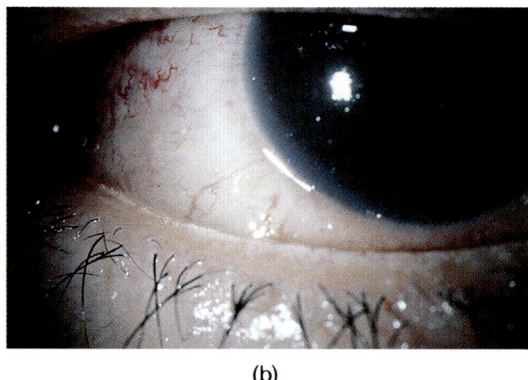

(b)

Figure 6.7  (a) Hyphaema with iridodialysis at 8 o'clock. (b) Total hyphaema (eight ball) filling the anterior chamber with dark red blood that is almost black.

damaged iris blood vessels. To minimise this risk, patients with a hyphaema should be admitted for bed rest. Cycloplegia (for example, homatropine 2%, three times a day) may reduce the incidence of secondary haemorrhage by preventing iris movement. Topical steroids (for example, dexamethasone 0·1%, four times a day) may also have a beneficial effect. Drugs with an antiplatelet action should be avoided.

### *Reduce complications*
- Control IOP—topical β blockers, acetazolamide, and glycerol may be required
- Surgical removal—if the IOP remains above 35 mm Hg for more than one week (or above 25 mm Hg for more than one day for patients with sickle cell trait or disease), the hyphaema should be washed out
- Prevention of corneal blood staining is a further indication for such surgery.

### *Screen for other ocular injuries*
- Retinal dialysis or tear—until the retina can be visualised, serial ultrasound scans should be performed to exclude a retinal detachment. Do not carry out indentation during indirect ophthalmoscopy because it may provoke further bleeding. Therefore, unless there is evidence of a retinal detachment, examination of the ora serrata should be deferred for 2–3 weeks. If it is apparent that the vitreous base is detached ("washing line" sign), a dialysis or an impending one must be presumed.
- Traumatic glaucoma—once the hyphaema has cleared the drainage angle should be examined by gonioscopy. If there is more than 90° of angle recession, long term glaucoma screening will be required.

## Iridodialysis and traumatic mydriasis

### *Iridodialysis*

A small one is not important as such and can be left. An iridodialysis can be repaired if it is disturbing vision by acting as a second pupil or if it is cosmetically unacceptable.

## Mydriasis

Traumatic mydriasis results from sphincter damage and may be temporary or permanent. It is important to inform the patient of the pupil's asymmetry to avoid unnecessary investigations later in life.

### Lens trauma

- Anterior dislocation—a lens dislocated anteriorly into the anterior chamber requires urgent removal to prevent permanent damage to the corneal endothelium. Instil a miotic to trap the lens there until the operation.
- Posteriorly dislocated lenses can often be left in the vitreous cavity unless they cause pupil block glaucoma, or inflammation resulting from the leakage of lens proteins.
- Partial dislocation or subluxation—if there is instability, particularly if there is vitreous herniation, there may be the risk of pupil block glaucoma. Requires close monitoring until a decision is reached as to whether surgery is needed.
- Cataract—sight limiting traumatic cataracts can be extracted later as an elective procedure.

### Retinal dialyses, tears and detachments, and macular holes

- Retinal dialysis—cryotherapy when hyphaema has absorbed.
- Peripheral tears—flat tears should be sealed with cryotherapy or laser photocoagulation.
- Tears with surrounding detachment—unless the elevated retina is very limited in extent some retinal procedure will be necessary. Large posterior tears, particularly those with associated vitreous haemorrhage, are better dealt with by an internal technique combined with vitrectomy.
- Macular holes rarely progress to detachment unless the eye is highly myopic; they do not require prophylactic treatment.

### Detachment of the vitreous base (Fig 6.8)

**Signs** The detached vitreous base takes with it patches of retinal pigment epithelium and gives the appearance of clothes hanging on a line ("washing line" sign).

**Action** Indent involved section of ora serrata to detect dialysis

# TRAUMA

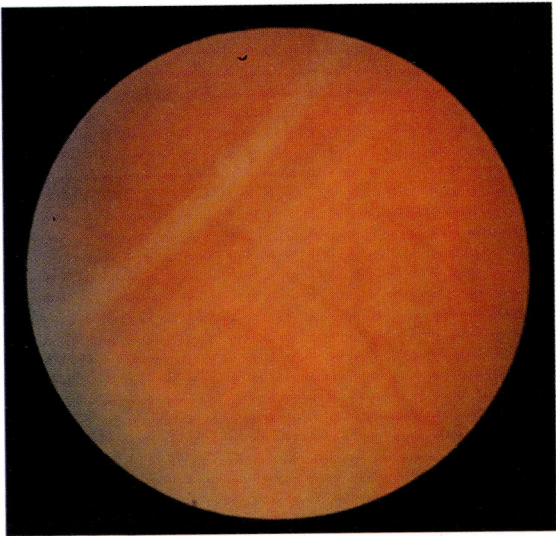

Figure 6.8 Detachment of vitreous base: "the washing line" is seen from 9 to 12 o'clock. This often looks more segmented as a result of patches of pigment epithelium being attached to the torn base.

which nearly always follows. Follow closely, and treat dialysis with cryotherapy or buckling.

## Vitreous haemorrhage

Vitreous haemorrhage usually absorbs over a period of weeks or months. During this time serial retinal ultrasound/scans should be performed to exclude a retinal detachment. (See also Management of vitreous haemorrhage in Chapter 4, page 86.)

## Commotio retinae

Traumatic retinal oedema usually resolves spontaneously. Incomplete recovery of vision may be the result of development of a macular hole or epiretinal membrane. No special treatment is required.

## Choroidal rupture

Choroidal ruptures typically involve the macula, causing variable, but often severe, visual loss. Although they are untreatable, patients require regular follow up because they are at risk of further visual loss from a subretinal neovascular membrane (SRNVM) growing through the break in Bruch's membrane. Patients should be advised to re-present if they notice further loss of vision because laser photocoagulation of an SRNVM is a theoretical option which may preserve vision.

## Scleral rupture

Although ultrasonography, MRI, and computed tomography (CT) may confirm the presence of a scleral rupture, they cannot exclude one. Surgical exploration is required if this diagnosis is suspected.

The IOP is usually low if the sclera is ruptured, but low pressure is not necessarily indicative of rupture.

## Blowout fracture

The indications for surgical repair of a fractured orbital floor are diplopia resulting from muscle entrapment and cosmetically unacceptable enophthalmos, but the timing of such surgery is debatable. Diplopia at presentation may result from haematoma and general bruising, which will resolve spontaneously over a few weeks. Similarly, orbital bruising may delay the development of enophthalmos. Some surgeons prefer to delay surgery by 10–14 days to allow soft tissue swelling to settle. Others prefer to operate within the first few days hoping that it is easier to reduce the prolapsed tissue without ensuing fibrosis.

### Investigations
- Suspected cases should all have either orbital floor plain radiograph or orbital CT scans. Remember that the medial wall is also very thin and not uncommonly involved.
- Full orthoptic assessment + Hess chart to plot progress.

### Action

***Indications for "immediate" intervention*** Where there is gross enophthalmos and marked displacement of the globe, early repair of the fracture and reduction of the prolapse are indicated. This should be planned with the oculo-plastic or faciomaxillary surgeon.

***Delayed intervention*** Those with less severe signs or enophthalmos of less than 2 mm should have their ocular movements recorded, including a Hess chart, and then be reviewed initially every 2–3 days. The need for repair of the fracture depends mainly on the degree of enophthalmos and, to some extent, on the amount of diplopia.

***Muscle surgery only*** This is reserved for less severe cases with little displacement and minor degrees of diplopia. Wait for orbital signs to settle and for the oculomotor abnormality to stabilise.

## Penetrating trauma and intraocular foreign bodies

Penetrating injuries and intraocular foreign bodies (IOFBs) may cause ocular damage by:

- Disruption of ocular tissues at the time of injury.
- Introduction of infection.
- Scar tissue formation, for example, contraction of scar tissue in the vitreous cavity may cause a tractional retinal detachment several weeks after the original injury.
- Reaction to a retained foreign body: retained iron particles gradually disperse throughout the eye and accumulate particularly in the retina, iris, lens, and trabecular meshwork. Over several years permanent degenerative changes occur in these tissues. Intraocular copper provokes an immediate and severe inflammatory reaction. The main risk from organic material is that of introducing infection, but the material itself will cause a granulomatous inflammation. By contrast intraocular glass, plastics, gold, silver, and lead are relatively inert.

### Assessment

***History*** (see also Preliminary assessment of ocular trauma on page 133)

It is essential to determine the precise circumstances of the injury because lack of symptoms does not exclude a serious injury. Although a wind blown foreign body on the surface of the globe will cause a sharp pain, an intraocular foreign body caused by hammering metal may only cause slight pain on entry and no immediate loss of vision.

## Examination

If an eye has obviously sustained a major penetrating injury, or this is suspected from the history, it is important not to cause further damage by doing a rigorous examination. The purpose of the examination is to categorise the type of injury and to obtain sufficient information to formulate a course of immediate action. For example, if there is a lacerated cornea with prolapsed iris, that information alone is sufficient to take the decision of surgical repair. More information gained at a price is redundant if it is not going to improve management of the immediate situation, because a more detailed examination of the eye can be made during surgery. Pressure on the globe, either directly or indirectly by forceful opening of swollen eyelids, is likely to cause extrusion of ocular contents. Similarly, foreign bodies or "blood clots" should not be removed from the eye. It is usually possible to obtain some indication of visual function, even if this is limited to "can see a bright light through closed eyelids".

## Symptoms and signs

### Penetrating injury with retention of an IOFB

This depends on the site of entry, type of foreign body, and the force of impact:

- Loss of vision from damage to the axial part of the cornea, lens, retina, or intraocular bleeding
- Pain suggesting an associated endophthalmitis or an inflammatory reaction to the foreign body
- Asymptomatic or minimal sysmptoms if a sharp and small foreign body enters through the limbus without damaging the lens
- Corneal perforation always leaves a full thickness scar
- Limbal or scleral perforation may leave a subconjunctival haemorrhage which, in this situation, should never be ignored
- A small hole in the iris is best seen by retroillumination
- Always dilate the pupil to look for matching localised lens opacity, or focal retinal haemorrhages. Gonioscopy and three mirror examination of the posterior segment are essential when searching for an IOFB.

## TRAUMA

### *Penetrating injury without IOFB*

Likewise, this will depend on the type of object and force causing the injury. Large injuries are obvious but small ones can be missed:

- Perforations through the cornea will tend to cause prolapsed iris and pupil distortion (Fig 6.9a)
- Axial wounds will cause reduced vision by damage to the cornea or lens
- Wounds posterior to the limbus may be masked by haemorrhage
- Prolapsed uvea (iris root or ciliary body) presents as a knuckle of pigmented tissue, sometimes only slight because of loss of the pigment layer (Fig 6.9b)
- Vitreous presents as a blob of jelly either mixed with uvea or by itself, when it can be easily missed
- The anterior chamber may not be shallow or the IOP low if the wound is plugged by iris.

Note that in posterior scleral perforations the length of the posterior wound may be much longer than the visible portion, because the side of the globe is being seen end on.

### *Penetrating injury with an ocular laceration*

It is important to differentiate between partial and full thickness corneal lacerations because the full thickness ones may be complicated by endophthalmitis or a retained IOFB. A full thickness injury is obvious when the anterior chamber is shallow or if there is iris plugging of the wound, but small self sealing lacerations are more difficult to recognise. If there is any doubt, perform Seidel's test and, if negative, attempt to open the wound by applying pressure on the globe with a glass rod or cotton bud.

### Investigations

- Plain radiograph with both posteroanterior and lateral views if there is any suggestion of a metallic foreign body (Fig 6.10)
- Ultrasound scan or computed tomography is required for a non-metallic foreign body.

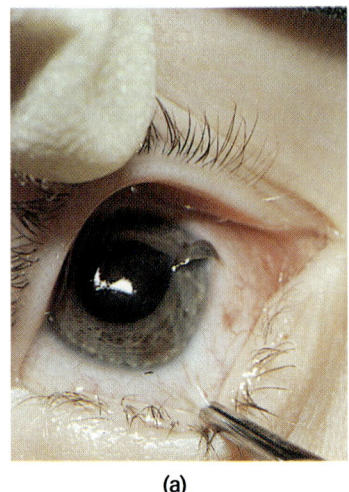

(a)

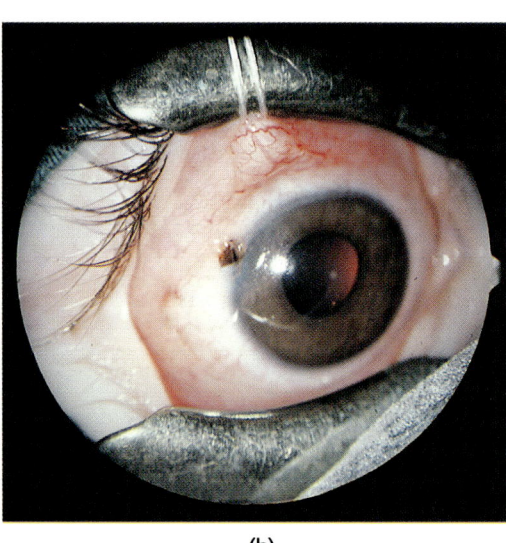

(b)

Figure 6.9  Perforation of the cornea with prolapsed iris: (a) the prolapsed tissue and distorted pupil is only fully seen when the lid is lifted; (b) prolapsed uveal tissue at the limbus with no pupil distortion.

# TRAUMA

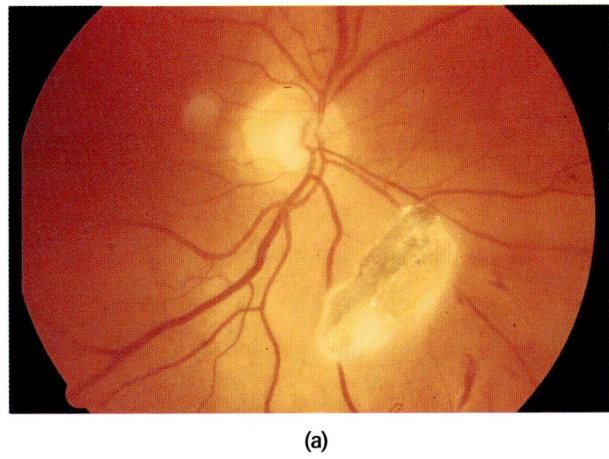

(a)

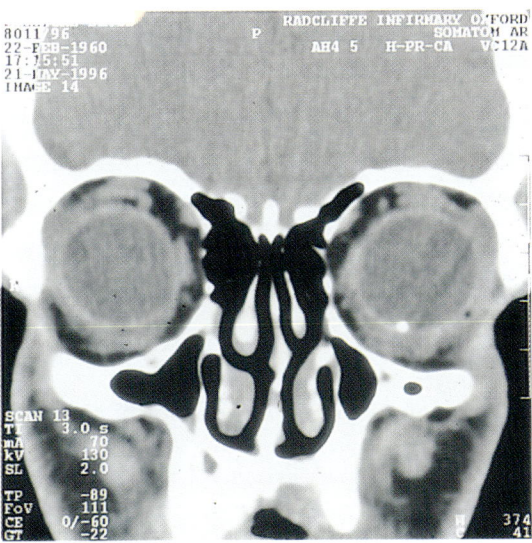

Figure 6.10 (a) Large metallic intraocular foreign body lying in the vitreous inferonasal to the disc. Two small haemorrhages are seen more peripherally. (b) CT of IOFB—one of a series of cuts to locate foreign body lying near the inferior equator of the globe.

EMERGENCY OPHTHALMOLOGY

## Management of penetrating injuries and intraocular foreign bodies

### *Perforated globe*

#### Preoperative management
- The eye should be protected from further injury by covering it with a shield that does not put pressure on the globe
- Analgesics and antiemetics should be prescribed
- If there is any chance of an intraocular foreign body, appropriate imaging should be arranged
- An urgent request for corneal graft donor material should be made if examination suggests that corneal tissue has been lost
- Consider prophylactic antibiotics if surgery is likely to be delayed for some hours.

**Primary surgery** The initial aim of surgery is to restore the structural integrity of the globe by identifying and suturing all corneal and scleral lacerations. Tissue thought to be non-viable or contaminated should be excised. An immediate enucleation is rarely justified because the eye can often make an astonishing recovery. During surgery samples of aqueous fluid, excised material, and vitreous (if the posterior segment is involved) should be sent for culture. Subconjunctival antibiotics (for example, gentamicin and cefuroxime) should be administered at the end of surgery.

#### Further management
- Antibiotic therapy: prophylactic topical and intravenous antibiotics should be prescribed for at least three days (often much longer) and the eye monitored for evidence of endophthalmitis (see page 270) which complicates 1–2% of perforating ocular injuries. Further treatment depends on the response.
- Further surgery is often required in posterior perforation if there is intravitreal blood, vitreous fibrosis, or retinal detachment. Intravitreal blood increases the likelihood of tractional detachment and early rather than late intervention is desirable if there is increasing vitreous fibrosis.
- Elective surgery to replace a scarred cornea or to remove a damage lens should wait for the eye to become quiet and to have regained a settled state.
- Sympathetic ophthalmitis and enucleation: an eye may have to

be enucleated if it develops endophthalmitis, or becomes blind and painful or cosmetically unacceptable. In the past up to 50% of perforated globes were removed to prevent the development of sympathetic ophthalmitis in the other eye. Sympathetic ophthalmitis is a severe bilateral inflammation that occasionally follows an injury to one eye and, although it can be prevented by early removal of the damaged eye, its incidence is decreasing and is usually responsive to high dose immunosuppression. Therefore perforated eyes are no longer removed if they have any visual potential.

### *Intraocular foreign body*

**Removal** This should be as soon as possible and foreign bodies should be sent for culture.

#### Surgical options
- Vitrectomy and removal with instruments; this is increasingly favoured and is obligatory for non-magnetic foreign bodies.
- Removal with a magnet directly over the foreign body or at the nearest point. This is not possible for posterior lesions.
- Magnetic removal through the pars plana by drawing the foreign body to a chosen point.

The argument against the magnet is that it may tear more tissue through disimpaction and again through the exit wound, especially for large particles. Vitrectomy and removal under direct visual guide are, however, a task for the specially trained. In general, a large perforation will require vitrectomy to prevent fibrosis and traction detachment.

Prophylactic intravitreal antibiotics should be administered (see page 270) if the foreign body was retrieved from the posterior segment.

**Waiting and watching** Some materials are inert (for example, glass) and if there is no obvious inflammation there may be a case for prophylactic treatment of possible infection and waiting to see if there is a reaction.

## Chemical burns

Chemical burns are a common cause of ocular injury because of the widespread use of strong alkalis and acids for both domestic and industrial purposes (Table 6.1). The severity of the burn depends both on the nature of the chemical and on how rapidly treatment is started. Detailed history taking and examination should be *deferred* until after irrigation of the eye.

Alkalis tend to cause more severe injuries than acids because they break down the epithelium and the alkali radical rapidly penetrates deeper into the tissues of the eye. By contrast, the epithelium provides an effective defence against weak acids, whereas stronger acids cause protein precipitation which creates a barrier to further tissue penetration.

Table 6.1 Common alkalis and acids

|  | Typical use |
| --- | --- |
| *Alkalis* | |
| Calcium hydroxide (lime) | Mortar and plaster |
| Sodium hydroxide (lye) | Drain and oven cleaners |
| Ammonium hydroxide | Household cleaners |
| *Acids* | |
| Sulphuric acid | Car batteries and toilet cleaners |
| Sodium hypochlorite | Swimming pool cleaners |

## Immediate treatment—irrigation and removal of foreign material

The eye is irrigated with physiological saline using an intravenous delivery tube for at least 30 min (2 litres of fluid), after which the pH in the fornices should be tested with litmus paper. Further irrigation is required if the pH is not neutral. Topical anaesthesia and a lid speculum are usually required to allow adequate access to the eye.

Retained material such as plaster or mortar must be looked for in the fornices and removed or it will gradually dissolve, causing further chemical injury. The eyelids should be doubly everted with a retractor and the conjunctival fornices swabbed with cotton tipped applicators moistened with ointment.

## Assessment
### Symptoms and signs

- Pain, watering, and loss of vision
- Signs of ocular damage are usually confined to the anterior segment:
    cornea—epithelial loss (staining with fluorescein), stromal

# TRAUMA

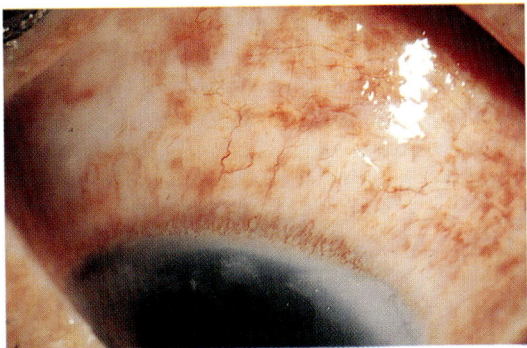

Figure 6.11   Acid burn showing widespread subconjunctival haemorrhages.

   opacification
conjunctiva—chemosis and injection, limbal ischaemia (Fig. 6.11), epithelial loss (Fig 6.12)
sclera—ischaemia and loss of vessels in severe cases
anterior chamber—possible flare and cells depending on severity
the IOP is frequently elevated for several hours after a severe chemical burn because of shrinkage of collagen; therefore the IOP is balanced between damage to the trabecular meshwork and that to the ciliary body
lid erythema, swelling, and varying loss of epithelium.

## Classification of chemical burns

   The prognosis and further management of a chemical burn depend on its severity (Table 6.2). Mild burns will heal rapidly without scarring. By contrast, severe burns initiate a significant

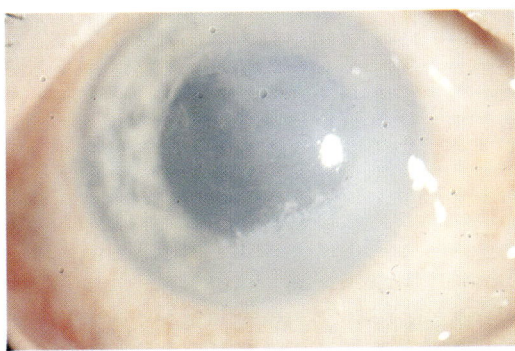

Figure 6.12   Alkali burn showing marked corneal haze and oedema.

acute inflammatory response during which the cornea is at risk of perforation as a result of the release of collagenase from neutrophils. In the later stages of healing, scar formation may cause opacification and vascularisation of the cornea, trichiasis from scarring of the hair follicles, cicatricial entropion, symblepharon, and reduced tear secretion caused by obliteration of lacrimal ducts and loss of globlet cells.

Table 6.2   Classification of the severity of a chemical burn

| Grade | Corneal findings | Limbal ischaemia | Prognosis |
|---|---|---|---|
| I | Epithelial damage only | None | Good |
| II | Hazy, but iris details visible | Less than one third | Good |
| III | Hazy; iris details obscured | One third to a half | Some loss of vision |
| IV | Opaque; pupil not seen | More than half | Poor |

## Further mangagement
### Mild chemical burns

Patients with epithelial damage including less than a third of the cornea or an equivalent area of conjunctiva can be treated in the same way as a corneal abrasion (see page 141).

### Severe chemical burns

Patients with extensive epithelial loss or grades II–IV chemical burns should be admitted. Their initial treatment includes:

- Prophylactic topical antibiotics.
- Cycloplegia with atropine drops 1% twice daily to relieve pain associated with ciliary spasm, and to prevent posterior synechiae. *Phenylephrine* should *not* be used because it may exacerbate limbal ischaemia.
- Topical corticosteroid for one week only to reduce inflammation (for example, dexamethasone 0·1% four times daily). By seven days collagenase activity is maximal and, as corticosteroid reduces collagen synthesis, its continued use beyond one week will tend to promote corneal thinning and perforation.
- Inhibition of collagenase: there is evidence that oral doxycycline 100 mg twice a day and topical acetylcysteine drops 20% every hour are inhibitors of this enzyme.
- Promotion of collagen synthesis: topical ascorbic acid (10% drops hourly) has been shown experimentally to decrease the

risk of corneal perforation. It is often prescribed orally (1 gram daily) as well.
- Control of intraocular pressure with oral acetazolamide or timolol drops as necessary.

## Superglue injuries

Cyanoacrylate based contact adhesives are usually accidentally instilled into the eye because their bottles (or containers) resemble those of a variety of eye drops (or ointment).

### Symptoms and signs

Patients present with pain and their lids stuck together. Fortunately, the glue does not penetrate deeply, and the tear film helps to prevent extensive adhesion betweeen the cornea and lids.

### Management

Adults can be treated at the slitlamp under topical anaesthesia applied through a gap between the lids. Children may require general anaesthesia. The glue, which is brittle when dry, is fractured using a pair of forceps or suture holders and the lids gradually parted. Once the lids have been opened any remaining glue is removed from the lids and fornices. An associated corneal epithelial defect is treated in the same way as a corneal abrasion (see page 141).

## Thermal burns

The eye is protected relatively well from thermal burns by the eyelids and the rapidity of the blink reflex, but it is still vulnerable to flash burns, sparks, or splashes from molten metals. The lower half of the globe and the inferior fornix are most at risk. Thermal burns frequently cause more severe injury to the eyelids.

### Symptoms and signs

Minor burns to the cornea cause pain, whitening and loss of epithelium. Severe burns may result in necrosis of the lower lid, cornea, and sclera.

Partial thickness burns of the eyelid skin cause pain, erythema with or without blistering, and marked oedema. By contrast, full thickness burns are often relatively painless because of extensive destruction of subcutaneous nerve endings. They produce a black or white coagulum with little oedema.

### Management

Minor corneal epithelial burns are treated in the same way as a corneal abrasion (see page 141). More severe ocular injuries require admission. Complications include corneal scarring, perforation, and symblepharon. Partial thickness burns of the skin of the eyelid only require adequate analgesia. As the dermis is not completely destroyed, healing usually occurs rapidly with mild, if any, scarring. If there is blistering, a non-adherent dressing should be applied. Patients with full thickness burns should be admitted. Healing is slow with extensive scar formation which may cause corneal exposure, ectropion, trichiasis, and punctal occlusion. Early skin grafting may be required.

## Radiation burn—arc eye

Unprotected exposure to ultraviolet radiation, most commonly from welding arcs or sunbeds, causes delayed loss of corneal epithelial cells.

### Symptoms and signs

Patients typically present 6–8 hours after exposure with bilateral severe ocular pain, photophobia, watering, and blurring of vision. Findings include a mild reduction of visual acuity, conjunctival chemosis and injection, and a generalised punctate corneal epithelial loss. Lid oedema and erythema may also be present.

### Management

Fortunately, the prognosis is that of complete recovery, usually within 24 hours. The eyes should be treated in the same way as a corneal abrasion (see page 141). If the patient's circumstances preclude bilateral padding, the less affected eye can alternatively be treated with frequent application of the antibiotic ointment. The use of a mydriatic reduces pain from ciliary spasm and minimises unwanted visits.

# 7 Diplopia

> **Definition**
> Diplopia exists when a patient is seeing two images of a single object

## Types of diplopia

- Binocular
- Monocular
- Physiological.

## Causes of diplopia

### Binocular diplopia

Typically this occurs when there is a deviation of the visual axes of the two eyes so that the points of interest do not fall on corresponding points of the retina.

*Causes* (Table 7.1)

- Nerve palsies affecting one of the three cranial nerves which supply the six extraocular muscles
- A breakdown of phorias or old muscle imbalance
- Tethering of the muscle or globe by fibrous tissue caused by trauma or inflammation
- Myositis and orbital disease
- Neuromuscular junction disease.

### Monocular diplopia

This is a form of pseudodiplopia in which the images are seldom entirely separate and are seen even when the other eye is covered. This commonly results from a refractive abnormality

Table 7.1 Typical presenting symptoms and signs of the different causes of binocular diplopia

| Condition | Symptoms |
|---|---|
| Breakdown of phorias or muscle imbalance especially as a result of congenital nerve palsy or weakness | Long history of intermittent diplopia when tired Deviation similar in all positions of gaze |
| Nerve palsies | |
|   Ischaemic lesions | Sudden onset, non-progressive Commonly a history of diabetes mellitus, hypertension, or microvascular disease |
|   Compressive lesions | Gradual onset with progressive worsening of symptoms |
| Muscle tethering | |
|   Old trauma | History of orbital injury Inferior rectus, medial rectus most often involved |
|   Thyroid eye disease (TED) | Intermittent onset becoming constant later Associated signs of TED Inferior rectus most often affected restricting upgaze |
| Inflammation Myositis, pseudotumour | Pain in direction of action of muscle signs of orbital inflammation |
| Orbital tumours | Displacement of globe Mechanical restriction of movement against tumour mass Orbital apex lesions may affect the nerves supplying the muscle and cause variety of diplopia, including total ophthalmoplegia |
| Neuromuscular junction Myasthenia | Intermittent at onset but becoming constant later Varies during the day but worse with fatigue Can mimic any cause of diplopia |

caused by astigmatism, cataract, corneal opacities, and a displaced lens or lens implant. The cause is duplication of an edge or edges as a result of lack of a sharp focus.

Monocular diplopia of sensory origin occurs rarely. It is sometimes seen after brain trauma or cerebrovascular accident. It may also occur during treatment of amblyopia, or in an amblyopic patient after loss of the good eye. This diplopia is not eliminated by using the pinhole.

Monocular diplopia can also be a functional symptom in a completely healthy individual, for example, in litigation cases.

## Physiological diplopia

This occurs normally and is commonly complained of by children. This happens when one becomes aware of the two images formed outside areas where the retinal points correspond. This can be illustrated by an example: hold a finger in front of the eyes when looking at a large object across the room. Two fingers are seen if the focus is on the object, or two objects if the focus is on the finger.

## Definitions of strabismus/squint

### Concomitant strabismus

In concomitant or manifest squint, the angle of deviation is constant regardless of the position of gaze. This is a typical picture of childhood strabismus and patients do not appreciate double vision, because the image of one eye is suppressed.

### Concomitant heterophoria

Many people have a concomitant heterophoria or latent squint where there is a tendency for the eyes to deviate into a squinting position, but this is normally prevented by central fusional mechanisms.

### Incomitant strabismus

The angle of the squint varies according to the direction of gaze and whether the right or left eye is fixing. They are usually caused by paresis or muscle underaction.

## History

When trying to establish the diagnosis, it is important to differentiate between new and potentially serious pathology from breakdown of muscle balance in longstanding disease.

*Ask the patient directly if the diplopia is monocular or binocular*

If monocular diplopia is eliminated when testing pinhole visual acuity, the cause is probably refractive.

*Determine if the diplopia is purely horizontal (that is, side by side), or if there is a vertical or torsional element*

**Horizontal diplopia** This indicates involvement of the horizontal recti. The common causes of horizontal diplopia are:

- Muscle balance problems such as breakdown of phorias, convergence, and accommodation insufficiency
- Lateral rectus weakness in palsies of nerve VI
- Medial rectus restriction in thyroid eye disease, medial wall orbital blowout fractures
- Orbital inflammatory processes (for example, myositis) involving the horizontal recti
- Myasthenia gravis.

**Vertical diplopia** This is usually secondary to disorders of the vertical recti or obliques. Common causes of vertical diplopia are:

- Muscle imbalance such as longstanding weakness of the superior oblique in congenital palsy of nerve IV
- Third, fourth, or multiple cranial nerve palsies
- Restriction of the inferior rectus in thyroid eye disease and inferior wall orbital blowout fracture
- Inflammatory disease
    direct involvement of muscles: pseudotumour and orbital myositis
    indirect cause of diplopia through cranial nerves: superior orbital fissure and cavernus sinus inflammation
- Local lesions, for example, tumours; orbital apex syndrome involving multiple cranial nerves (from inflammation, tumour, thyroid eye disease)
- Myasthenia gravis.

*Did the diplopia start suddenly? Are symptoms intermittent, progressive or stationary?*

Much of the pathology causing diplopia has a typical history of onset and progression (see Table 7.1).

*Is there any pain associated with the diplopia?*

Examples of painful conditions:

- Inflammatory lesions, for example, pseudotumour
- Ischaemic lesions, for example, cranial nerve infarction
- Compressive lesions, for example, aneurysm of the posterior communicating artery with a pupil involving palsy of nerve III.

*Are there any other neurological symptoms?*

Problems with gait, balance, muscle power, urinary problems, and headache may all be related. Think of multiple sclerosis, brainstem ischaemia, raised intracranial pressure, and space occupying lesions.

### Is there any relevant medical history?

**Single cranial nerve palsies** Diabetes, smoking, hypertension, and being aged over 55 years are risk factors.

**Other diplopia** Cerebral vascular accident, thyroid disease, herpes zoster.

### Is there any relevant ocular history?

- Previous ocular surgery such as retinal detachment or squint surgery
- Thyroid eye disease
- Orbital trauma.

## Examination of the patient with diplopia

A systematic approach is needed to avoid missing relevant signs. The following are the recommended sequences.

### Monocular diplopia

- Pinhole testing: diplopia eliminated in nearly all cases
- Slitlamp examination for cornea or lenticular abnormalities
- Refraction for astigmatism and ametropia.

### Binocular diplopia
#### Inspection

**Abdominal head postures** These are used by the patient to put the head into such a position that the weak muscle is used to the minimum. The simplest example is a head turn to the left for a left lateral rectus weakness which obviates the need for extreme left gaze. If there is an abnormal head posture, ask how long the posture has been adopted. Old photographs are often helpful.

#### Eye alignment and lid position
- Globe displacement, for example, tumour, thyroid eye disease
- Proptosis, for example, tumour, thyroid eye disease

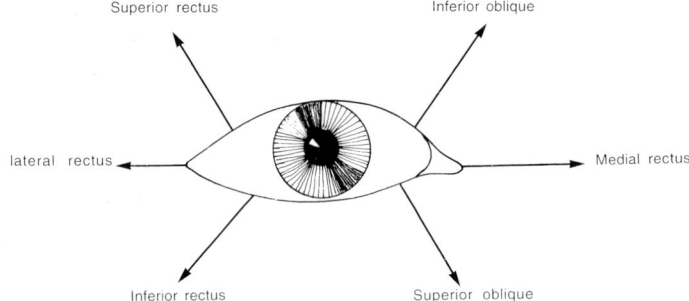

Figure 7.1 Directions of principal action of the six muscles of the right eye.

- Enophthalmos, for example, old blowout fracture, sclerosing breast carcinoma in the orbit
- Ptosis, for example, palsy of nerve III, myasthenia
- Eyelid retraction, for example, thyroid eye disease.

**Globe injection and chemosis** These suggest orbital disease, such as thyroid eye disease or a pseudotumour.

### Examination of eye movements

There are six positions for each eye in which one can best isolate the action of a single muscle (Fig 7.1). Note the vertical acting recti are most effective in abduction and the obliques in adduction.

**Test versional movements with both eyes open** Examine eye movements in the nine positions of gaze (Fig 7.2), noting any limitation of movement which can result either from weakness or from restriction of the extraocular muscles. In incomitant squint

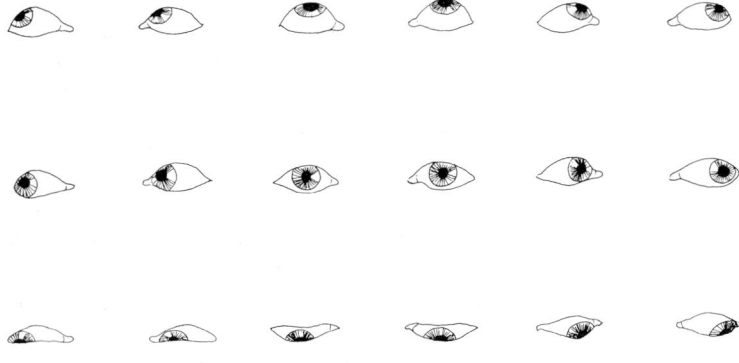

Figure 7.2 Nine positions of gaze.

# DIPLOPIA

(see Definition, page 161), the angle of deviation is dependent upon the position of gaze and there will be a position in which diplopia is maximal. The double vision will be worse when a patient with a weak muscle attempts to look in the direction of the field of action of that muscle. Alternatively, a patient with a tight, fibrosed, or restricted muscle will exerience worsening of the diplopia when an attempt is made to look away from the field of action of the affected muscle.

> **Example**
>
> If a patient complains that the double vision is always worse when looking to the right, this could be secondary to:
>
> - A right lateral rectus or left medial rectus palsy, or
> - A right medial rectus restriction, for example, from thyroid eye disease or medial wall blowout fracture

Test convergence by getting the patient to fixate on a target that is brought closer and closer to the patient's nose. The eyes should turn inward equally and smoothly. This is a voluntary movement and requires patient cooperation.

**Test uniocular movements or ductions with one eye covered** In large concomitant squints one eye may give the false impression of having restricted movements by not fixing when both eyes are open. By occluding one eye and testing the movements uniocularly, it is possible to determine whether movements are genuinely restricted.

### *The diplopia test*

In cases where there is obvious restriction of ocular movement, it is relatively easy to identify the muscle at fault. In cases where limitation of movement is not obvious, use the position of maximum diplopia as a clue. Use a light source or point target for fixation:

- Ascertain the position of maximum diplopia by moving a fixation target in the six positions corresponding to the directions of principal action of the six muscles (see Fig 7.1)
- Holding the fixation target in the position of maximum diplopia, occlude one eye at a time and ask the patient when the more peripheral and weaker image disappears

- The peripheral image belongs to the eye with the underacting muscle.

### *The cover–uncover test*

In concomitant squints, the angle of the deviation remains the same regardless of position of gaze. This is typical of childhood squints (usually no diplopia) and breakdown of phorias in adults.

The cover–uncover test is done with the patient fixing on a near target, a distant target, and then one in the far distance. Using a near target with fine detail will induce both accommodation and convergence. To avoid accommodation use a light such as a pen torch.

The test is as follows—cover and then uncover the eye that appears to be fixating. Use an occluder that completely covers the eye; it is important to prevent the patient from looking round the occluder.

When covering the fixating eye, observe the uncovered eye. If it moves to take up fixation there is a manifest squint.

### *The alternate cover test*

If there is no manifest squint the alternate cover test is used to reveal a latent deviation or phoria (that is, a tendency for the eyes to deviate into a squinting position normally prevented by central fusional mechanisms when both eyes are open):

- Occlude each eye alternately several times to dissociate the eyes
- Keeping the occluder over one eye, make sure that the uncovered eye is fixating by moving the fixation target from side to side
- The occluder is then taken away and the behaviour of the eye just uncovered is observed.

In a latent squint, the occluded eye drifts under the occluder and has to move to regain fixation and binocular single vision again. Exophoria denotes a tendency for the eye to drift outwards, esophoria inwards, hyperphoria upwards, and hypophoria downwards.

### *The three step test for vertical diplopia*

Elevation of the eye is carried out by the combined action of the superior rectus and inferior oblique. Depression of the eye is carried out by the combined action of the inferior rectus and the

# DIPLOPIA

superior oblique. Each of these four muscles has a main field of action which is illustrated in Fig 7.1.

The three step test is useful in some cases of vertical diplopia when it is difficult to determine which muscle is at fault or to confirm findings on examination of eye movements.

The rationale of the test is to halve the number of possibilities by each step, so that the eight possibles have been reduced to one after the final step (see Appendix A for more detailed explanation of how the test works).

- *Step 1:* observe which eye is higher in the primary position. Confirm by the cover test if in doubt.
- *Step 2:* determine if the vertical deviation increases in right or left gaze.
- *Step 3:* determine whether the maximum vertical deviation of the two eyes occurs when the head is tilted either to the right or the left shoulder (Bielschowsky's head tilt test).

The differentiation between the muscles involved in the three step test is demonstrated empirically in Fig 7.3 (see Appendix A for explanation).

## Forced duction test

This test is done to differentiate between a paretic or fibrotic muscle. Local anaesthetic is put in the eye and then the eye can be rolled from side to side with a cotton bud pressed firmly on the sclera. There is resistance to movement in cases of fibrosis, but not in cases of paresis. Alternatively, a toothed forceps can be used to hold the eye at the muscle insertions, but only after sufficient topical anaesthesia has been applied.

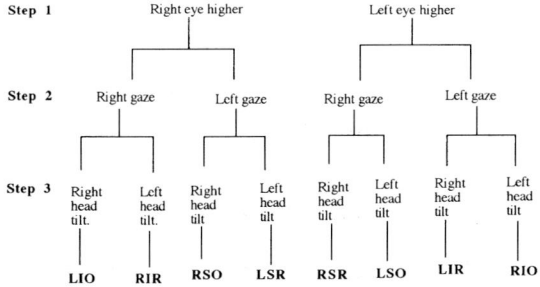

Figure 7.3  The three step test: L, left eye; R, right eye; IO, inferior oblique; IR, inferior rectus; SO, superior oblique; SR, superior rectus.

### Confirmation of the diagnosis

**The Hess chart** This is obtained by dissociating the two eyes either by red/green filters (the Hess screen test) or by a mirror (the Lees screen). The foveal projections of the non-fixing eye are plotted on to a chart to form an inner square of eight dots and an outer square of sixteen dots. Muscle underaction in the defective eye and the corresponding overaction in the fellow eye can be plotted. Provided that the patient is cooperative, these tests are precise and repeatable on different occasions.

## Diagnosis and management of horizontal diplopia

Horizontal diplopia indicates an inability of the horizontal recti to function normally caused by either weakness or restriction from a variety of causes (Fig 7.4). (See also Table 7.2 and box.)

Table 7.2  Differential diagnosis of horizontal diplopia

| Muscle affected | Nerve supply |
| --- | --- |
| Lateral rectus | Sixth cranial nerve |
| Medial rectus | Inferior division of third cranial nerve which also supplies inferior rectus, inferior oblique, and the pupil |

### Causes of horizontal diplopia

*Orthoptic*
   Decompensating phorias
   Convergence and divergence insufficiency
   Convergence spasm
   Acute squints
*Vascular/demyelination*
   Palsy of nerve VI
   Internuclear ophthalmoplegia
*Immunological/inflammatory*
   Myasthenia gravis
   Thyroid eye disease
   Orbital myositis
*Trauma*
   Muscle haematoma
   Media wall blowout fracture of the orbit
*Raised intracranial pressure*
   Palsy of nerve VI

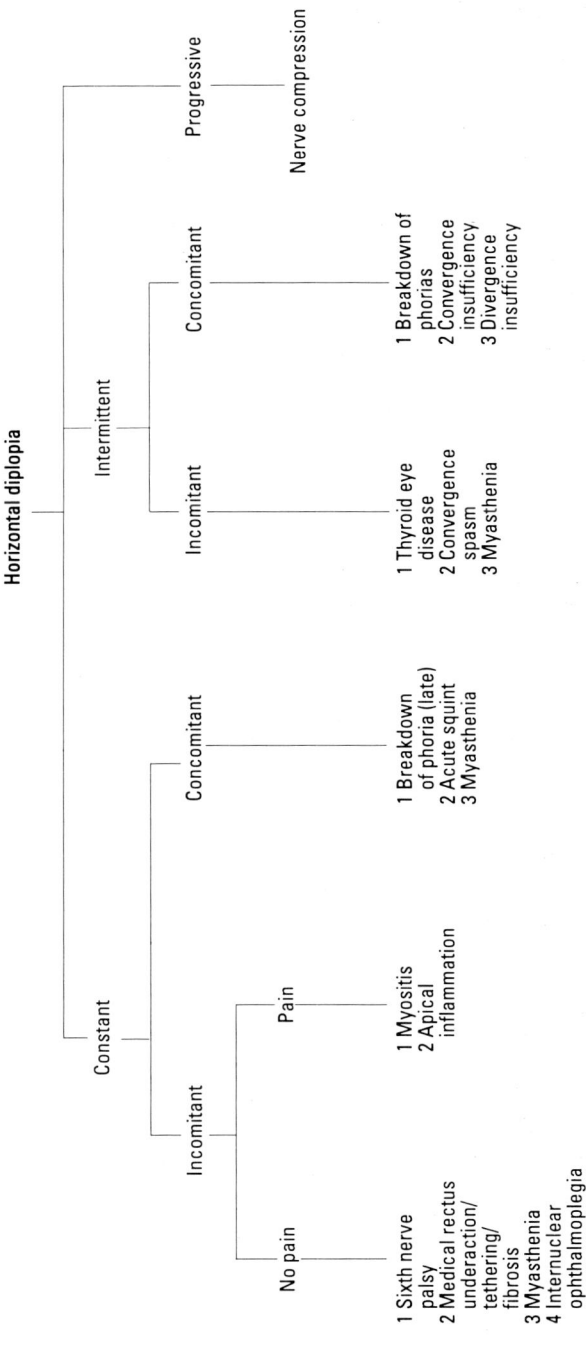

Figure 7.4 Systemic approach to diagnosis of horizontal diplopia.

## Intermittent or variable during the day
### Horizontal decompensating phorias

Phorias (latent squint, see Definition, page 166) can be horizontal or vertical in nature. Only horizontal phorias are discussed here.

Many people have a concomitant heterophoria or latent squint in which there is a tendency for the eyes to deviate into a squinting position; this is normally prevented by central fusional mechanism.

In general an esophoria is found in individuals with uncorrected hypermetropia, and an exophoria is found in those with uncorrected myopia. Only if the fusional amplitudes are inadequate, or if there is some sensory obstacle interrupting fusional mechanisms, will the phoria break down. Once fusion has broken down, other factors, such as the excessive accommodation used by hypermetropic individuals, will help establish a permanent squint. At first the phoria will be intermittent, but in time it will become constant.

#### Symptoms and signs
- Intermittent diplopia
- Heterophoria on cover testing
- Frontal headache, asthenopic symptoms, and a history of shutting one eye.

#### Associated factors
- Increasing symptoms with age, fatigue, and illness
- Uncorrected refractive error.

#### Management
- Check eye movements to eliminate a neurological or mechanical cause
- Do the cover–uncover test to detect any latent squint
- Refraction and appropriate spectacles
- Orthoptic exercises
- Prisms
- Surgery only if necessary (diplopia may persist or change after surgery).

### Convergence insufficiency

This is defined as an inability to maintain or obtain adequate binocular convergence.

### Symptoms and signs
- Frontal headaches and eye strain associated with close work
- Blurred vision and intermittent diplopia for near fixation
- Exophoria for near fixation
- Near point of convergence is reduced, being greater than 10 cm.

If the uniocular accommodation is better than binocular accommodation, convergence insufficiency is the probable diagnosis. If accommodation insufficiency is present, both uniocular and binocular accommodation will be below normal for the patient's age.

### Management
- Any significant refractive error should be corrected
- Suitable patients will respond to orthoptic exercises such as simple convergence exercises
- In patients who are unwilling to do the exercises, or in whom there is no improvement, prisms may help
- In severe cases, surgery may help although there is a risk of persistent diplopia.

## Convergence spasm

### Symptoms and signs
- Intermittent
- Painful horizontal versions
- Miosis of pupils on lateral gaze
- Usually bilateral, although sometimes there is a unilateral abduction deficit.

### Associated factors
- Strong degree of convergence, which is sustained through repeated examinations
- More cases are not pathological, although occasionally they may be associated with underlying disorders of the vestibular system or brain stem.

**Management** The patient is using convergence as a mechanism to prevent the eye from moving laterally. Full abduction may be noted on testing saccades or oculocephalic movements. Patching or cycloplegic drops may inhibit the reflex enough to allow the examiner to elicit normal abduction.

These are difficult patients to treat. First ensure that the symptoms do not mask a genuine pathology. Symptoms may be purely functional and can follow minimal head trauma where litigation is involved. In these patients, discussion with the patient about all their other "problems" may help.

## Divergence insufficiency

### Symptoms and signs
- Rare
- Intermittent diplopia for distance
- Esotropia/esophoria for distance
- The eso deviation is greater for distance than for near.

### Associated factors
- Prolonged and excessive convergence.

### Management
- Refraction
- If there is excessive convergence, use orthoptic exercises
- Prisms
- Rarely, surgery.

## Myasthenia

For a cause of intermittent diplopia in any direction, see page 179.


## Constant diplopia

### Palsy of nerve VI

The sixth nerve has the longest course at the base of the brain. It supplies the lateral rectus muscle; a palsy causes double vision, increasing on lateral gaze to the side of the lesion. Most palsies of nerve VI do not localise, because a variety of intracranial processes can stretch and damage the nerve as it passes over the tip of the petrous bone.

### Symptoms and signs
- The affected eye turns in and abducts poorly
- Abnormal head posture with a head turn to the side of the lesion
- Mild retro-orbital pain in some cases.

### Associated factors
- Microvascular disease

- Trauma
- Raised intracranial pressure
- Intracranial tumours
- Meningitis.

## Differential diagnosis
- Thyroid eye disease
- Medial wall blowout fracture of the orbit
- Myasthenia gravis
- Orbital myositis
- Convergence spasm.

**Prognosis** The prognosis for recovery of palsies of nerve VI is good when the cause is: microvascular, increased ICP, after lumbar puncture, or postviral. Such palsies secondary to severe head trauma or longstanding compression have a poorer prognosis.

**Management** Check for other neurological signs. Brainstem lesions are nearly always associated with other neurological symptoms, such as an ipsilateral facial palsy.

In children, postviral syndromes, trauma, and neoplastic disease are the usual causes of palsies of nerve VI. Up to one third of children with brainstem glioma are reported to present with a unilateral isolated palsy of nerve VI, so neuroimaging is mandatory. Most postviral palsies of nerve VI recover but can be recurrent.

Unilateral palsies in young adults should also be investigated fully with a vascular work up, neuroimaging, and lumbar puncture.

As an isolated finding in a patient over the age of 50, microvascular disease is the most frequent cause. An ESR should be taken to exclude temporal arteritis. These patients can be followed expectantly in the clinic with neuroimaging if there is no resolution after 3 months.

Bilateral palsies of nerve VI almost never result from vascular disease; they need neuroimaging and lumbar puncture.

To alleviate diplopia occlude one eye. Prisms can be tried for small deviations. In children, the eyes should be patched alternately to avoid amblyopia ("lazy eye"). Botulinum toxin injected into the medial rectus prevents contracture while waiting for recovery of lateral rectus function. After six months of stable deviation, surgery can be considered.

The management of individual cranial palsies is summarised in Table 7.3.

### Acute squint

An acute esotropia (convergent squint) of sudden onset and the complaint of diplopia should always be evaluated for neurological problems. Unilateral or bilateral palsies of nerve VI may quickly compensate and become concomitant in nature, in which case it may be difficult to recognise the paretic muscle.

There are, however, two forms of acute concomitant strabismus which occur without obvious neurological causes.

**Acute strabismus after artificial interruption of fusion**
This occurs after occlusion to one eye, for example, after padding for corneal abrasion, occlusion for amblyopia, or after trauma has closed the lids for several days. In children the occluded eye tends to be in an esotropic position, and in adults with a large angle exophoria, an exotropic position.

Management involves the following:

- Correction of any refractive error
- Resolution will be spontaneous in some
- Surgery.

**Acute strabismus without any interruption of fusion**
There is acute onset of a relatively large angle esotropia and diplopia. The refractive and accommodative contribution is minimal. It may be precipitated by illness or stress, but could also occur spontaneously. It would appear to result from the patients having a mild esophoria, but with only very slim fusional reserve.

Management involves the following:

- Check refraction
- Surgery: prognosis good.

### Internuclear ophthalmoplegia

Internuclear ophthalmoplegia (INO) is a lesion in the medial longitudinal fasciculus (MLF) between the nucleus of cranial nerve III on one side and the contralateral nucleus of nerve VI.

Table 7.3 Table of management of cranial nerve problems causing diplopia

| Cranial neve palsy of | Symptoms and signs | Causal factors | Management |
|---|---|---|---|
| Nerve III | Ptosis, eye down and out<br>Pupil sparing<br><br>Ptosis, eye down and out<br>Pupil dilated | Microvascular disease:<br>  hypertension<br>  diabetes<br>  temporal arteritis<br>Older age group<br>Compressive lesions<br>Posterior communicating artery aneurysm | Microvascular investigations (BP, glucose, ESR)<br>Neuroimaging if atypical<br><br>Immediate admission<br>Neuroimaging<br>Angiography<br>Lumbar puncture |
| Nerve IV | Vertical diplopia<br>Compensatory head tilt to opposite side with chin depression<br>Congenital=intermittent history; large vertical phorias, tilt in old photograph | Trauma<br>Viral in children<br>Congenital 20–40 year age group<br>Microvascular in older age group<br>Tumour is rare | *Congenital palsy*: no investigations unless atypical<br>*Younger patients*: neuroimaging and systemic evaluation<br>*Older patients*: microvascular investigations<br>Neuroimaging |
| Nerve VI | Horizontal diplopia<br>Loss of abduction<br>Compensatory head turn to the side of the lesion | Trauma<br>Raised intracranial pressure<br>Tumours<br>Viral—younger age<br>Microvascular—older age | *Unilateral sixths*: children and young adults: neuroimaging and full systemic investigations<br>*Older patients*: microvascular investigations<br>Neuroimaging if atypical<br>*Bilateral sixths*: full evaluation with neuroimaging and lumbar puncture |

### Symptoms and signs
- Relatively rare
- Patients may not complain of diplopia
- Typically, there is an apparent medial rectus paresis in the eye on the side of the lesion
- There is nystagmus of the contralateral abducting eye
- To accentuate the signs of a partial INO, ask the patient to look rapidly from side to side from targets (for example, pen, fingers), held up on the right and left; the adducting eye will appear to lag behind.

### Associated factors
- Multiple sclerosis
- History of urinary frequency or urgency
- Previous resolving neurological deficits
- Microvascular disease: hypertension or diabetes
- Head trauma.

### Differential diagnosis
- Pseudo-INO from myasthenia gravis
- Other causes of an adduction defect: thyroid eye disease, orbital myositis, or, very rarely, a lesion of nerve III involving only the medial rectus.

**Prognosis** Cases secondary to multiple sclerosis can be expected to show spontaneous improvement with time. The amount of recovery for other causes depends on the amount of structural damage to the neuronal circuits.

**Management** Bilateral INO is most frequently seen in demyelinating disease (multiple sclerosis). Brainstem vascular disease is associated more commonly with a unilateral INO, although it is not unusual for a bilateral INO to occur.

Magnetic resonance imaging is the neuroimaging modality of choice for evaluating the posterior fossa. Not only is the brain stem depicted more clearly, but it also provides evidence of multiple sclerosis.

### *Myasthenia gravis, thyroid eye disease, orbital myositis, and trauma*

These can cause vertical as well as horizontal diplopia and are described in more detail in the next section.

## Diagnosis and management of vertical diplopia with or without a horizontal component

Vertical diplopia indicates abnormal function of the vertical recti or oblique muscles as a result of weakness (for example, palsy) or restriction (for example, tethering) (Fig 7.5). (See also Table 7.4 and box.)

Table 7.4 Differential diagnosis of vertical diplopia with or without a horizontal element

|  | Muscles involved | Nerve supply |
| --- | --- | --- |
| Elevators | Superior rectus | Superior division of cranial nerve III (also supplies the levator muscle) |
|  | Inferior oblique | Inferior division of cranial nerve III (also supplies medial rectus, inferior rectus, and pupil) |
| Depressors | Inferior rectus | Inferior division of cranial nerve III (also supplies medial rectus, inferior oblique, and pupil) |
|  | Superior oblique | Cranial nerve IV |

---

**Causes of vertical diplopia**

**Orthoptic**
  Decompensating phorias
  Longstanding superior oblique underaction; congenital palsy of nerve IV
**Vascular/demyelination**
  Palsy: of nerves III or IV, or multiple
  Skew deviation
**Immunological/inflammatory**
  Myasthenia gravis
  Thyroid eye disease
  Orbital myositis
**Infection**
  Orbital cellulitis
**Trauma**
  Muscle haematoma
  Orbital wall blowout fracture
  Previous ocular surgery
**Compressive/infiltrative**
  Multiple oculomotor nerve palsies/orbital apex syndrome
  Orbital tumours

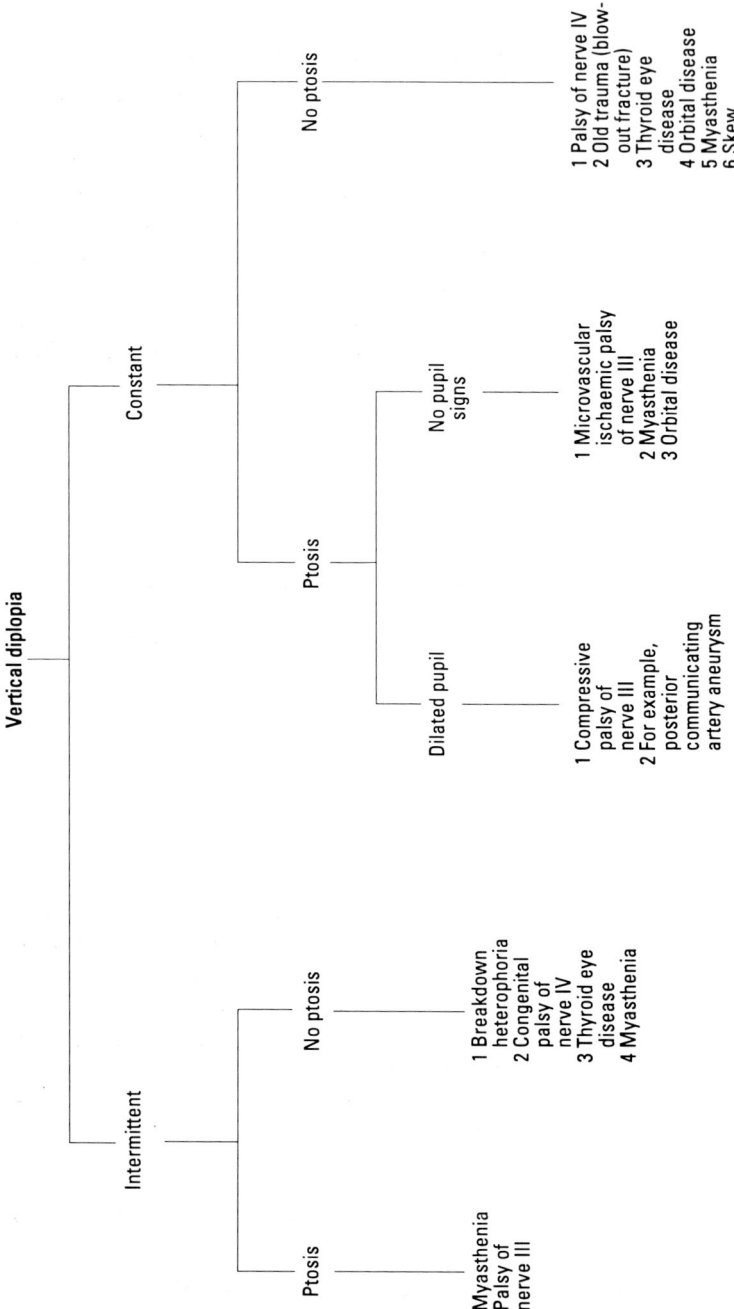

Figure 7.5  Systemic approach to diagnosis of vertical diplopia.

## Intermittent or variable during the day
### Breakdown of existing ocular muscle imbalance

The most common cause of a vertical ocular muscle imbalance is longstanding superior oblique weakness or a congenital palsy of nerve IV (see Palsy of nerve IV on page 183). There is often an associated abnormal head posture which may have been present for some time and is evident on reviewing old photographs. The patient complains of increasing problems with diplopia, asthenopic symptoms, and headache, especially when using the eyes.

A hypo- or hyperphoria may decompensate to give symptoms of headache, "eye strain", and intermittent diplopia, especially with prolonged close work.

#### Associated factors
- Increasing symptoms with age, fatigue, and illness
- Uncorrected refractive error.

#### Management
- Check eye movements to eliminate a neurological or mechanical cause
- Do the cover–uncover test to detect any latent squint
- Bielschowsky's three step test
- Refraction and appropriate spectacles
- Orthoptic exercises
- Prisms
- Surgery.

### Myasthenia gravis

Myasthenia gravis is an immunologically mediated disorder in which antibodies bind to acetylcholine receptors of striate muscle in such a way that they block the normal synaptic transmission of acetylcholine. Fifty per cent of patients present with ocular symptoms and over 90% eventually develop eye movement abnormalities. "Ocular myasthenia" refers to myasthenia limited to the eyes on clinical examination, and, in 40% of patients presenting with eye signs alone, systemic disease is never manifested.

#### Symptoms and signs
- Myasthenia may mimic any cause of diplopia, including ocular nerve palsies
- Variable ptosis and lid fatiguability on sustained upward or lateral gaze

- Cogan's lid twitch sign occurs when the patient looks down and then straight ahead; as the eyes move from the down position to straight ahead, there is a transient eyelid flick upwards before the lids settle into their usual ptotic position.

### Associated factors
- Symptoms of general myasthenia
- Thymoma.

### Management
- Any oculomotor disturbance without obvious explanation should be investigated for the possibility of myasthenia.
- Take blood for acetylcholine receptor antibodies. In cases of doubt the Tensilon test will help confirm the diagnosis. Refer the patient to a neurologist.
- Before doing a Tensilon test, have resuscitation equipment to hand. Either give atropine 0·4 mg 15 min before the test or have it ready to counter unwanted cholinergic side effects. Give a test dose of 2 mg Tensilon intravenously and, if there is no adverse reaction after one minute, inject a further 8 mg. The response can either be charted subjectively with a momentary improvement in symptoms or objectively with Hess charts.
- Computed tomography or MRI of the chest to look for lymphoepithelial thymoma, present in 10–15% of patients with myasthenia gravis.
- Treatment is with acetylcholinesterase inhibitors, systemic steroids, and thymectomy.

## *Thyroid eye disease*

The most commonly involved muscle is the inferior rectus causing vertical diplopia. The second most commonly involved muscle is the medical rectus causing horizontal diplopia.

For symptoms and signs and management see Chapter 10.

When the diplopia has been stable for at least six months on Hess chart testing, extraocular muscle surgery can be considered.

### Constant diplopia
#### *Palsy of nerve III*

Cranial nerve III supplies the superior, medial, and inferior rectus muscles, and the inferior oblique. The nerve also carries

# DIPLOPIA

pupillomotor fibres for pupil constriction, and fibres to the ciliary muscles for accommodation and innervation to the levator muscle of the upper eyelid.

Palsies of nerve III can be total or partial. The position of an eye with a total palsy of nerve III is down and out with ptosis and a dilated pupil.

### Symptoms and signs
- Pain in the face, headache, and retro-orbital pain are characteristic of palsies associated with a posterior communicating aneurysm, but they can also occur with pupil sparing palsies
- The patient may complain of a droopy lid, unequal pupil size, and/or diplopia
- Diplopia is not a problem if there is a total ptosis
- Up to 3 mm of proptosis may be associated with a total palsy.

### Associated factors
- Isolated palsy involving the pupil is associated with a posterior communicating aneurysm
- Pain is usually a predominant symptom
- Pupil sparing palsies tend to be associated with microvascular disease, for example, diabetes.

Less common causes include trauma, tumour compression, migraine, infection (meningitis), and vasculitis. There may be accompanying neurological signs.

Aberrant regeneration of nerve III occurs with chronic compressive lesions. It is characterised by lid retraction or pupillary constriction on attempted downgaze or adduction.

Table 7.5 shows the major clinical findings that help to differentiate between compressive and ischaemic paresis of nerve III.

Table 7.5 Differentiating features between ischaemic and compressive palsies of nerve III

| Feature | Ischaemic | Compressive |
| --- | --- | --- |
| Associated neurological signs | Seldom seen | Usually present |
| Pain | Variable | Usually pesent |
| Pupillary involvement (%) | 5 | 95 |
| Age at onset | Over 40 years | Any age |
| Aberrant regeneration | Not present | Chronic progressive compressive lesions |

### Prognosis
- In palsies of nerve III secondary to microvascular disease, the prognosis is good with recovery in 2–3 months
- In compressive lesions, the amount of recovery depends on persisting neuronal damage.

### Differential diagnosis
- Myasthenia gravis
- Orbital disease
- Thyroid eye disease.

### Management (see box)

---

**Management**

**Evaluation of potential underlying causes**
*Pupillary involvement with a palsy of nerve III*
Admit to hospital with computed tomography or MRI to exclude a space occupying lesion. If these studies are inconclusive the patient needs angiography and lumbar puncture

*Pupil sparing palsy of nerve III*
Presence of vascular disease
- In the diabetic, hypertensive, or elderly patient, exclude serious related disease from the history and clinical examination
- ESR for giant cell arteritis
- Follow the patient weekly for several weeks; arrange neuroimaging if the palsy progresses or associated neurological signs develop

Absence of obvious vascular disease
- Investigate for vascular and vasculitic disease
- Neuroimaging is on an individual basis depending on symptoms

**Alleviation of patient symptoms**
- As a result of the multiple extraocular muscles involved, only partial palsies may be amenable to treatment with prisms
- If the ptosis is *complete*, the patient will have no diplopia
- If there is *diplopia*, then *occlusion* of the paretic eye will give symptomatic relief
- If the *dilated pupil* causes visual symptoms, weak *pilocarpine* drops can be tried

---

The patient should be followed in the orthoptic department with Hess charts and, if the deficit is stable for a minimum of six months, then surgery to improve cosmetic appearance can be considered. Often the best that can be achieved is a small area of binocular single vision in the primary position.

The management of individual cranial palsies is summarised in Table 7.3.

## Palsy of nerve IV

Nerve IV supplies the superior oblique muscle; it is the cranial nerve with the longest intracranial course and the one most frequently involved by trauma. Palsies of nerve IV are the most common cause of acquired vertical strabismus.

### Symptoms and signs
- Torsional vertical double vision
- Diplopia maximal on looking down, causing symptoms with reading and going down stairs
- Compensatory head tilt to the opposite side to the lesion with chin depression
- Head tilt on old photographs with congenital palsy of nerve IV
- Large phorias may be demonstrated in congenital cases.

### Associated factors
- Congenital nerve palsies are the most common cause of a palsy of nerve IV
- Severe head trauma with loss of consciousness
- Bilateral palsies of nerve IV occur following trauma, presumably secondary to damage in the anterior medullary velum where the two nerves cross
- Minor head injuries producing a palsy suggest a possible tumour
- Recent viral illness in children
- Microvascular disease, smoking, hypertension, and diabetes in the over 50 age group
- Compressive lesions causing palsies of nerve IV are rare.

### Differential diagnosis
- Thyroid eye disease
- Myasthenia gravis
- Orbital trauma.

**Prognosis** If secondary to ischaemia, mild head trauma, and compression of short duration, the prognosis for recovery is good. In severe head injury and longstanding compression, prognosis is poor.

**Management** Superior oblique muscle weakness can be difficult to pick up on examination of eye movements, especially in bilateral partial palsies.

Bielschowsky's three step test and orthoptic evaluation with Hess charts can help in the diagnosis.

Occlusion of the paretic eye or the use of prisms with small deviations can give symptomatic alleviation of the diplopia. Surgery is only contemplated when the deviation has been stable for six months.

The work up of an isolated palsy of nerve IV depends on the age of the patient:

- In all patients without a history of trauma, esecially those between the ages of 20 and 40 years, consider a congenital palsy of nerve IV. Patients with a congenital palsy of neve IV are able to fuse large degrees of vertical deviation which would cause symptomatic diplopia in normal subjects.
- Up to the age of 50 with no evidence of congenital palsy, there should be neuroimaging and investigations for vascular and vasculitic disease.
- Over the age of 50, the most probable cause of an isolated palsy of nerve IV will be vascular occlusion. Neuroimaging is delayed unless the palsy is progressive or non-resolving.
- In all age groups, consider a Tensilon test to exclude myasthenia.

The management of individual cranial palsies is summarised in Table 7.3.

### Multiple oculomotor nerve palsies

#### Symptoms and signs
- The pathology is either in the brain stem or peripheral
- Brainstem pathology will have other neurological signs
- Peripheral pathology lies at or in front of the cavernous sinus
- Lesions causing mutiple oculomotor nerve palsies are usually compressive, infiltrative, or traumatic
- Toxic motor nerve palsies have no distinguishing characteristics; a good history is essential for suspecting the diagnosis.

#### Differential diagnosis
- Myasthenia
- Ocular myopathies

- Cavernous sinus processes: aneurysm, pituitary tumour, meningioma, arteriovenous fistula
- Orbital: orbital apex syndrome, for example, from orbital metastases, thyroid eye disease, pseudotumour, myositis, and Tolosa–Hunt syndromes
- Rare disorders affecting multiple cranial nerves include amyloid, arteritis (especially temporal arteritis), and tumour infiltration of the muscles.

### Management
- Neuroimaging of the orbital apex region; computed tomography is superior to MRI for bony involvement
- General medical evaluation looking for a primary tumour
- Thyroid function
- Angiography if an aneurysm if suspected.

## *Skew deviation*

Skew deviation is a vertical misalignment of the eyes secondary to disruption of supranuclear input, commonly caused by brainstem or cerebellar disease.

### Symptoms and signs
- The vertical deviation may be constant, vary, or even alternate with direction of gaze
- Usually *no* associated torsional diplopia
- Other brainstem findings such as internuclear ophthalmoplegia
- Occipital or retro-orbital head pain.

### Associated factors
- Ischaemic brainstem disease
- Multiple sclerosis.

### Management
- Neuroimaging.

## *Orbital trauma*

Orbital injuries are almost always caused by blunt trauma, either from an object striking the face, for example, a fist, or through the patient being thrown against a hard surface.

In the acute stage, orbital and muscle haematoma may cause diplopia in any direction.

Orbital wall fracture causes limitation of movement secondary to prolapse of orbital tissue and subsequent fibrosis. Blowout fractures of the floor of the orbit typically cause a vertical diplopia; those of the medial wall cause a horizontal diplopia.

For details on management see Blunt trauma (page 146).

### Idiopathic orbital inflammatory disease (pseudotumour, orbital myositis, Tolosa–Hunt syndrome)

These poorly understood inflammatory diseases of the orbit may preferentially affect the muscles (orbital myositis), the superior orbital fissure (Tolosa–Hunt syndrome), or the cavernous sinus. Any combination of muscle palsies may occur.

Involvement of the orbital apex may adversely affect the optic nerve. Pain will be a prominent feature of any severe inflammation. For more details see Chapter 10.

### Orbital tumours

Occasionally, orbital tumours present as a primary limitation of ocular motility, the direction of limitation depending on the location of the tumour.

For more information see Chapter 10.

### Orbital cellulitis

For more details see Chapter 10.

### Previous periocular surgery

In retinal detachment surgery, silicone rubber tires and sponges are sutured to the sclera and may interfere with eye movement. This is especially true if the explant has been placed under an extraocular muscle, or if there has been repeated surgery. Damage to a muscle or its nerve supply may result in a more neurogenic type of palsy. Similar problems with muscle function can follow other extraocular surgery, such as squint surgery.

**Management** Most retinal detachment explants can be safely removed three months after surgery. Unfortunately, diplopia may persist secondary to fibrosis, and squint surgery may be necessary on the unaffected eye.

# 8 Headache

It is difficult to separate out "pain" from an "ache" because patients often use the words loosely to mean an unpleasant sensation. Most people would accept that there is a difference in the meaning of the two words even though it is only a question of degree. Headache is used to describe a persisting aching sensation, whereas pain tends to be more easily localised, sharper, and more acute in nature. There will always be some overlap in the presentation of some conditions as well as the response of patients as a result of variation. In addition, it is important to remember that headache and pain are subjective and the severity of the patient's complaint is not always proportional to the seriousness of the disease.

The patient complaining of headache is frequently referred to the ophthalmologist because of the widely held belief that headaches may have an ocular cause. Although muscle imbalance and refractive problems such as presbyopia can give rise to "eye strain", most headaches are benign in nature with no obvious ocular or systemic cause. Headache and ocular pain may, however, be the manifestations of potentially sight or life threatening disease and it is important to know how to recognise these serious conditions.

The diagnostic approach to the subject of headache is shown in Figs 8.1–8.4. The A&E department is not the ideal place for treating headache, but it is the place for identifying those serious conditions for which a delay in recognition would be detrimental.

## History taking

History taking is the most important part of the assessment of a patient with headache because there are often no clinical signs and the only clues to the aetiology lie in the history. The following highlights characteristic symptoms of certain types of headache.

EMERGENCY OPHTHALMOLOGY

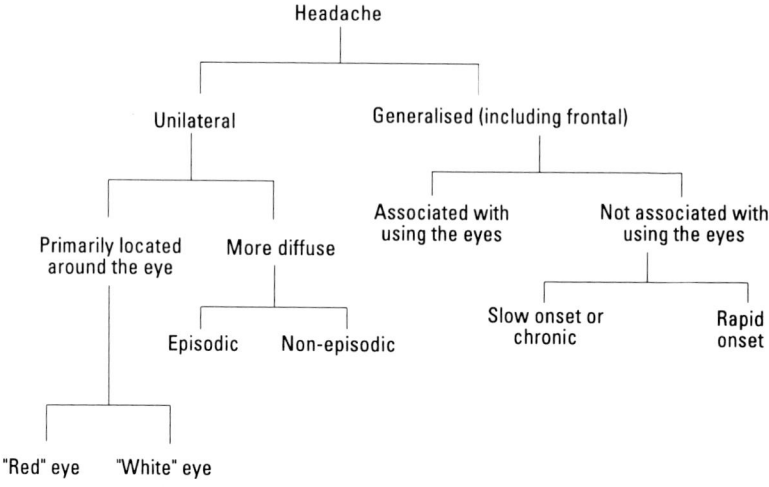

Figure 8.1 A symptomatic approach to classification of headache.

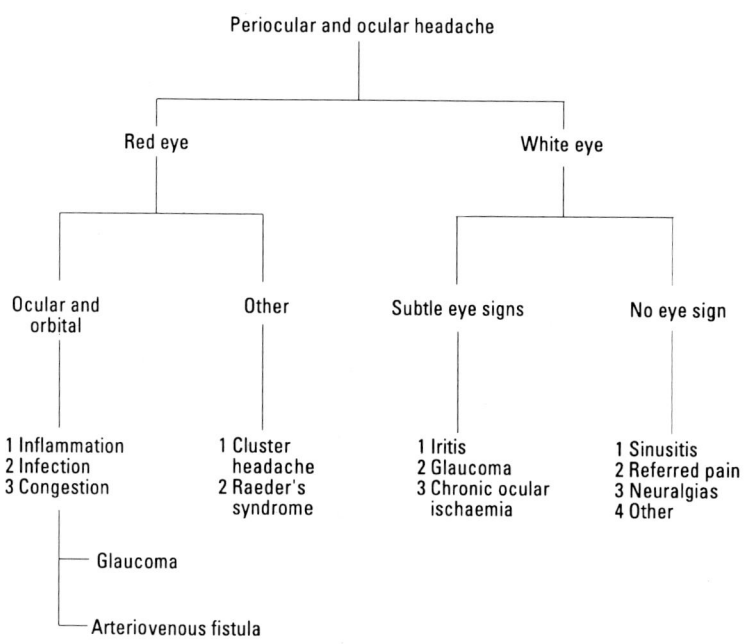

Figure 8.2 Periocular and ocular headache.

# HEADACHE

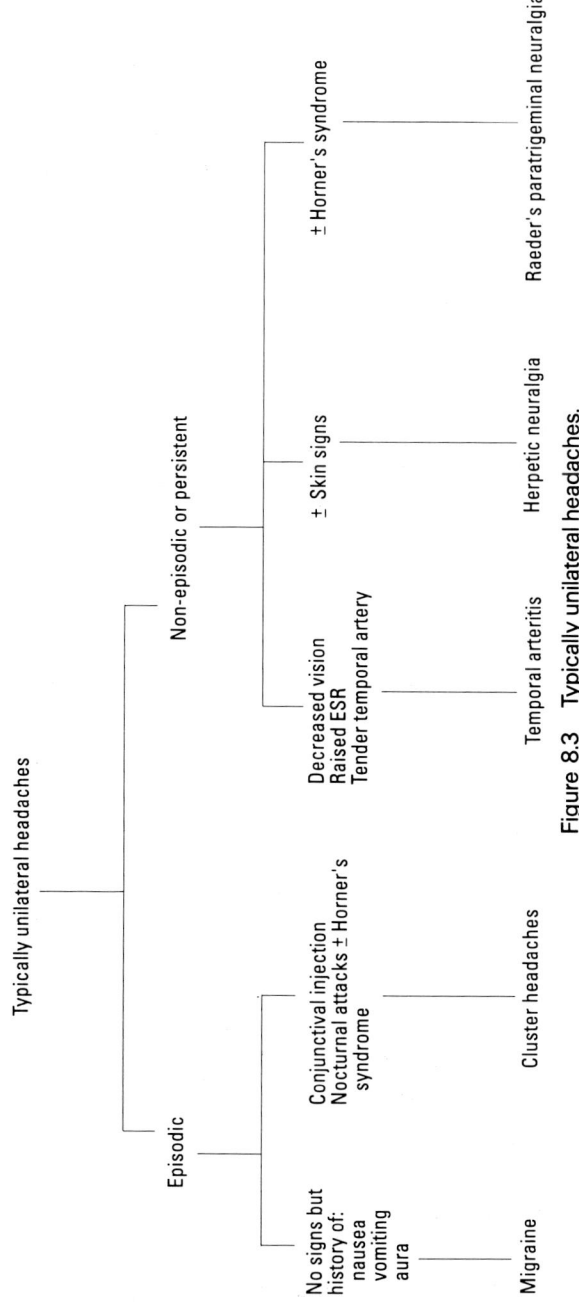

Figure 8.3 Typically unilateral headaches.

# EMERGENCY OPHTHALMOLOGY

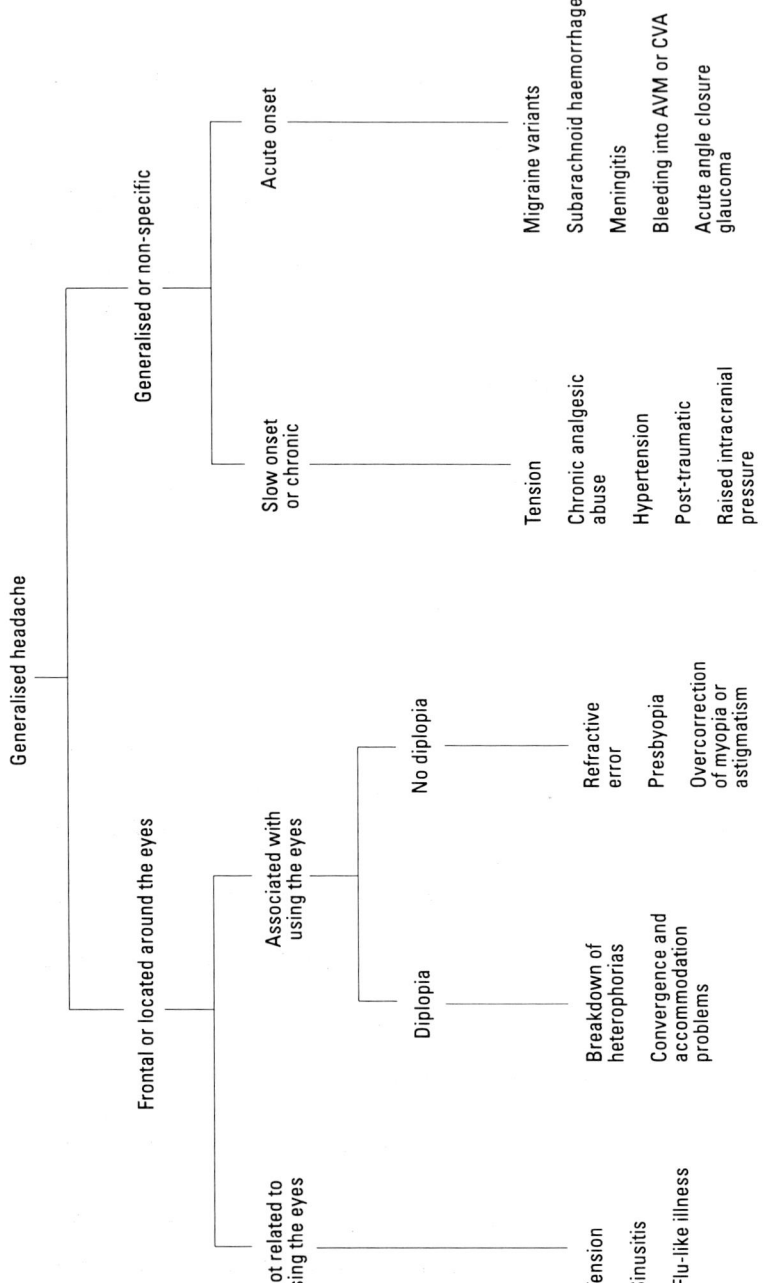

Figure 8.4 Generalised headaches: CVA, cerebrovascular accident; AVM, arteriovenous malformation.

## Characteristics of the headache
### Location
- Unilateral: migraine, temporal arteritis, trigeminal neuralgia, herpes zoster
- Frontal/periorbital: "eye strain", sinusitis, retrobulbar neuritis, referred pain
- Facial/anterior neck: trigeminal neuralgia, atypical facial pain, herpes zoster (see Chapter 9).

Pain always occurring in the same location suggests an intracranial stuctural problem, for example, arteriovenous malformation.

### Duration of the headache
- Short lived pains: typical of neuralgias
- Episodic, recurrent headaches: migraine, cluster headaches
- Chronic persistent temporal headache in an elderly person: temporal arteritis.

### Nature of the headache
- Sharp lancinating pains: neuralgias
- Throbbing pain: migraine, sinusitis
- Band like: tension headaches.

### Speed of onset
- Sudden and abrupt, usually vascular, for example, subarachnoid haemorrhage, bleeding into a tumour.

### Is the headache or pain present on wakening or does it occur at particular times of the day?
- Headache present on waking associated with vomiting: raised intracranial pressure (ICP), brain tumour
- Worse towards the end of the day: tension headaches, sinus headaches
- Nocturnal headaches: cluster headaches.

### Are there any precipitating factors?
- Food stuffs: migraine
- Stress, prolonged close work: tension, muscular, eye strain, migraine.

### Are there any aggravating factors that worsen the headache?
- Coughing, bending, sneezing, or climbing stairs: these may worsen the pain in raised ICP, sinusitis, migraine

- Pain on moving the eye: retrobulbar neuritis.

### What drugs is the patient taking?

Some drugs cause headaches, for example, nitrates, ergotamine. Other drugs such as analgesics can also cause headaches when taken on a daily basis.

### Is there a family history of headaches?

Migraine is commonly familial and a family history is important when the diagnosis is first made.

### Is the patient ill and are there any general health problems or systemic disease?

- Malaise, weight loss, jaw claudication, and arthralgias: temporal arteritis
- Fever: meningitis and general systemic infection such as 'flu
- Raised blood pressure: hypertension
- Psychological illness: depression is a relatively common cause of headache but may be difficult to diagnose.

## Examination of the patient with headache

1 Visual assessment, best corrected visual acuity, and pinhole acuity. Reduced vision—think of temporal arteritis, retrobulbar neuritis.
2 Look at the optic discs for evidence of disc swelling: raised ICP, malignant hypertension, temporal arteritis.
3 Check eyes and orbits for signs of inflammation, raised intraocular pressure, or proptosis. Tap over the sinuses to look for tenderness, although do not tap directly over the infraorbital nerve (or too firmly), as this may in itself cause pain. Consider sinus radiographs and refer to the ENT department if necessary.
4 Look for thickened temporal arteries, absent pulsation, and scalp tenderness in the over 55 age group. Check both ESR and C-reactive protein (CRP) for confirmation of giant cell arteritis. Temporal arteritis can occur in patients under 55 years of age but is rare.
5 Look for evidence of hypertension and infection. Check blood pressure and temperature and look for signs of meningeal irritation.
6 Look for neck stiffness or muscle tenderness: indicative of

muscular spasm, cervical spondylosis, or meningeal irritation caused by either blood or infection.
7 Look for other neurological signs—altered mentation, disturbance of gait, muscle power, tone and reflexes, cranial nerve and pupil function, visual fields, and colour vision defects.
8 Children commonly complain of headaches. Childhood headaches are usually associated with systemic infections, tension or stress (for example, problems at school or in the family), and migraine. Ask about a family history of migraine, social problems, and schooling; look for papilloedema; check blood pressure; and refer to the paediatrician if there is any suspicion of a serious cause.

## Headaches in or around the eye

### Differential diagnosis of ocular and periocular headache, and pain

**Red eye**
Infection
  Endophthalmitis, corneal abscess, orbital cellulitis
Inflammation
  Iritis, scleritis, pseudotumour
Congestion
  Acute glaucoma
  Orbital vascular problems, for example, arteriovenous fistula, cavernous sinus thrombosis
Other
  Cluster headaches; Raeder's syndrome

**White eye**

*Minimal eye signs*
Inflammation
  Low grade iritis
  Posner–Schlossman
  Retrobulbar neuritis (see Visual loss)
  Posterior scleritis
Raised intraocular pressure
  Rarely, chronic angle closure and open angle glaucoma
  Posner–Schlossman
Vascular
  Chronic ocular ischaemia

*No eye signs*
Infection
  Sinusitis
Referred pain
  Greater occipital neuralgia
  Meningeal ischaemia
Neuralgias
  Trigeminal; zoster (see Pain)
Vascular
  Migraine, cluster headache
Idiopathic
  Effort headache
  Pain with no known cause

## Associated with a red eye (see Chapter 5)

The cause is usually ocular or orbital. Variants of migraine headaches (for example, cluster headaches) can be associated with an injected eye (see box).

## Associated with a "white" eye

An apparent white eye does not completely rule out inflammation or raised intraocular pressure.

## Minimal eye signs
### Iritis

Low grade inflammation—cells and flare in anterior chamber (see Red eye).

## Glaucomatocyclitic crisis (Posner–Schlossman syndrome)

A recurrent secondary open angle glaucoma with a mild iritis.

### Symptoms and signs
- Slight blurring of vision and haloes around lights
- Surprisingly little pain; may have ocular discomfort or unilateral headache
- Open angles
- Intraocular pressure can be up to 70 mm Hg and stays there for a few hours up to a few days
- Occasional keratic precipitates and a few cells in the anterior chamber.

**Management** Reduce the intraocular pressure with systemic acetazolamide. Recent reports suggest topical aproclonidine may be just as effective. The benefit of topical steroids is debatable.

### Posterior scleritis

This is inflammation of the posterior sclera.

### Symptoms and signs
- Moderately severe periorbital pain
- Can keep the patient awake at night
- Vision reduced if there is macular oedema or optic nerve involvement

- Proptosis in 50% of patients
- White eye in the absence of any other eye disorders.

### Management
- Ultrasonography and computed tomography show thickened sclera
- Most patients require systemic steroids, but some resolve on non-steroidal anti-inflammatory drugs alone.

### *Glaucoma*

Any type of glaucoma giving rise to asymmetrical involvement, especially of relatively gradual onset, may be associated with a unilateral headache with little evidence of congestion and redness. Raised pressure may be secondary to intraocular inflammation, for example, ophthalmic zoster, Posner–Schlossman syndrome. The glaucoma is sometimes bilateral and symmetrical.

**Management** Check the intraocular pressure, look for inflammatory signs in the anterior chamber, and perform gonioscopy to determine if open or closed angle glaucoma.

Open angle glaucoma is treated primarily with topical medication, for example, topical β blockers.

Chronic angle closure may be helped by YAG laser iridotomy, and with topical treatment such as β blockers and miotics.

The management of acute angle closure glaucoma is discussed in Chapter 5.

### *Chronic ocular ischaemia*

#### Symptoms and signs
- Persistent pain and ache in and above the eye
- Chronic ocular ischaemia: rubeosis, retinal haemorrhages, low intraocular pressure.

#### Associated factors
- Carotid artery occlusion
- Potential cerebral infarction.

#### Management
- Listen for carotid bruit
- Computed tomography, Doppler ultrasonography, and angiography
- Anticoagulation, consider vascular intervention.

### No eye signs

*Sinusitis* (see Frontal headaches, page 203)

Frequently, sinus pain localises around one or both eyes. There may be symptoms of a postnasal drip and tenderness over the sinuses.

#### Greater occipital neuralgia

This is a headache syndrome that involves the eye and orbit, often causing the patient to seek advice from the ophthalmologist.

Branches of the second cervical nerve (from vertebra C2) emerge through the tendinous fascia of the semispinalis capitis and trapezius near their attachment to the external occipital protuberance. Centrally, in the spinal cord, C2 fibres mix with fibres of the descending tract of nerve V.

Tension in the posterior neck muscles irritates the greater occipital nerve and afferent impulses stimulate nerve V, giving rise to painful sensations as if they are coming from the first division of nerve V.

There are no eye signs but there is often localised tenderness over the inferior aspect of the occipital protuberance of the affected side.

Treatment consists of heat, massage, soft collars (for example, for cervical spondylosis), alterations in lifestyle to avoid stooping, etc., injections of local anaesthetic with or without steroid into the sensitive area, and muscle relaxation techniques.

#### Referred pain from dural or meningeal ischaemia

The trigeminal nerve provides branches to the pain sensitive structures, such as dura, venous sinuses, and blood vessels, as it passes through the cranial cavity. Pain can then be referred to the eye and orbit from intracranial lesions.

Occipital lobe infarcts cause referred pain to the inner canthus. Coexisting field defects may help confirm the diagnosis. Meningeal ischaemia may cause a vague headache or pain on the same side.

There is often a history of associated risk factors, for example, raised blood pressure, diabetes mellitus, and previous cerebrovascular accidents.

#### Migraine

This can cause a pain and headache which is localised around one eye. Migraine patients often complain of a pain behind the eye and may find that placing digital pressure on the eye relieves some of the pain, through stimulation of the afferent pathway, depressing the activity of the pain fibres.

Forty two per cent of migrainous patients and 3% of the non-migrainous population are prone to sudden jabs of pain in the head, eye, or orbit without warning (ice-pick pains). These pains coincide with the usual site of the patient's migraine headache in 40% of patients. These pains seem to be entirely benign and the patient can be reassured.

### Exertion or exercise induced headache

This is a headache that primarily affects men from 10 to 70 years of age, and comes on suddenly after a period of intense exercise. Although disconcerting, the headache is benign and 30% of those who experience it are free from symptoms in five years and 70% within ten years. The aetiology is unknown.

#### Symptoms and signs
- Unilateral retro-orbital pain
- Nausea or vomiting
- Prostration may occur
- Visual scotomata
- Often a family history of migraine.

## Typically unilateral, episodic, severe throbbing headache

---

#### Differential diagnosis of episodic headache

Vascular
  Migraine
  Cluster headaches
  Intracranial arteriovenous malformation (AVM) or leaking aneurysms (see "Generalised headaches", page 205)

---

### Migraine

- Common
- Affects 20% of the population, women twice as often as men
- Aetiology unknown.

### Symptoms and signs
- Headache can be severe and tends to be throbbing
- Usually unilateral, episodic, but may affect the other side
- Duration 2–3 hours although can be up to 18–36 hours
- Nausea or vomiting.

### Associated factors
- Family history of migraine
- Age of onset: childhood to teens
- Often precipitating factors are cheese, red wine, chocolate and coffee, lack of sleep, missing meals, and stress.

There are several distinct migraine entities.

#### *Common migraine*

This is the most common form of headache caused by migraine. There are no distinctive premonitory symptoms or associated neurological signs.

#### *Classic migraine*

This is associated with *aura preceding the headache*. Visual aura commonly consists of scintillating scotoma or fortification spectra in the visual field of both eyes lasting 15–20 minutes. As the aura disappears the headache begins.

#### *Complicated migraine*

In this form focal neurological symptoms accompany or follow rather than precede the headache. The neurological symptoms can be permanent. There are several types of complicated migraine.

#### *Retinal migraine*

A unilateral visual loss usually described as a "white out", followed by a typical migraine headache. Vascular and embolic disease need to be excluded if there is no history of migraine.

#### *Ophthalmoplegic migraine*

This commonly affects children in the first decade and nerve III is the most frequently involved followed by nerve VI. The pupil may be spared and paresis usually follows a migraine headache. The ophthalmoplegia can last for weeks and may be permanent.

### Cerebral migraine

This migraine headache is associated with motor, visual, and other sensory deficits (such as hemiplegia and hemianopia) which occur during the headache and can be permanent.

### Basilar migraine

Involvement of the vertebral basilar system causes a bioccipital headache, tinnitus, vertigo, ataxia, and diplopia, and sometimes total blindness. Neurological symptoms usually clear but permanent deficits can occur in rare instances.

### Migraine equivalents

Focal neurological deficits without headache occur in older patients with a migraine history. It is the repetitive and benign nature of the symptoms that suggests the diagnosis. If the symptoms become atypical or occur in a patient with no migraine history, computed tomography is needed to exclude a structural problem.

**Differential diagnosis of migraine** The history is all important in the diagnosis.

Migraine headaches often affect one side predominantly but do shift sides, unlike headaches caused by arteriovenous malformations or leaking aneurysms.

Leaking occipital arteriovenous malformations, transient ischaemic attacks, or carotid artery occlusion can all duplicate the scintillating scotomata of classic migraine. In migraine, however, the headache typically *follows* the visual aura, unlike other pathologies causing visual symptoms.

**Management.** There is no test for migraine and the diagnosis is made on the history. If there is any doubt, arrange neuroimaging, Doppler vascular ultrasonography, or carotid angiography.

For ophthalmoplegic migraine there has to be a strict criterion for diagnosis: the onset must be in the first decade with a history of typical migraine or a strong family history.

Ninety per cent of patients obtain relief with medical treatment. Simple analgesics are the first line of treatment. Prophylactic drugs are used if the attacks are frequent and severe.

### Cluster headaches

#### Symptoms and signs
- Unilateral, periorbital, severe, boring pain
- Redness and watering of the ipsilateral eye and nasal stuffiness
- Rapid onset; duration 1–4 hours
- Fifty per cent of the attacks occur at night
- An ipsilateral Horner's syndrome occurs in about 50% of patients and may persist between attacks
- The pattern of the headaches is one of recurrent bouts; symptoms occur daily for periods with completely symptom free periods in between
- More common in middle aged men.

#### Associated factors
- May be a family history of migraine
- Can be precipitated by alcohol.

**Differential diagnosis** Few headaches mimic this. Carotid dissection can be associated with Horner's syndrome, but the pain on carotid dissection is more persistent in nature.

**Management** Treatment is either vigorous exercise or inhalation of 100% oxygen at the very first sign of attack. Some normal anti-migraine treatments can be effective as can treatment with lithium.

## Chronic unilateral headache

---

### Differential diagnosis of unilateral head pain of a constant or persistent nature

Vascular
    Temporal arteritis (see also Chapter 2)
    Chronic paroxysmal hemicrania
    Raeder's paratrigeminal syndrome (rare)
Degenerative
    Temporomandibular joint dysfunction
Neuralgias
    Herpes zoster pain (see Chapter 9)
Intracranial structure lesion
    Raeder's paratrigeminal syndrome
    Arteriovenous malformation (see Generalised headaches, page 205)

---

## HEADACHE

### *Temporal arteritis*

This affects nearly one in 1000 of those aged 60 years or over. It is more predominant in white European women.

**Symptoms and signs**
- A variable headache but can be severe and persistent
- Usually unilateral and located to the temple
- Visual symptoms: transient visual loss, progressive field loss, homonymous field defects, and sudden irrecoverable visual loss from ischaemic optic neuropathy
- Diplopia if oculomotor nerves are involved.

**Associated signs**
- Temporal arteries may be thickened and tender with absent pulsation
- Jaw claudication, shoulder and hip girdle arthralgias, general malaise, and fever
- High ESR, commonly above 80 mm/h, although a normal ESR does not exclude temporal arteritis; CRP may be raised in cases where ESR is normal.

**Management** Untreated severe visual loss occurs in more than half and in about 80% of these the loss is bilateral. For details on treatment see Chapter 2.

### *Temporomandibular joint dysfunction*

Pain in the temple and region of the temporomandibular joint is more common as people start to lose their natural teeth, and is suspected of being related to occlusal instability.

**Symptoms and signs**
- Pain in the face, jaws, and ears, and headache
- Joint noise
- Pain on opening the mouth
- Difficulty in opening the mouth wide and in chewing
- Clicking and crepitation of the temporomandibular joint
- Tenderness on palpation of the masseter muscle and over the temporomandibular joint
- Impaired mandibular mobility, irregularity, deviation, and locking of the mandible.

**Management** Some of the above symptoms overlap with those of temporal arteritis. Usually the elderly patient with temporal arteritis complains of systemic symptoms and shoulder arthralgias. Once temporal arteritis has been eliminated as a possible diagnosis, refer the patient to an orthodontist for advice.

### Chronic paroxysmal hemicrania

This is a rare variant of cluster headaches typically affecting women.

#### Signs and symptoms
- Chronic unilateral hemicranial pain with daily superimposed recurrent focal head pain
- Associated with nasal stuffiness, rhinorrhea, tearing, and conjunctival injection.

**Management** The curative effect of indomethacin is so dramatic, it is almost diagnostic.

### Raeder's paratrigeminal syndrome

A rare headache predominantly affecting middle aged to elderly men.

#### Signs and symptoms
- Severe unilateral persistent pain in the region supplied by the ophthalmic division of the trigeminal nerve
- There is an ipsilateral Horner's syndrome, nasal stuffiness, and red eye
- Other neurological signs suggest a parasellar mass or aneurysm.

#### Management
- Neurological and radiological evaluation
- In the absence of a parasellar mass, treat as if a variant of cluster headaches with ergotamine, methysergide, lithium, and steroids.

## Frontal headaches

> **Differential diagnosis of frontal headaches and their relationship to ocular use and double vision**
>
> *Associated with ocular use*
> Intermittent diplopia
>  Heterophoria (see Chapter 7)
>  Convergence weakness (see Chapter 7)
>  Convergence spasm (see Chapter 7)
> No diplopia
>  Refractive errors
>  Muscle contraction headaches/tension headaches (see Generalised headaches, page 205)
> *Not associated with ocular use*
> Infections
>  Sinusitis
>  Infections, influenza
> Muscular
>  Greater occipital neuralgia (see Periocular headaches, page 196)
>  Tension headaches

## Frontal headaches associated with use of the eyes

### Intermittent diplopia

*Heterophoria, convergence, and/or accommodation insufficiency*

The effort needed to maintain binocular vision, convergence, or accommodation causes a frontal headache on prolonged close work (see Chapter 7).

*Convergence and/or accommodative spasm*

#### Symptoms and signs
- Intermittent diplopia, blurred vision, frontal headache, and ocular pain
- There is a variable convergent squint with miosis of pupils on lateral gaze; it can mimic palsy of nerve VI and cause unnecessary alarm (see Chapter 7).

## No diplopia
### Refractive errors

- Although uncommon, headaches can be caused by uncorrected presbyopia, hyperopia, or astigmatism
- Myopia hardly ever causes symptoms unless over corrected.

#### Symptoms and signs
- Bilateral frontal headaches occurring regularly after use of the eyes.

**Management** Despite correcting the refractive error, symptoms may not always be relieved, and these patients may be otherwise prone to muscular tension or migraine headaches

## Frontal headaches not related to ocular use
### Sinus disease

#### Symptoms and signs
- Moderate, aching in nature, and frontal in location, occurring later in the day
- Tends to localise around one or both eyes
- Tenderness on tapping over the sinuses
- Increased pain on bending over
- General malaise.

#### Associated factors
- Postnasal drip and a history of sinus disease.

#### Management
- Radiograh or computed tomography of the sinuses
- Systemic antibiotics
- Referral to ENT department.

### Infections, fevers, and influenza

#### Symptoms and signs
- Moderate in nature, throbbing, frontal, and constant.

#### Management
- Look for pyrexia, other symptoms or signs of infection, or influenza.

## Generalised and non-specific headaches (Table 8.1)

Table 8.1  Differential diagnosis of headaches that tend to cause a generalised, non-localised type of head pain, or have variable symptoms on presentation

|  | Chronic or slow onset | Rapid onset of symptoms |
|---|---|---|
| Muscular | Tension headaches<br>Cervical spondylosis |  |
| Vascular | High blood pressure<br>Temporal arteritis | Subarachnoid haemorrhage<br>Pituitary apoplexy (rare) |
| Trauma | Post-traumatic headache |  |
| Intracranial lesions | Brain tumour<br>Arteriovenous malformations<br>Benign intracranial hypertension |  |
| Infection |  | Systemic fever<br>Meningitis |
| Other | Depression<br>Other<br>Chronic analgesic abuse<br>Idiopathic | Migraine variants |

## Chronic
### Tension headaches

There is, unfortunately, ambiguity as to the definition of tension headache. "Tension" may refer to anxiety related to stressful events, or to muscle contraction. Thus, a heterogeneous group of patients has come together under this label by virtue of the fact that their headaches are not the result of migraine or other causes.

#### Symptoms and signs
- Bilateral dull band like sensation that may affect any part of the head
- Occurring on an almost daily basis with symptoms worse at the end of the day
- Simple analgesics may have little effect, and in fact these patients may also be analgesic abusers.

#### Associated factors
- Frequently associated with tenderness of the trapezius and occipital ridge
- Prolonged close work may precipitate the headache
- Linked with stress, anxiety, or depression although a direct link to stress is not always clear
- Cervical spine disease.

### Management
- For situational stress try psychotherapy and relaxation techniques
- If simple analgesics do not provide relief, daily amitriptyline may help.

### *Chronic analgesic abuse*

Chronic overuse of analgesics and opiates leads, in turn, to chronic headache, initiating further analgesic ingestion. Forty per cent of headache patients attending hospital clinics complain of a chronic type of headache. Seventy five per cent of chronic headache sufferers consume painkillers every day. It is estimated that "medication misuse headache" may affect 1% of the entire population.

### Symptoms and signs
- Refractory headache
- Occurs daily
- Varies in severity, type, and location
- Can wake the patient at night, typically between 2 and 5 am
- Usually there is a history of a primary type of headache (for example, migraine) which has been transformed into what the patient recognises as a different form of chronic headache.

**Management** Once the headache has been recognised, the patient has to be taken off the painkillers. Unfortunately 50% relapse after one year.

### *Raised blood pressure*

Up to 50% of those with chronic hypertension complain of headaches, although the mechanism for the pain is uncertain. Headache often accompanies malignant or accelerated hypertension where the diastolic blood pressure is over 140 mm Hg.

### Symptoms and signs
- Retinal signs: arteriovenous crossing changes, branch vein occlusions, macular oedema and exudates, and papilloedema
- Papilloedema which can be associated with fleeting obscurations of vision.

### Associated factors
- Proteinuria

- Cardiovascular problems: swollen ankles, shortness of breath
- Eighty per cent of patients with phaeochromocytoma experience a crescendo headache associated with pallor, tachycardia, and sweating during paroxysmal increases in blood pressure.

**Management** Refer to general physician or family doctor for blood pressure control and investigations.

### Post-traumatic headaches

About half the patients hospitalised for closed head injury have headaches lasting up to one year.

#### Symptoms and signs
- Dull, aching, generalised, headaches which occur daily, and do not correlate to the severity of the trauma
- Associated with poor concentration, memory problems, and irritability.

**Management** Therapy consists of reassurance and relaxation therapy. Ergot preparations may help.

### Benign intracranial hypertension

This is more common in obese women of child bearing age. Fifty per cent of patients will have some visual loss and 25% will have severe visual loss.

#### Symptoms and signs
- Moderate, relatively constant headache
- Occasionally visual obscurations or intracranial noises
- Optic nerve papilloedema and sometimes palsies of nerve VI
- Lumbar punctures show a high opening pressure above the normal range of 50–200 mm $H_2O$.

#### Associated factors
- Tetracycline
- Vitamin A
- Systemic steroids
- Oral contraceptive.

**Management** Neuroimaging is necessary to rule out a space occupying lesion and then lumbar puncture establishes the diagnosis.

Treatment is with acetazolamide, frusemide, steroids, and repeated lumbar punctures. Hypertension, high intraocular pressure, and uraemia should be controlled because these all appear to be risk factors in visual loss. The patients must be followed with *regular fields* and contrast sensitivity tests. Optic nerve sheath fenestration or lumbar–peritoneal shunting is undertaken when visual function deteriorates or headaches cannot be controlled medically.

### *Brain tumour headaches*

About three quarters of brain tumour patients have a headache and, in about half of brain tumour patients, headache is the first complaint. Twenty per cent of pituitary tumours present with headache.

#### Symptoms and signs
- The common brain tumour headache is a boring pain present on waking; coexisting vomiting is a sign of raised ICP
- Exacerbated by exertion, change in posture, or cough
- There may be other neurological signs and papilloedema.

More rarely a brain tumour presents with a paroxysmal type of headache. The pain is maximum in 1–2 seconds and lasts 1–2 hours. It can be associated with loss of consciousness or drop attacks.

Rarely a bleed into a pituitary tumour (pituitary apoplexy) can cause a headache of sudden onset with visual loss and ophthalmoplegia.

**Management** If the headache is at all suspicious neuroimaging is mandatory.

### *Arteriovenous malformations*

Intracranial arteriovenous malformations (AVMs) are *rare* anomalous communications between arteries and veins, usually lying within the cerebral tissues.

#### Symptoms and signs
- Before rupture, there is a chronic nondescript headache which may mimic migraine
- Slowly progressive neurological defects or focal seizures
- Cranial bruit

- Symptoms with rupture are similar to subarachnoid haemorrhage although permanent neurological deficit is more likely
- The 20–30 year age group, although a few are delayed to around 50 years.

**Management**
- Listen for a bruit
- Computed tomography and angiography
- Surgical and radiological intervention.

*Other causes of generalised headaches* (see box)

---

Depression
  This may account for 9–10% of headache sufferers. Ask about mood, sleep patterns, eating and weight loss, motivation, and social factors
Alcohol intoxication
  The "hangover" of the following day!
Carbon dioxide retention
  Chronic lung disease with hypercapnia
Drugs
  For example, nitrates, ergotamine, oral contaceptives
Altitudinal headache
Nocturnal teeth clenching or grinding
  Postulated as a cause of early morning migraine and other headaches

---

### Acute onset
#### Subarachnoid haemorrhage

This is caused by rupture of a berry aneurysm, usually in the anterior circulation, in relation to the circle of Willis. In about one third of patients, aneurysms are multiple.

**Symptoms and signs**
- More common in the 35–65 year age group
- Usually no premonitory signs or headaches
- The headache is dramatic, abrupt, and excruciating ("thunderclap")
- It is associated with a stiff neck and vomiting
- Neurological signs such as a pupil involving palsy of nerve III

- Half the patients become unconscious at the outset, another 25% within 15 min, and overall 45% die
- Partial rupture results in "sentinel" headaches in up to 50% of patients, which may herald a total rupture at a later date.

**Management** Immediate admission and neuroimaging are necessary. Computed tomography should show blood in the CSF space. Lumbar puncture will confirm the presence of blood in the CSF if needed.

Angiography is necessary to look for other aneurysms.

### *Meningitis*

#### Symptoms and signs
- Any age group
- Severe intermittent to constant pain
- There may be referred pain to the anterior face
- Associated malaise, pyrexia, neurological signs, and cervical rigidity
- Rapid deterioration.

**Management** There should be immediate admission by general physician, neuroimaging, and lumbar puncture, and administration of intravenous antibiotics.

### *Cerebrovascular accident* (actual or impending)

- Pain is caused by meningeal ischaemia
- Signs are related to position.

#### Management
- Neuroimaging
- Referral to physician.

### *Acute angle closure glaucoma*

See Chapters 5 and 2.

# 9 Pain

As stated in Chapter 8, the distinction between a "pain" and "ache" is a matter of degree. As pain is subjective, pain thresholds vary and the same stimulus will produce very different reactions in different individuals. Sherrington regarded pain as an integral component of nervous activity and described it as "the psychical adjunct of an imperative protective reflex". There is also an emotive component: in 1979 the International Association for the Study of Pain defined pain as ". . . an unpleasant sensory and emotional experience associated with actual or potential tissue damage, or described in terms of such damage". Thus pain is insistent and disabling, and the patient in pain will go on seeking relief until the problem is resolved. Action is expected of the doctor who needs to know the scope of the problem and how to deal with it. This chapter aims to provide a logical framework for managing a patient presenting with pain in the A&E department.

Pain can arise from a lesion intrinsic to the eye and orbit or it can be referred. Lesions arising in the eye and orbit will have signs evident on examination. Absence of signs suggest a referred pain which may have a characteristic pattern. A detailed history is therefore important.

## History taking

### Loss of vision

Pain associated with loss of vision tends to be associated with severe inflammatory, infective, or ischaemic processes or acute glaucoma. The vision can be lost through cloudy media, for example, corneal oedema with acute glaucoma, or through involvement of the optic nerve in an inflammatory process, for example, retrobulbar neuritis—orbital inflammation causing an apical syndrome.

# EMERGENCY OPHTHALMOLOGY

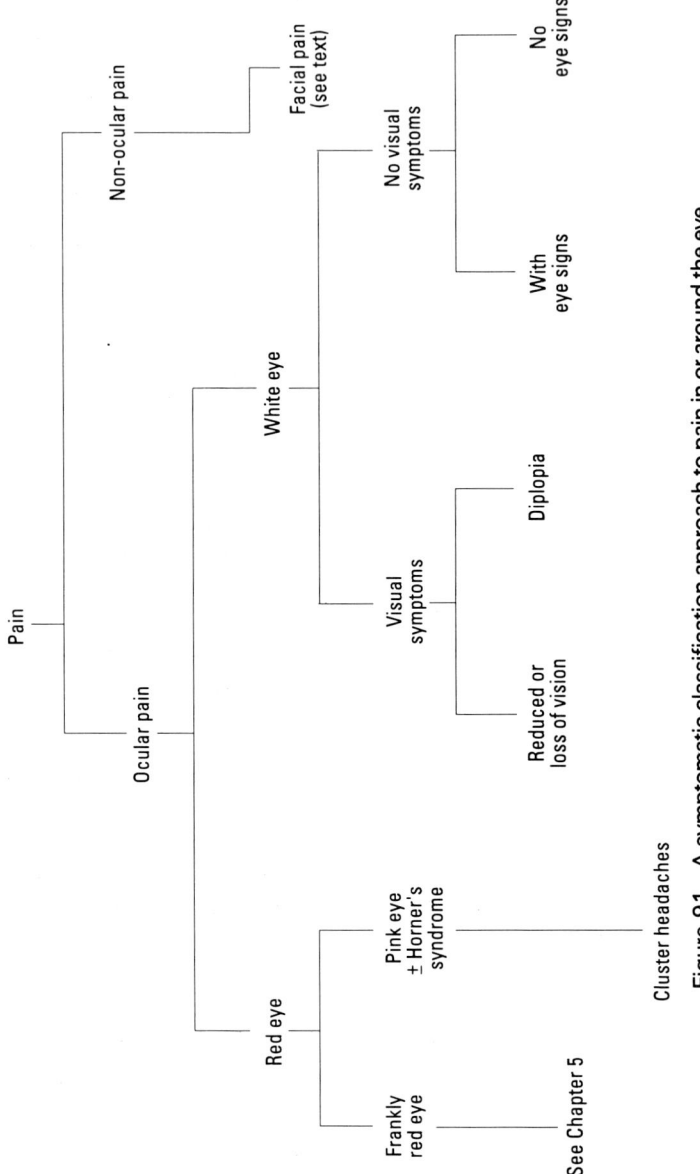

Figure 9.1 A symptomatic classification approach to pain in or around the eye.

## Nature of the pain

The characteristics of the pain should match the pathology found. If not, there may be another undiscovered cause for the pain.

Certain types of pain and their associated symptoms can be quite characteristic, as outlined in Table 9.1.

Table 9.1  Pain histories and their relationships to possible diagnoses

| Symptoms | Possible diagnoses |
|---|---|
| Severe aching ocular pain<br>Can wake the patient at night | Endophthalmitis<br>Anterior and posterior scleritis<br>Orbital pseudotumour<br>Cluster headaches |
| Aching, throbbing pain varying from mild to severe in a blind eye | Phthisis bulbi<br>Rubeotic glaucoma |
| Sharp ocular pain, photophobia, and watering<br>Foreign body feeling | Corneal abrasions, foreign bodies<br>Viral and bacterial keratitis<br>Contact lens problems |
| Throbbing pain and photophobia | Acute iritis<br>Corneal ulcers and abscesses |
| Severe throbbing pain not necessarily described by the patient as ocular, nausea, vomiting | Acute glaucoma<br>Migraine |
| Retrobulbar aching pain on moving the eye | Retrobulbar neuritis |
| Excrutiating lancinating facial pains | Trigeminal neuralgia |
| Burning facial pain<br>Previous history of ophthalmic herpes zoster | Postherpetic neuralgia |

## Associated photophobia

Pain from iritis, corneal lesions, and foreign bodies is typically associated with photophobia from ciliary spasm in bright lights.

## Diplopia

This indicates involvement of the muscles, nerves, or orbital apex.

## Previous ocular history and surgery

Some eye conditions are recurrent, for example, iritis. Inflammation and infection may complicate all forms of ocular surgery.

213

### Associated systemic symptoms?

- Nausea and vomiting—acute glaucoma
- General malaise, arthralgias, jaw claudication—temporal arteritis
- Rheumatoid arthritis—anterior scleritis.

## Examination

1 Visual assessment, best corrected visual acuity, and pinhole acuity.
2 Check for a relative afferent pupil defect.
3 Look at the pattern of redness of the eye (see Chapter 5).
4 Examine the eye for clarity of the cornea, and stain with fluorescein to look for epithelial loss. Look at the anterior segment for activity and whether a hypopyon is present. Check intraocular pressure. Dilate and check the posterior segment.
5 In suspected orbital disease palpate each quadrant of the orbit for masses and look for proptosis.

## Painful red eye (Fig 9.2) (see Chapters 5, 10, and 11)

Conditions causng a severe pain result from ocular trauma, corneal ulcers, abscesses, endophthalmitis, inflammatory eye disease, acute glaucoma, and orbital inflammatory disease.

A description of the pain typical of these conditions is summarised in Table 9.1.

### Ophthalmic signs: visual disturbance or visual loss

All the above conditions can cause some degree of visual loss, but corneal ulcers and abscesses, endophthalmitis, severe uveitis, and acute glaucoma may dramatically reduce vision.

#### Painful blind eye

The pain can vary from a mild nagging ache to a severe life dominating pain. The eye is usually red to a varying degree, but occasionally there are no overt signs of ocular inflammation.

#### Phthisis bulbi

The eye may be disorganised from old trauma or previous

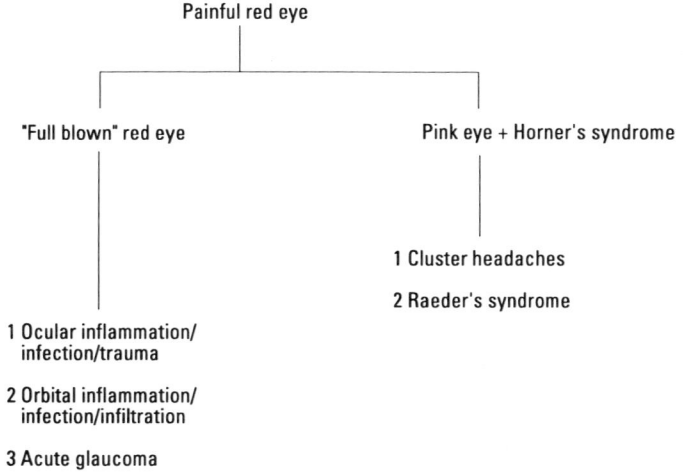

Figure 9.2  Differential diagnosis of painful red eye.

surgery (for example, failed vitreoretinal surgery), and be hypotonic and visibly smaller than the normal eye.

### *Rubeotic glaucoma*

Rubeotic eyes with very high pressures can cause pain. The eyes may become inflamed or the cornea may decompensate with the formation of bullae, abrasions, or ulcers.

**Management**  Always look at the other eye for disease and the possibility of sympathetic ophthalmitis. The affected eye is blind so the rationale of treatment is to make the patient comfortable with topical steroid and atropine drops. If this fails retrobulbar alcohol or evisceration may be the only solution to alleviate the symptoms.

## Ophthalmic signs: red eye and painful diplopia

Pseudotumour and orbital myositis can cause a painful diplopia with injection over enlarged inflamed muscles, and orbital congestion. Involvement of the superior orbital fissure or cavernous sinus gives a variety of ophthalmoplegias. It is a very painful condition with a gnawing, boring pain.

Acute thyroid ophthalmopathy is less painful, with orbital congestion, variable proptosis, and lid retraction. Cavernous sinus thrombosis and arteriovenous fistula cause ophthalmoplegia, red eye, proptosis, and retro-orbital pain.

For management see Chapter 10.

### Ophthalmic signs: red eye and Horner's syndrome

The pain of cluster headaches and Raeder's syndrome is also severe, with a unilateral pain behind the eye or in the first division of the trigeminal nerve. There is often an associated Horner's syndrome with nasal congestion and a red eye on the side of the pain. See Chapter 8 for more details.

## Painful white eye (Fig 9.3)

Table 9.2 Differential diagnosis of a white painful eye

| Ophthalmic signs | No ophthalmic signs |
| --- | --- |
| Ocular inflammation | Infection |
|   Retrobulbar neuritis |   Sinusitis |
|   Posterior seleritis | Vascular or structural lesions |
|   Iritis |   Referred pain |
| Vascular |   Migraine (see Chapter 8) |
|   Chronic ocular ischaemia | Muscular |
|   Subarachnoid haemorrhage |   Tension headaches (see Chapter 8) |
|   Microvascular infarction cranial nerves | Other |
|   Aneurysm of the posterior communicating artery |   Idiopathic |
| Orbital | |
|   Orbital tumours | |
|   Orbital apex syndrome (infiltration, inflammation) | |
| Other | |
|   Chronic glaucoma | |
|   Ophthalmic herpes zoster | |

### Ophthalmic signs: visual disturbance

***Retrobulbar neuritis*** (see Chapter 2)

Typically a rapid onset of visual loss is associated with periocular pain worsened by eye movement. The visual loss usually recovers after 6–8 weeks.

***Posterior scleritis*** (see Chapter 8)

A moderately severe periorbital pain can keep the patient awake

# PAIN

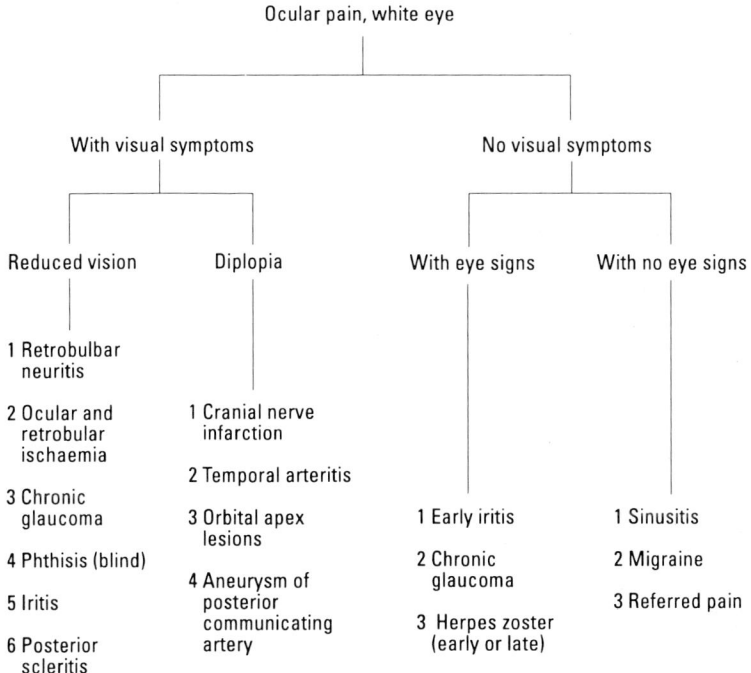

Figure 9.3 Differential diagnosis of painful white eye.

at night. Vision is reduced if there is macular oedema or optic nerve involvement, and there is proptosis in 50% of patients.

## Chronic ocular ischaemia (see Chapter 8)

Persistent pain in and above the eye is associated with rubeosis, retinal haemorrhages, and low intraocular pressure. Vision may be reduced.

## Anterior and retrobulbar optic nerve ischaemia

Ocular and orbital pain may precede anterior and retrobulbar ischaemic optic neuropathy.

## Ophthalmic signs: painful diplopia
### Cranial nerve infarction (see Chapter 7)

This is usually unilateral. Microvascular disease causing infarction of cranial nerves VI, IV, III, and II may be accompanied by periorbital, retro-ocular, or frontal pain. Ophthalmic herpes zoster may be associated with cranial nerve palsies.

### *Temporal arteritis* (see Chapter 2)

This does not normally cause an ocular or orbital pain, but must be considered in any differential diagnosis of diplopia particularly in the elderly patient. It may cause diplopia as part of a widespread ischaemia, by affecting oculomotor nerves either peripherally or centrally. Always check the erythrocyte sedimentation rate (ESR) and C-reactive protein (CRP) of an elderly person with diplopia.

### *Subarachnoid haemorrhage* (see Chapter 7)

Aneurysms of the posterior communicating artery cause a pupil involving palsy of nerve III. Blood in the subarachnoid space is an irritant and is accompanied by a severe headache.

### *Cavernous sinus lesions*

There is pituitary apoplexy and inflammatory masses in the cavernous sinus. Involvement of cranial nerve V causes retro-orbital and ocular pain.

The bleeds into a pituitary tumour can cause total ophthalmoplegia of both eyes and visual loss.

### *Orbital tumours*

Orbital signs are usually present (see Chapter 10).

### *Orbital apex syndrome*

Involvement of the orbit with inflammatory masses can cause varying ophthalmoplegia and a deep boring pain in the orbit.

### *Aneurysm of the posterior communicating artery*

This typically causes severe unilateral frontal headache with a pain around the eye. Compression of nerve III causes ptosis and gives diplopia from palsy of nerve III, either partial or complete.

Management is immediate admission for neuroimaging and referral to neurosurgery.

## No eye signs
### Sinusitis

The headache from sinusitis can localise around the eyes (see Chapter 8).

### Referred pain from dural or meningeal ischaemia

The trigeminal nerve provides branches to the pain sensitive structures such as dura, venous sinuses, and blood vessels as it passes through the cranial cavity. Pain can then be referred to the eye and orbit from intracranial lesions.

### Greater occiptal neuralgia

There is referred retro-orbital pain from irritation of C2, either from cervical spine disease and C2 root problems, or from irritation of the peripheral branches of the greater occipital nerve.

### Migraine

Migraine headaches are variable and may be located around or behind one of the eyes.

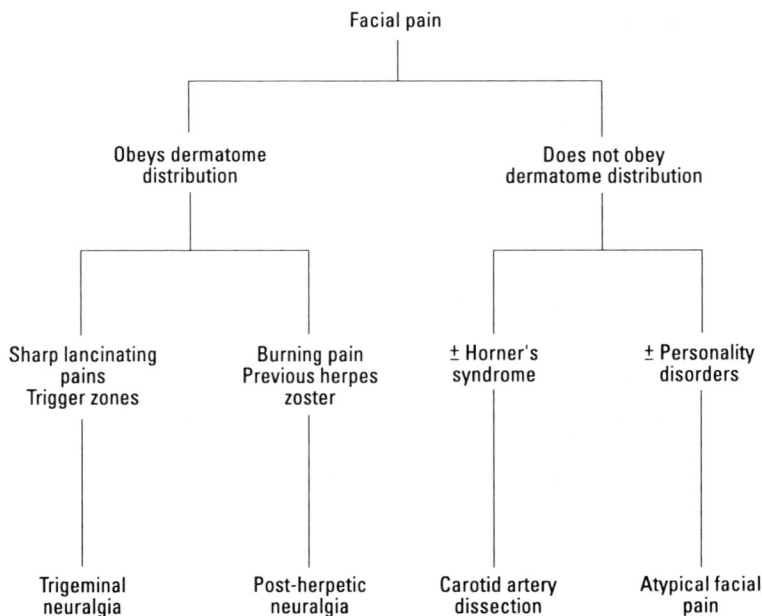

Figure 9.4 Differential diagnosis of facial pain.

## Idiopathic

There will always be a group of patients who present complaining of pain in the eyes, for whom no identifiable cause can be found. The vast majority of these pains are benign in nature. The important point is to exclude serious and treatable disease.

## Facial pain (Fig 9.4)

Facial pain may present to the ophthalmologist if the trigeminal nerve is involved, because this gives a pain around the eye. In addition, the ocular effects of ophthalmic zoster are well known, resulting in the referral of these patients to an eye department for assessment.

---

**Differential diagnosis of facial pain**

Neurological
   Trigeminal neuralgia
   Herpes zoster neuralgia
Vascular
   Carotid artery dissection
Psychological
   Atypical facial pain
Local causes
   Sinusitis
   Dental problems

---

## Herpetic neuralgia (see also Chapter 5)

### Symptoms and signs
- Herpes zoster pain is a burning recurrent pain
- The pain is localised in a skin dermatome or cranial nerve, for example, the first division of nerve V
- Redness confined to the dermatome may precede diagnostic vesicles
- The pain precedes the rash by 3–4 days, and may persist for months or years.

### Management
- Refer to a specialist in pain control

- There is no entirely successful medical treatment of the neuralgia
- Prompt recognition of the acute attack and treatment with systemic acyclovir may be beneficial.

## Trigeminal neuralgia

There are three divisions of the trigeminal nerve:

1. The first division of nerve V (V1), or the ophthalmic, supplies the eye, conjunctiva, upper lid and forehead, sphenoid and ethmoid sinuses, nasal mucosa, and the skin of the tip of the nose
2. The second division of nerve V (V2), or the maxillary division, supplies the skin of the lower lid and midface
3. The third division of nerve V (V3), or the mandibular division, supplies both sensory function to the lower face and motor function to the muscles of mastication.

### Symptoms and signs
- Paroxysms of unilateral excruciating pain lasting seconds to minutes
- V2 and V3 are more often affected than V1
- There may be autonomic signs (lacrimation, conjunctival injection, salivation, flushing)
- Sensation to touch is normal
- Trigger zones can exist near the eye, nose, or mouth, and attacks are precipitated by cold air or touch
- Predominantly occurs in 50–60 year age group
- Spontaneous remissions do occur.

### Associated factors
- Multiple sclerosis especially in patients under the age of 50
- Cross compression of nerve roots by aberrant blood vessels
- If there is associated hyperaesthesia and atrophy of the muscles of mastication, suspect a posterior fossa tumour.

**Management** Refer to a neurologist for evaluation and management. Neuroimaging (MRI is the most useful) will help exclude multiple sclerosis, tumour, and other possible causes of facial pain.

Management is initially medical with agents such as carbamazepine. Surgery to destroy the pain fibres in the trigeminal ganglion is only undertaken when medical treatment fails. There are long term problems with corneal anaesthesia in a significant number of patients after surgical intervention.

### *Atypical facial pain*

#### Symptoms and signs
- A chronic, constant, boring, deep, non-dermatomal pain which may have trigger points
- Usually located in the maxillary areas
- Rarely associated with a pathological process
- Occurs in personality disorders.

#### Management
- Organic disease must be ruled out with neuroimaging
- The differential diagnosis includes temporal arteritis, carotid occlusion or dissection, and temporomandibular joint problems
- Treatment is with low doses of tricyclic antidepressants and counselling.

### *Carotid artery dissection*

A rare cause of headache.

#### Symptoms and signs
- Moderate persistent pain in the neck, throat, and face with an ipsilateral Horner's syndrome
- Trauma may initiate dissection.

#### Management
- Computed tomography scan, Doppler ultrasonography, and angiography
- Immediate anticoagulation to prevent total thrombosis or emboli.

# 10 Swellings around the eye

Patients present with swellings around the eye to the A&E department surprisingly frequently because of either an acute condition or anxiety over a chronic one.

Whatever the cause, swellings arise from one of the following five anatomical sites:

1 The orbit
2 The lids
3 The lacrimal gland
4 The lacrimal drainage system
5 The conjunctiva.

## The orbit

"Localised" lesions produce symptoms and signs by causing compression or displacement, and they can arise from any of the tissues of the orbit or adjacent structures.

"Diffuse" swellings are caused primarily by a more diffuse process or are the secondary effects of a more remote disease. Table 10.1 provides a working classification.

The *direction of displacement* of proptosis depends on the position of the primary orbital disease: axial displacement occurs in intraconal lesions and sideways displacement in paraglobal disease.

## The lids

"Localised" swellings will mostly be obvious and common pathologies are listed in Table 10.2.

Table 10.1  Classification of swellings

| Unilateral | | Bilateral | |
|---|---|---|---|
| No proptosis | Proptosis | No proptosis | Proptosis |
| Preseptal cellulitis | TED<br>Cellulitis (orbital)<br>Pseudotumour<br>Tumour<br>CCF<br>Vascular tumour or varices | Preseptal cellulitis<br>Allergy<br>Early TED | TED<br>Infiltrative lesion, for example, lymphoma<br>Inflammation, for example, acute sinusitis<br>Cavernous sinus thrombosis |

TED, thyroid eye disease.
CCE, carotid–cavernous fistula.

Table 10.2  Localised swelling of the lids

| Retention cyst | Infection | Allergy | Tumours | |
|---|---|---|---|---|
| | | | Benign | Malignant |
| Zeiss | Styes | Medication | Any skin tumour | Basal cell carcinoma |
| Moll | Meibomian | Insect bite | | Squamous carcinoma |
| Meibomian | Molluscum contagiosum | | Seborrheic keratosis | Meibomian gland carcinoma<br>Malignant melanoma |

"Diffuse" swellings are one of the following:

- Infective
- Allergic—acute
- Infiltrative (for example, neoplasm)—slowly progressive.

Lacrimal gland pathology consists chiefly of three types:

- Inflammation
- Tumour
- Cysts.

*Pain* is caused by either *inflammation* or an *invasive tumour*.

Lacrimal sac and drainage systems have a limited number of pathologies, most of which result in blockage of the tear duct, giving rise to problems secondary to the obstruction. These problems are:

- Watering

- Infection
    reflux conjunctivitis
    dacryocystitis ± mucocele.

Tumours of the lacrimal sac are very rare.
Conjunctival swellings are rare as such and are caused by:

- Subconjunctival retention of fluid
- Infiltrative lesions, for examples, lymphoma
- Inflammatory process which would give rise to a red eye (see Chapter 5).

---

### Important points in history taking and examination

1 *General well being:* as a good many orbital problems are manifestations of a systemic disease, it is important to ask questions about the general health. This is particularly important in children.
2 *Duration:* an acute onset favours infection or allergy, but not tumour or congenital abnormality.
3 *Pain* will favour inflammation unless there is orbital infiltration involving the periosteum.
4 *Diplopia* signals muscle involvement or restraints caused by fibrosis after trauma or Graves' ophthalmopathy.
5 *Allergy* is often supported by previous history or other known allergies.
6 *Visual deterioration* needs to be checked by refraction or a pinhole test and indicates possible nerve compression in orbital disease.
7 *Relative afferent pupil defect* is a confirmatory sign of nerve damage in diminished vision.
8 *Proptosis* should be measured by Hertel's exophthalmometer.
9 *Displacement* is gauged by drawing an imaginary cross through the centre of the bridge of the nose to compare the two sides.

---

## Symptoms and signs of orbital disease

### Eyelid swelling

- Oedema is variable and depends on the cause
- Erythema and tenderness are common in inflammatory disease
- Check for lid retraction and lid lag on downgaze, if thyroid eye disease (TED) is suspected
- It is important to differentiate between preseptal oedema (in

which there is no proptosis) and postseptal oedema, particularly in infection.

## Proptosis

Patients may complain of bulging eyes, pressure, or that one eye seems bigger/smaller than the other.

Measure protrusion using a Hertel's exophthalmometer. A difference of more than 2 mm between the two eyes is significant. Normal values lie between 16 and 19 mm and values exceeding that are abnormal.

Differentiate a large globe (for example, axial myopia), contralateral enophthalmos, and proptosis.

### *Double vision*

This indicates restriction of movements as a result of tethering or myositis or from cranial nerve involvement.

The inferior rectus is commonly involved in thyroid eye disease, resulting in limitation and increasing diplopia on upgaze.

Confirm by orthoptic assessment and Hess chart.

## Pain

Pain is a sign of acute inflammation of any orbital tissue including the globe (for example, sclera). It is also caused by infiltrations of the periosteum.

It is a non-specific symptom which is present in a variety of conditions, ranging from pseudotumour, orbital myositis, posterior scleritis, invading tumours, to apical arteritis. The pain caused by inflammation is moderate to severe and it may wake the patient at night.

## Reduced vision

Varying degrees of loss of vision can occur depending on the disease process. Blurred vision from refractive changes or exposure keratopathy as a result of proptosis should be improved with a pinhole; loss of vision, especially colour vision, is a sign of optic nerve compression from increased intraorbital pressure. A relative afferent pupillary defect (RAPD) would be a confirmatory sign and field tests should be carried out to plot the defect or relative scotomata.

Visual evoked potentials would be useful in doubtful cases.

## Displacement of globe

The direction of displacement indicates the origin of the lesion, for example, a lacrimal gland mass causes the globe to be displaced downwards and nasally, a mucocele downwards and laterally, and a maxillary antral mass will displace upwards. A retrobulbar lesion within the muscle cone results in forward displacement and axial proptosis.

## Globe retropulsion

This compares the ease with which a proptosed eye can be gently but firmly pushed back into the orbit, compared with the normal eye. Increase resistance is felt in patients with thyroid eye disease and orbital tumors.

This is a difficult test to interpret and is of limited value.

## Auscultation of the globe

A bruit may be present in a patient with a carotid–cavernous fistula and may be heard by placing the bell of a stethoscope over the closed upper lid or the side of the orbit.

# Painful pathology of orbital disease: management

### Orbital cellulitis (Fig 10.1)

#### Definition
- Infection involving the soft tissues of the orbit
- Often occurs in young adults or children.

#### Causes
- Spread of infection from surrounding sinuses, for example, ethmoidal, maxillary
- Orbital trauma or surgery
- Secondary to bacteraemia.

#### Symptoms and signs
- Systemically unwell, febrile patient
- Headache; pain, redness, and swelling of the lids
- Difficulty in opening the eyes as a result of swelling; conjunctival chemosis
- Painful, limited eye movements; diplopia
- Decreased vision

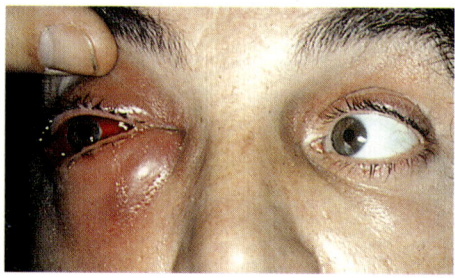

Figure 10.1 Orbital cellulitis: note generalised erythema, oedema, and ophthalmoplegia.

- Acutely tender over the inflamed sinus.

### Management
- Emergency admission; baseline computed tomography (CT) to demonstrate sinusitis and to exclude abscess
- ENT opinion regarding drainage of abscess and treatment of sinusitis
- Baseline full blood count and blood cultures
- Intravenous antibiotics; cover Gram positive, Gram negative, and anaerobic organisms
- General monitoring, assessing progress with 4 hourly Snellen acuity, ocular motility, and proptosis.

### *Inflammatory pseudotumour* (Fig 10.2)

#### Definition
- Non-specific orbital inflammatory syndromes characterised by a mass like lesion simulating a primary orbital neoplasm
- Range from a diffuse process affecting a part of or the entire orbit to a localised process affecting a specific orbital tissue, for example, myositis or dacryoadenitis.

#### Clinical features
- Age: second to eighth decade; can be bilateral in children
- Onset: commonly acute or subacute with severe orbital pain
- Signs of orbital congestion: proptosis, lid oedema, erythema, and marked conjunctival chemosis
- Double vision is common and reduced vision is a serious feature
- Associated uveitis if anterior involvement; raised intraocular pressure (IOP)

# SWELLINGS AROUND THE EYE

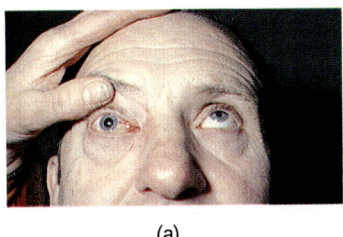

(a)

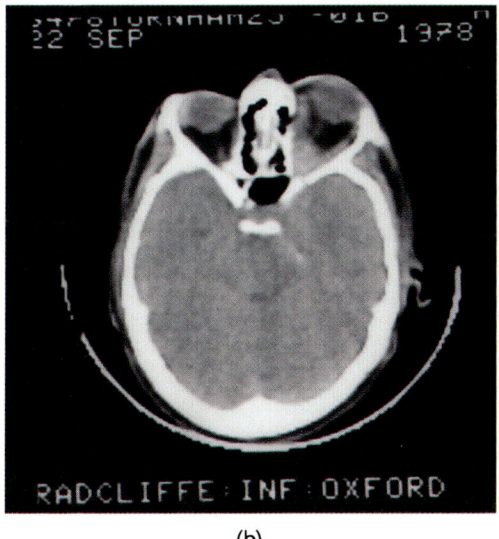

(b)

Figure 10.2 (a) Pseudotumour of right orbit: note injection and restriction of eye movement; (b) CT scan showing a mass in the orbital apex.

- Papillitis and optic neuropathy if posterior involvement.

### Differential diagnosis
- Orbital cellulitis, but no sinus involvement or systemic features; bear in mind mucormycosis in diabetic or immunocompromised patients
- Children—think of rhabdomyosarcomas, metastatic neuroblastoma, or leukaemic infiltration of the orbit
- Do ANCA (antineutrophil cytoplasm antibody) test for Wegener's granulomatosis (usually more chronic) and test for vasculitis.

### Management
- CT scan as soon as possible ± magnetic resonance imaging (MRI)
- Show an irregularly circumscribed enhancing mass which may obliterate normal orbital structures ± enlargement of adjacent extraocular muscle
- Admit for systemic investigation and possible biopsy
- Systemic corticosteroids ± cytotoxic drugs.

## Pathology associated with discomfort in orbital disease: management

### Carotid–cavernous fistula (Fig 10.3)
### *Direct fistula*

**Definition** An abnormal communication between the cavernous sinus and the carotid arterial system.

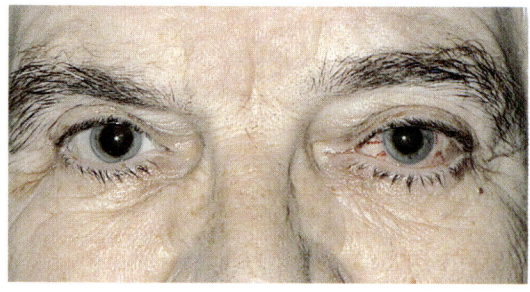

(a)

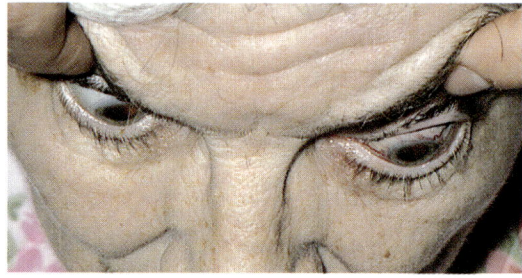

(b)

Figure 10.3 Caroticocavernous fistula causing a sudden red eye, chemosis and dilated conjunctival vessels: (a) front view; (b) showing proptosis.

### Symptoms and signs
- Sudden onset of red eye that may be painful or uncomfortable
- Lid and orbital congestion with dilated episcleral veins and raised intraocular pressure (IOP)
- Blurred vision; double vision; ophthalmoplegia or nerve VI involvement is common
- Pulsatile exophthalmos and bruit in fast flow form
- Fundus signs include retinal haemorrhages, dilated retinal veins, and disc oedema
- Anterior segment hypoxia may develop with rubeosis, cells and flare, and cloudy media.

### Associated factors
- Trauma to the base of the skull (resulting in a fracture) and tearing of the internal carotid artery within the surrounding cavernous sinus
- Spontaneous rupture of an intracavernous aneurysm in a hypertensive patient.

### Management
- Computed tomography shows dilated superior ophthalmic vein
- Angiography
- Radiological embolisation or neurosurgical intervention.

## *Indirect fistula*

### Definition
- Communication between the dural arteries and veins
- Intracavernous part of the carotid artery remains intact
- Arterial blood flows through the meningeal branches and enters the cavernous sinus indirectly.

### Symptoms and signs
- Dilated episcleral veins and mild congestion
- Dull ache
- Mild proptosis, ptosis; diplopia; no bruit
- Chronic fistula results in raised IOP and disc cupping.

### Associated factors
- Hypertension
- Postmenopausal women
- Congenital malformation.

### Management
- Computed tomography and angiography
- May close spontaneously
- Surgical or radiological intervention if troublesome.

### *Thyroid eye disease or Graves' ophthalmopathy* (Figs 10.4 and 10.5)

#### Terminology
- Graves' disease is a syndrome of hyperthyroidism, diffuse goitre, ophthalmopathy, pre-tibial dermopathy, and thyroid acropathy. Hyperthyroidism is caused by a family of thyroid stimulatory immunoglobulins active towards the thyroid stimulating hormone (TSH) receptor.
- Graves' ophthalmopathy is synonymous with thyroid eye disease and most affected patients will have hyperthyroidism.
- Ophthalmic Graves' disease or euthyroid Graves' disease affects patients with typical signs of Graves' ophthalmopathy, but who have no signs of demonstrable thyroid disease. This affects about 10% of patients.
- About 80% of patients with TED have overt or subtle signs of hyperthyroidism, 10% will have Hashimoto's thyroiditis, and 10% will have no signs.

#### Clinical features
- Patients complain of discomfort, foreign body sensation, and photophobia.
- They may have noticed "bulging eyes", puffy lids, diplopia, or abnormal lid position, for example, ptosis or lid retraction.

#### General symptoms
- History of weight loss, palpitations, nervous irritability, and heat intolerance

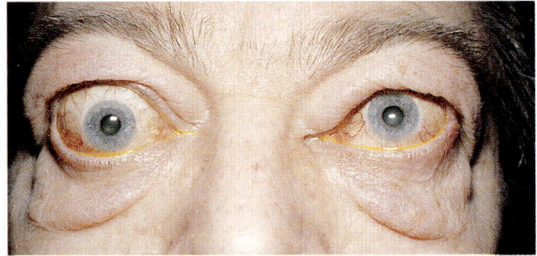

Figure 10.4 Patient with thyroid eye disease (Graves' ophthalmopathy) showing swollen, puffy lids, lid retraction, and conjunctival injection.

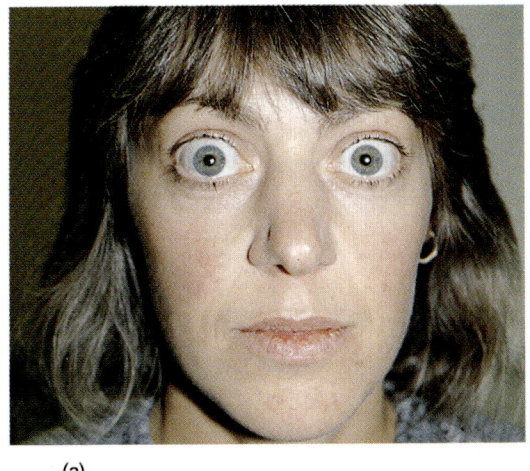

(a)

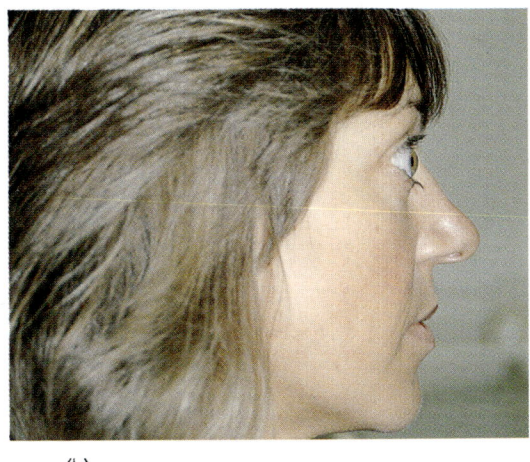

(b)

Figure 10.5 (a) Thyroid eye disease with marked lid retraction and (b) exophthalmos.

- Systemic features: tachycardia, tremor, goitre, and pre-tibial myxoedema.

### Ocular features
#### Lid disease
- Lid retraction (Dalrymple's sign); characteristic sign of Graves' disease; may be unilateral, bilateral, or asymmetrical

- Pseudo-lid retraction; caused by proptosis
- Lid lag (Von Graefe's sign); seen on downgaze when the position of the lid does not follow the globe
- Diffuse swelling and oedema; caused by orbital fat prolapse into lid.

### Soft tissue disease
- Conjunctival injection and chemosis are common; in florid cases the conjunctiva may prolapse over the lower lid.
- Superior limbic keratoconjunctivitis:
    usually found in women
    unilateral, bilateral or markedly asymmetrical
    changes are confined to the superior tarsal and bulbar conjunctiva with localised hyperaemia and papillary hypertrophy
    adjacent cornea may show punctate erosions and filamentary keratitis
    associated with dry eye conditions.
- Proptosis:
    indicates orbital disease
    TED is the most common cause of unilateral or bilateral proptosis
    can occasionally be marked
    corneal exposure is common and results from incomplete lid closure.
- Extraocular muscles:
    inflammation, fibrosis, and contraction result in limitation of movement and diplopia
    IOP is raised when measured with eyes in upgaze; an increase of 5 mm Hg is significant
    frozen globe results from extensive tethering
    most frequently involved muscles are inferior rectus and medial rectus.
- Optic nerve compression:
    apex of the orbit is the most common site
    look for abnormalities of visual acuity, colour vision, pupillary function (an afferent pupil defect), and the visual fields (a central or paracentral scotoma).

### Investigations
- Tests of thyroid function—including TSH levels and thyroid autoantibodies

## SWELLINGS AROUND THE EYE

- CT scan (including coronal views of orbit) shows swelling of one or more extraocular muscles with sparing of the tendons.

### Management
- This is best undertaken in a specialist endocrine clinic.

### *Patients with sore, gritty eyes*
- Symptomatic relief:
    topical lubricants, for example, frequent artificial tear drops during the day and lubricating ointment at night for dry $\pm$ eyes superior limbic keratitis
    5% acetylcysteine drops dissolves abnormal mucus in patients with filamentary keratitis.
- For corneal exposure:
    mild cases—taping the eye lids at night
    more severe cases—a lateral tarsorrhaphy will reduce exposure
    for severe lid retraction—recession of the levator muscles
    severe cases—see below.

### *Patients with diplopia*
Full orthoptic work up and investigations to eliminate other forms of acquired squint. Prisms are useful where the squint is relatively concomitant but will only help a small percentage of cases long term.

Patients should be referred to the clinic for further assessment and possible squint surgery once the deviation is stable.

### *Optic neuropathy*
Patients with signs of optic neuropathy require *urgent* assessment for one of the following treatment options:

- High dose systemic steriods
- Radiotherapy
- Surgical decompression.

Patients with severe inflammation, pain, and proptosis require systemic corticosteroids to bring the disease under control, that is, enteric coated prednisolone 80–100 mg daily or larger dose.

### *Corneal exposure caused by severe proptosis*
The severe proptosis is the result of very severe inflammation and congestion of the orbit. Persistent exposure leads to

ulceration and eventual perforation, and is as much an emergency as optic neuropathy.
Immediate treatment:

- Admit for frequent moistening and/or enclosing the eye by cling film to conserve moisture
- Medical decompression with high dose steroids
- Surgical decompression.

Radiotherapy as an alternative does not work fast enough in this situation and is for the longer term as either a supplement or replacement for steroids.

Mild exposure caused by incomplete excursion of the lid during blinking or in sleep is dealt with above.

## Painless pathology of orbital disease: management

### Vascular tumours
These are rare but many are treatable.

#### Symptoms and signs
*Capillary haemangioma* (Fig 10.6)
- Presents at birth or in infancy
- Soft, painless
- May be associated with discoloration of the eyelids
- Lump increases in size with crying.

*Cavernous haemangioma* (Fig 10.7)
- Presents in adulthood
- Slowly progressive, unilateral, painless, axial proptosis.

#### Management
*Capillary haemangioma*
- Watch out for ambylopia by having regular orthoptic reviews
- Lesion will regress and disappear by about five years
- Much reassurance is needed for usually distressed parents
- Intralesional injection of steroids if very unsightly or threatening amblyopia by covering pupil axis.

*Cavernous haemangioma*
- Orbital ultrasonography or computed tomography
- Surgery: excision for pronounced symptoms.

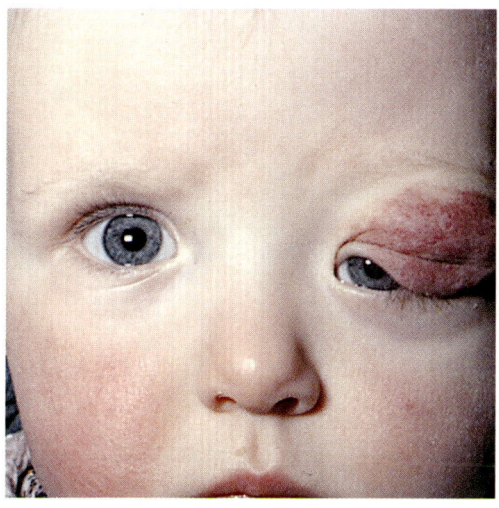

Figure 10.6 Capillary haemangioma causing ptosis but not obstructing visual axis.

## Cystic tumours
### *Dermoid cysts* (Fig 10.8)

- Present in small children as firm, painless, mobile lesions
- Usually, the location is in the upper temporal aspects of the orbit; sometimes it is nasal
- They can "leak", causing local inflammation or become infected
- Occasionally present in young adults with slowly progressive proptosis
- Intraorbital extension possible.

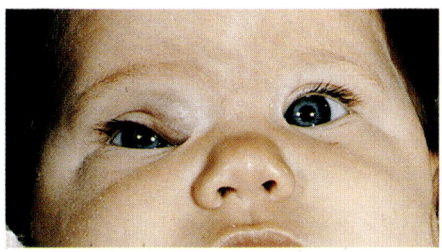

Figure 10.7 Cavernous haemangioma of medial part of right upper lid.

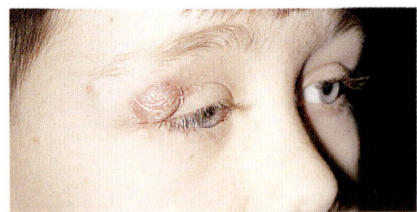

Figure 10.8 Infected dermoid cyst in a young boy arising in a typical (though not invariable) position.

### Management
- CT scan to exclude orbital involvement
- Surgical excision.

### *Mucocele*

- Caused by progressive accumulation of secretions from the sinus epithelium
- Invades the orbit as a cystic mass from either the frontal or ethmoid sinuses
- Feels firm if still covered by bone and painless if not infected.

### Management
- Usually undertaken by ENT surgeons
- Differentiate from an encephalocele in the young
- Indications for excision:
    infection
    nerve compression
- Leave alone if asymptomatic or in elderly patients.

## Malignant tumours
### *Rhabdomyosarcoma* (Fig 10.9)

- Rare
- Presents in young children in the first decade from five onwards, but may present in adolescence
- Rapid onset of painless, progressive proptosis
- Exclude an inflammatory or infective process
- CT scan will show a mass arising from an extraocular muscle with possible bony involvement.

### *Lymphoma/lymphoid hyperplasia*

- Adults; 60 years +

# SWELLINGS AROUND THE EYE

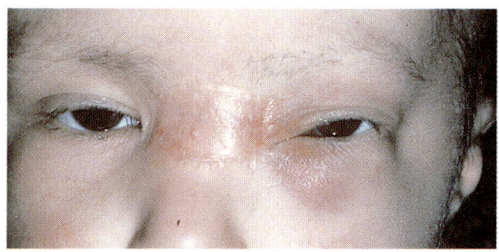

Figure 10.9  Rhabdomyosarcoma causing erythema, swelling, and proptosis.

- Present with rubbery mass palpable in either the superior or the inferior fornix
- Arises commonly from the anterior part of the orbit, including the lacrimal gland or conjunctiva
- The indolent form is more common, but lymphomas may be fulminant or spread from adjacent structures.

### Management
- Chest radiograph and blood specimens for serum electrophoresis
- CT scan of orbit
- Admit to define the disease/urgent referral to oncologist for further investigations.

## *Metastatic tumours*

### Differential diagnosis
- Adults—primary sites are the breast, bronchus, gastrointestinal tract, prostate, and kidney
- Children—primary sites are neuroblastoma, Ewing's sarcoma, Wilms' tumours, and leukaemic deposits.

**Management**  Admit for further investigations and determine site of primary.

# Symptoms and signs of lid disease

## Swelling of the lids

Localised swellings that involve the lids are usually easily identified by both the patient and the doctor. Diffuse swelling can involve one or all four lids and can be very asymmetrical.

### Differential diagnosis
- Local—cyst, stye, tumour
- Diffuse—allergy, preseptal cellulitis.

### Itching of the lids
Itching is commonly associated wih puffy swollen lids.

### Differential diagnosis
- Allergy to topical medication
- Contact dermatitis.

### Pain, redness, or tenderness
This is typical of infection of the lid.

## Management of lid swellings

### Painful pathology
***Preseptal cellulitis*** (Fig 10.10)

### Definition
- Infection confined to the tissues anterior to the orbital septum
- Does not penetrate the posterior aspect of the orbit (unlike orbital cellulitis), hence there is no proptosis
- Occurs in any age group but more common in younger people.

### Causes
- Trauma to the surrounding soft tissues; organisms: *Staphylococcus aureus*, streptococci
- Sinus infections; suspect *Haemophilus influenzae* in children.

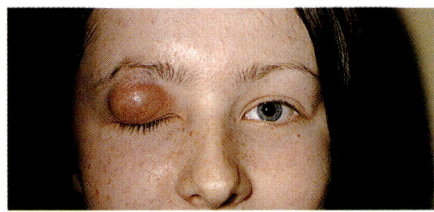

Figure 10.10 Preseptal cellulitis in a young girl, leading to an abscess of the upper lid. Note that the patient looks well.

# SWELLINGS AROUND THE EYE

### Symptoms and signs
- Unilateral swollen, red, and tender eyelid; sticky eye
- Lids tight but it is possible to open them easily; globe is quiet and white; no proptosis
- Vision normal
- The patient is generally well
- Consider viral aetiology if there is a skin rash.

### Management
- Exclude orbital involvement, sinusitis, and dental abscesses
- Bacterial swabs indicated if there is a skin wound or purulent discharge; broad spectrum oral antibiotics, for example, amoxycillin, erythromycin, 10–14 day course
- Review daily until clinically improved
- Good prognosis.

## Lid infections

### Diagnosis
- Painful lump on lid
- Style: infection of hair follicle
- Internal hordeolum: abscess of a meibomian gland.

### Management
- Exclude staphylococcal blepharitis
- Remove lash; bathe lid with hot compresses
- Topical chloramphenicol drops
- Subsequent incision and curettage of remaining chalazion.

## Painless pathology
### Cysts and benign tumours

#### Diagnosis
#### Meibomian cyst (chalazion)
- Firm, painless swelling in tarsal plate
- May be associated with conjunctival granuloma.

#### Retention cysts
- Small painless swelling containing either watery secretions (cyst of Moll) or lipid (cyst of Zeiss).

#### Squamous papilloma and seborrhoeic keratose
These are common in elderly people.

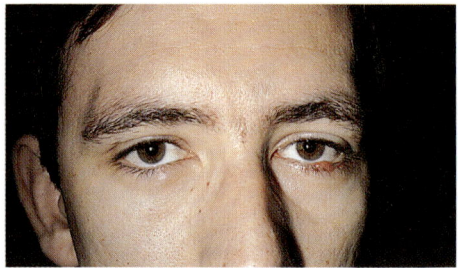

Figure 10.11 Chalazion of the right lower lid seen through the skin—a stye turned to chronic hordeolum on left lid margin.

### *Keratoacanthoma*
- Rapidly growing
- Histologically can mimic squamous cell carcinoma.

### Management
### *Chalazion* (Fig 10.11)
- Conservative: leave well alone (many resolve spontaneously), if not bothering patient
- Surgical: incision and curettage under local anaesthetic
- Commonly recur, especially in patients with chronic blepharitis
- If recurs in the *same site*, suspect underlying pathology, for example, basal cell carcinoma.

### *Retention cysts* (Fig 10.12)
- Cysts of Zeiss or Moll are located on the anterior lid margins
- Puncture with a needle is used as a temporary measure
- Excision is needed for a more permanent cure.

### *Squamous papillomas, seborrhoeic keratoses, and senile keratoses*
- Excision if unsightly or if the diagnosis is uncertain.

### *Keratoacanthoma* (Fig 10.13)
- Excise if persistent.

### Malignant tumours

#### Basal cell carcinoma (Figs 10.14 and 10.15)
#### *Clinical features*
- Most common primary malignant tumour of the lids

# SWELLINGS AROUND THE EYE

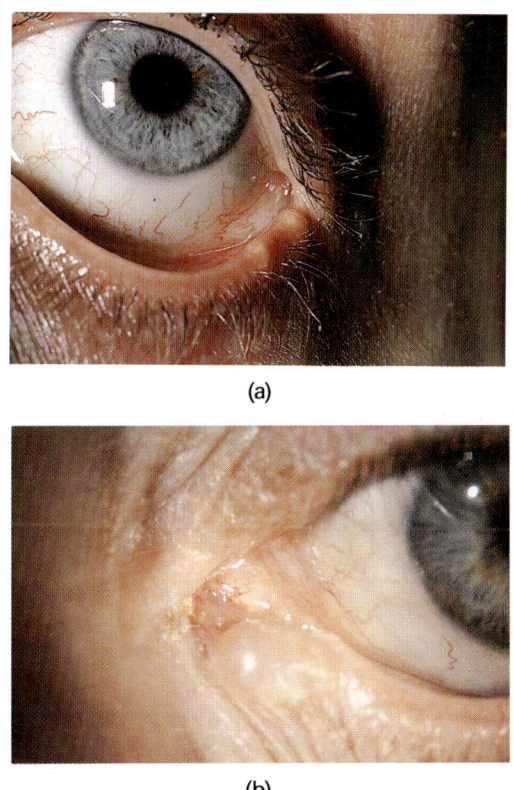

Figure 10.12 (a) Retention cysts of Zeiss (sebaceous material) on the lower lid. (b) Cyst of Moll (watery).

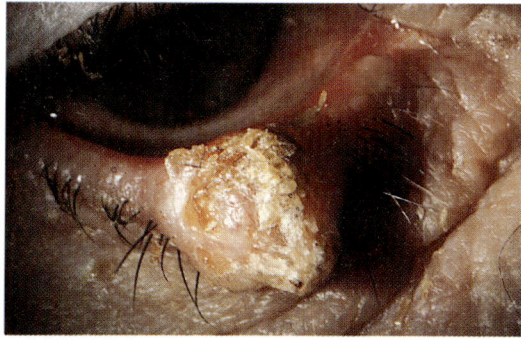

Figure 10.13 This warty, hyperkeratotic lesion of the lower lid is typical of a squamous papilloma. Histological examination showed a keratoacanthoma, however.

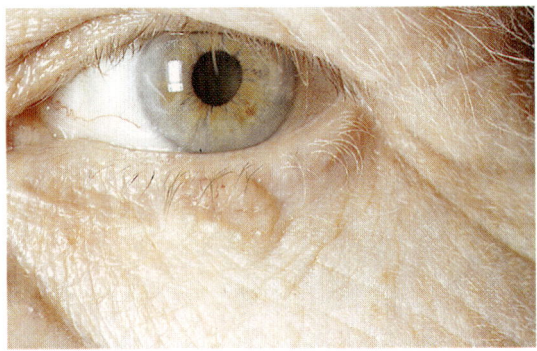

Figure 10.14 Basal cell carcinoma of the lower lid showing the classic appearance of a rodent ulcer.

- Risk factors: age and exposure to sunlight
- Commonly found on the lower lid
- Various forms: rodent ulcer is the most common:
    raised lesion which bleeds easily on touch
    ulcer margins have well defined rolled appearance
    surface looks pearly; the centre is vascular
    medial canthal lesions have worse prognosis
- Other forms are: (1) sclerosing and (2) cystic.

**Management**
- Surgical excision
- Radiotherapy.

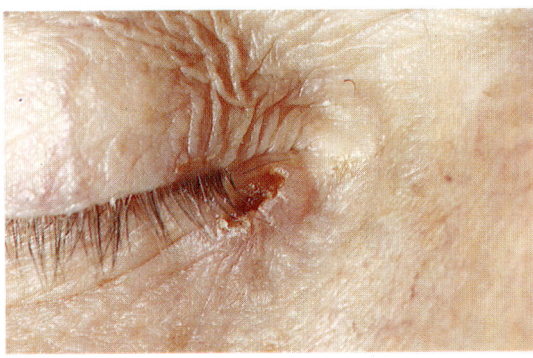

Figure 10.15 Basal cell carcinoma showing a scab formed over a bleeding centre.

# SWELLINGS AROUND THE EYE

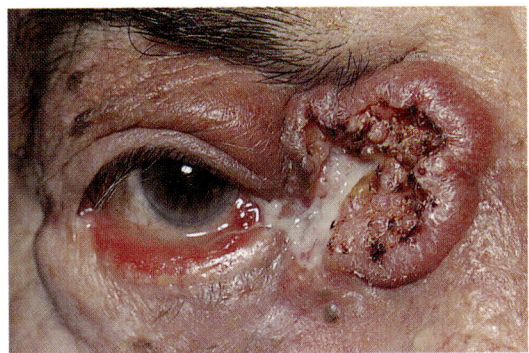

Figure 10.16   Squamous cell carcinoma.

## Squamous cell carcinoma (Fig 10.16)
### Diagnosis
- Less common than basal cell carcinoma but also has a very varied clinical appearance
- Fast growing; upper lids mostly affected
- Differential diagnosis is a keratoacanthoma which is rapidly growing and may have invasive appearance; metastasis to local lymph nodes.

### Management
- Referral for biopsy and surgical excision.


## Itchy irritable lids
### *Molluscum contagiosum* (Fig 10.17)

This is caused by a viral infection of the lids.

#### Symptoms
- Red, irritable, watering eye.

#### Signs
- Umbilicated nodule(s) at the lid margin
- Conjunctival injection
- Follicular conjunctivitis
- Punctate staining of the corneal epithelium caused by superficial keratitis.

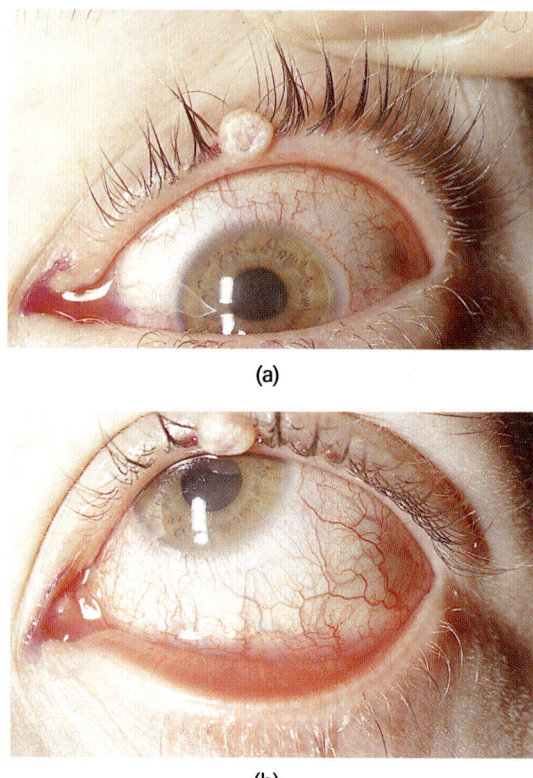

Figure 10.17 (a) Molluscum contagiosum with (b) conjunctivitis.

### Management
- Local cautery of the lesion.

### *Allergy*

See Chapter 5.

# Symptoms and signs of lacrimal gland disease
## Swelling

Disease of the lacrimal gland gives rise to swelling at the outer one third of the upper lid. It is usually unilateral and may be associated with tenderness and erythema.

For bilateral swellings, consider sarcoid, thyroid eye disease, or lymphoproliferative disease. The globe will be displaced and proptosed, and the patient may complain of double vision.

### Differential diagnosis
- Child: dermoid
- Adult:
  lacrimal gland tumour or granuloma—histologically, about 50% of tumours are epithelial cell tumours which may be either benign mixed cell tumours or carcinomas; the rest are inflammatory masses, for example, sarcoidosis, pseudotumour dacryoadenitis.

## *Pain*

Pain indicates (1) acute inflammation or (2) invasion of periosteum or surrounding tissue.

Chronic inflammation and slowly growing masses do not cause pain as a rule.

### Differential diagnosis
- Children—acute dacryoadenitis
- Young adults—acute dacryoadenitis or carcinoma
- Middle aged or elderly adults—dacryoadenitis, malignant mixed cell epithelial tumour, adenoid cystic tumour, or pseudotumour.

## *No pain*

The absence of pain indicates a slow process and the absence of inflammation or infiltration.

**Differential diagnosis.** Benign mixed cell tumour, lacrimal gland cyst, dermoid, or lymphoproliferation/lymphoma.

### Space occupying lesions of the lacrimal gland

| *Cysts* | *Inflammation* | *Tumours* |
|---|---|---|
| Dermoid | Non-specific adenitis | Lymphoproliferative disease |
| Lacrimal cyst | Infection | Epithelial tumour |
|  |  | Mixed cell adenoma |
|  |  | Adenoid cystic carcinoma |
|  |  | Other |

# Management of lacrimal gland swellings (Fig 10.18)

## Painful pathology
### Dacryoadenitis

This condition may be bacterial or viral in origin and typically occurs in children or young adults.

It may occur in association with mumps or glandular fever.

### Symptoms and signs
- Painful swelling over outer one third of the upper lid
- Watering eye
- Preauricular lymphadenopathy.

### Treatment
- Broad spectrum oral antibiotics for 7–14 days
- Analgesia.

### *Adenocarcinoma and adenoid cystic carcinoma*

These are malignant lacrimal gland tumours.

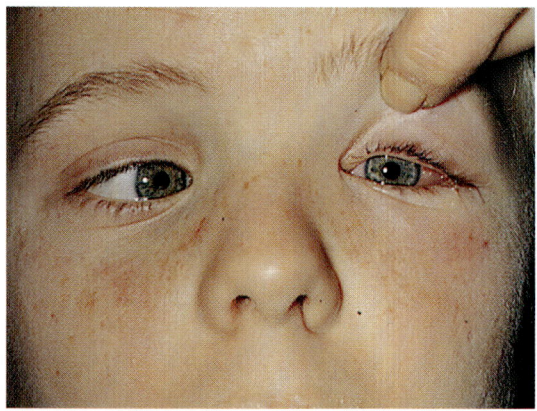

Figure 10.18 Lacrimal gland swelling: painful adenitis (viral) with chemosis and limitation of abduction.

### Symptoms and signs
- Rapid onset of a painful swelling of the outer one third of the upper lid
- Globe displacement and proptosis
- Double vision.

### Management
- CT scan of the orbit will reveal a mass in the lacrimal gland with possible adjacent bone involvement
- Refer for open biopsy to confirm the diagnosis
- Surgical exenteration and radiotherapy.

## Painless pathology
### *Mixed cell lacrimal gland tumour*

#### Symptoms
- Gradual onset of a swelling in the outer one third of the upper lid
- There may be a well defined painless mass
- Globe displacement downwards and medially
- Proptosis
- Double vision.

#### Management
- CT scan of the orbit will show enlargement of the lacrimal gland
- Referral for surgical excision with intact capsule to prevent local recurrence
- Biopsy *contraindicated* as with any lacrimal mass; a lacrimal gland mass should be exposed so that, if a well encapsulated mass exists, it can be removed *in toto*.

### *Lymphomas*
- Present as smooth, sausage shaped tumours of the upper lid
- Refer for further investigation and management.

### *Sarcoidosis*
- May have systemic disease
- Patients should have a chest radiograph—bilateral hilar lymphadenopathy

- Serum angiotensin converting enzyme may be elevated (see Sarcoid and diagnostic tests, page 84).

## Symptoms and signs of nasolacrimal disease

### Watering eye

Disease of the nasolacrimal system frequently leads to obstruction of the tear passages. Obstruction to flow may occur anywhere along the duct system and may be caused by: punctal stenosis, canalicular stenosis, lacrimal sac infection, lacrimal sac mass, or nasolacrimal duct obstruction.

It is important to exclude causes of excess tearing from irritation.

### Lacrimal sac swelling

Obstruction superior to the common canaliculus may have no signs besides watering. Distal or inferior to the lacrimal sac, obstruction could lead to distension of the sac, mucocele formation, and infection.

Acute infection leads to pain, erythema, and swelling of the sac which lies just inferomedial to the medial canthus. Pressure over the sac can result in regurgitation of purulent discharge through the punctum.

#### Differential diagnosis
- Dacryocystitis
- Mucocele
- Tumour of the lacrimal sac
- Ethmoid sinusitis.

## Management of nasolacrimal problems

### Painful pathology
***Dacryocystitis*** (Fig 10.19)

#### Definition
- Infection involving the nasolacrimal sac; may be recurrent
- Occurs in all age groups.

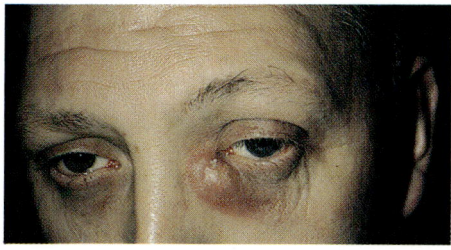

Figure 10.19   Dacryocystitis in an adult with an abscess of the lacrimal sac.

### Symptoms and signs
- Painful swelling over nasolacrimal sac; sticky eye; purulent discharge from punctum with pressure on sac
- Preceding history of epiphora.

### Management
- Either oral or parenteral broad spectrum antibiotics, for example, amoxycillin, cephalosporin
- Topical antibiotics
- Analgesia
- If there is a nasolacrimal sac abscess, consider incision and drainage under general anaesthetic, but this should be avoided if possible because of the likelihood of a subsequent lacrimal fistula
- Do not probe nasolacrimal system until infection has settled
- Definitive treatment is by dacryocystorhinostomy and internal drainage when infection is controlled.

## Painless pathology
### *Lacrimal sac mucocele*

Chronic dacrocystitis in adults can result in the development of a lacrimal sac mucocele. This is a distended, atonic sac filled with sterile mucopus.

### Symptoms
- Watering eye
- Painless palpable swelling at the innermost aspect of the lower lid
- Pressure over the swelling causes regurgitation of mucous discharge from the lower punctum.

## Management
- Refer for dacryocystorhinostomy.

### Lacrimal sac tumour
- Very rare.

#### Symptoms and signs
- Watering eye
- Previous episodes of dacrocystitis
- Irrigation causes the reflux of blood stained fluid
- Palpable mass below the medial canthal tendon.

#### Investigation
- Filling defect in dacryocystography; computed tomography to exclude bone invasion.

#### Management
- Refer for surgical excision and radiotherapy.

# Conjunctival swellings (Figs 10.20–10.22)

### Painful
Usually inflammatory and will have a red eye (see Chapter 5).

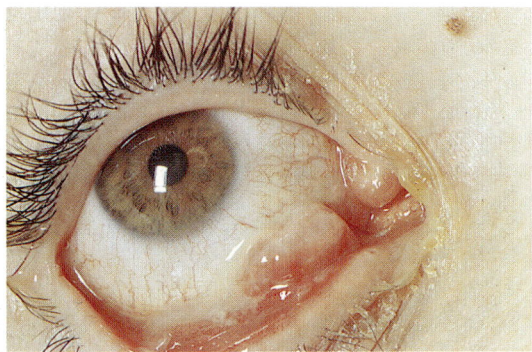

Figure 10.20 Conjunctival granuloma in the lower fornix with overlying mucopus.

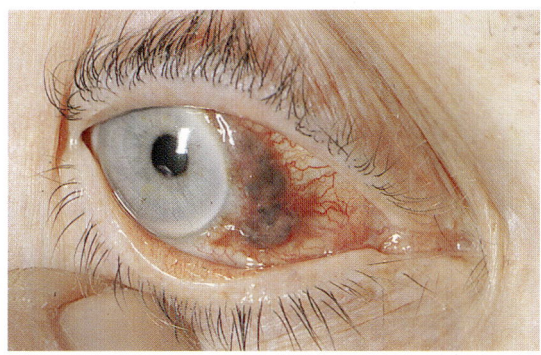

Figure 10.21   Conjunctival malignant melanoma arising at the limbus.

## Painless pathology
### Diffuse chemosis

- May occur after lid surgery
- Probably the result of damage to the lymphatic drainage.

### Localised cystic swellings

- Retention of clear fluid forming pseudocysts, which are usually discovered by a relative or incidentally by the patient when looking into the mirror
- No pathological significance and may disappear in a short time
- May have a history of chronic irritation.

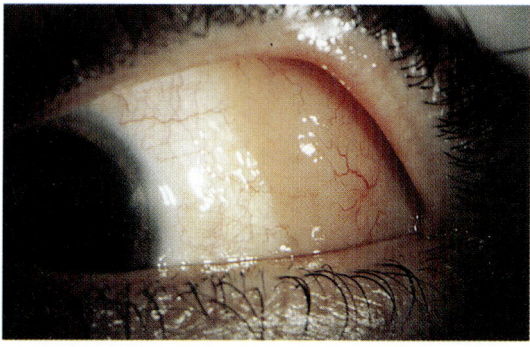

Figure 10.22   Lymphoma spreading from the upper fornix—it is soft and painless.

### Management
- Reassurance
- Puncture with sterile hypodermic needle
- Treat allied symptoms, for example, those of blepharitis.

### Dermolipomas or lipomas (localised swelling nesting in the anterior orbit)

- Smooth contour with no posterior border; superolateral fornix more often affected
- Yellowish fatty material usually visible
- Soft, indefinite outline to touch
- Benign, long-standing, and usually non-progressive.

### Management
- Leave alone unless exceptional symptoms
- Removal can be difficult and need not be complete
- The levator and the lacrimal ductules can be easily damaged on removal.

### *Conjunctival tumours*

- Rare
- Intrinsic tumours usually cause an associated red eye
- Pigmented tumours may not do so in the early stages, but any tumour will have bulk and its own blood supply
- Lymphoid infiltrations develop slowly and may remain asymptomatic for some time apart from the diffuse pinkish mass; usually extend from the fornices.

**Management** Refer for consideration of surgical excision and radiotherapy.

### *Granulomata* (Fig 10.20)

These are caused by retained suture material most commonly after retinal detachment or squint surgery

### Symptoms and signs
- Soreness; gritty sensation
- Small, fleshy lumps involving the bulbar conjunctiva
- Local conjunctival injection.

**Management** Topical steroids will reduce inflammation and, if this is insufficient, excision can be performed under local or general anaesthesia.

# 11 Contact lens problems

The contact lens wearing population in developed countries is steadily increasing. Large numbers of people are wearing contact lenses because of their ready availability. As many patients only become aware of their problems when the lenses are removed, they usually resort to the A&E department for advice if complications occur out of hours.

## Common problems

There are five main reasons for presentation of contact lens wearers in the A&E department:

1 Pain
2 Reduced vision
3 Redness
4 Lost lens within the eye
5 Optician referral, for example, infection, inflammation, and neovascularisation.

## Causes of eye pathology and symptoms

- Overwear/tight fit, leading to hypoxia and epithelial breakdown
- Malfitting, foreign body, or damaged lens leading to corneal abrasion
- Corneal infiltrates (especially soft lens wearers, probably caused by debris)
- Corneal infection—bacterial or *Acanthamoeba* sp.
- Trauma from poor handling
- Chemical toxicity from cleaning solution.

All of the above can give rise to symptoms ranging from severe discomfort to pain, photophobia, and watering.

- Allergy to the solution or preservative
- Giant papillary conjunctivitis—probably an allergy to protein deposits.

Itching and irritation will be the primary symptoms which will tend to be bilateral.

Reduced vision will depend on the location of the corneal pathology and therefore on the condition of the lenses if still on the eye.

## Diagnosis of the problem

### History

Enquire about the following.

### *What type of lens is the patient wearing?*

There are three basic types in general use: (1) hard, (2) gas permeable, and (3) soft. Both the "hard" and gas permeable lenses are rigid and ride on a cushion of tears. Fitting of these lenses needs to be exact and the posterior surface of the lens needs to conform to the curvature of the cornea. Soft lenses mould on to the shape of the cornea (and are in direct contact with the epithelium). Although soft lenses are more easily tolerated in the short term, especially those with a high water content, they are more prone to breakage, surface deposits, and bacterial colonisation. There is a higher risk of microbial keratitis with soft than with rigid lenses.

Soft disposable lenses are now widely fitted. They are changed frequently, but unless disposed of daily, require daily cleaning and disinfection.

### *What cleansing routine is the patient following?*

The cleansing method depends on the type of lens. For *hard lenses* the standard regimen is

- Cleaning in a commercial cleanser
- Rinsing in saline
- Storing and soaking in a wetting solution containing a preservative.

For *soft lenses* the regimen is more involved and there is a higher incidence of sensitivity to preservatives than with rigid lenses. Rigid contact lens solutions are *not* compatible with soft lenses:

- Clean in recommended cleaning solution
- Rinse with saline
- Disinfect with either (1) cold disinfection method or (2) hydrogen peroxide system with neutralisation.

Multipurpose solutions incorporating macromolecules include a cleaner in the disinfecting solution. Patients should rub and rinse their lenses and soak in fresh solution each day.

Protein removal tablets are indicated when lenses are changed infrequently.

### Points in the history
- Ascertain whether there is a departure from routine
- Check if there has been neglect in sterilisation of the lens
- Check if inappropriate solution or tap water has been used
- Check if solutions are still in date.

### What is the contact lens wearing schedule?

- What is the maximum wearing time?
- What is the usual wearing time?
- Have the lenses been worn overnight or during a cat-nap?
- Were there any special circumstances such as a long flight which may lead to excessive dehydration?

### Is there an allergic tendency?

Allergy to the chemical agents, including the preservatives, is common:

- Does the patient have any known allergy?
- Is there a history of atopy in the family?
- Has there been a previous allergic reaction?

### How old are the lenses?

There is a relationship between proneness to sensitivity and lens age, probably because the preservative concentrates within the soft lens matrix. High water content lenses may produce an allergic type of reaction after prolonged soaking in protein removing solution.

## Examination

The following are specific points to look for.

- Lid swelling and signs of contact dermatitis.
- Conjunctival signs including eversion of the upper lid to check for giant papillae.
- Surface changes of the cornea and limbus, for example, neovascularisation. Best seen with the contact lens out and using oblique illumination or retroillumination. Do not instil fluorescein with a soft lens in place to avoid permanent discoloration. Where possible get the patient to remove the contact lens to avoid dispute in case of lens damage.
- Contact lens movement on blinking:
  excessive movement gives rise to irritation and instability—for soft lens this means exposure of the limbus in any direction of gaze; for hard lens it means moving across the lateral limbus. Common causes for a soft lens include (1) wearing the lens inside out and (2) giant papillary conjunctivitis (evert upper lid); for a hard lens (1) poor fit and (2) lens put in the wrong eye.
  Too tight a fit will prevent circulation of the tear and give rise to symptoms. Common causes for a soft lens include mild conjunctival injection or oedema; for a hard lens (1) falling asleep wearing the lens, for example, during a siesta, or (2) initial poor fit.
- Staining patterns with fluorescein: clinically, staining at the 3 and 9 o'clock positions indicates incomplete blinking and localised drying of the corneal epithelium. Diffuse fine (superficial) corneal staining suggests hypoxia or a chemical sensitivity reaction.

## Management of specific problems
### Hypoxia

All lenses reduce the transmission of oxygen to the cornea to some extent. Extended wear in an unaccustomed patient can result in acute hypoxia (Fig 11.1).

**Cause** Usually there is a history of excessive wearing time.

#### Symptoms and signs
- Blurred vision, pain, photophobia, and watering 2–3 hours after removal of the lenses

# EMERGENCY OPHTHALMOLOGY

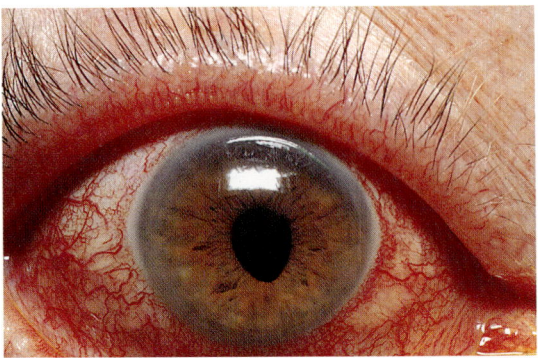

Figure 11.1  Injected, painful eye from contact lens overwear.

- Examination shows epithelial and stromal oedema
- Epithelial irregularities stain with fluorescein.

### Management
- Remove the lens—the corneal oedema usually clears within 24–48 hours
- Pain relief with oral analgesia
- Topical antibiotic and a mydriatic to relieve ciliary spasm should be prescribed for 2–3 days or until symptoms clear.

## Toxicity

**Cause**  Commonly results from insertion of lenses without having rinsed them properly, or having rinsed them in some solution other than the correct agent.

### Symptoms and signs
- Painful red eye
- Corneal staining with fluorescein—ranges from being punctate to large corneal abrasions.

### Management
- Remove the lenses
- Pain relief with oral analgesia
- Cycloplegic drops and antibiotic ointment
- The patient can apply eye pads and lie in a darkened room at home
- The lenses must be thoroughly rinsed before further use.

# CONTACT LENS PROBLEMS

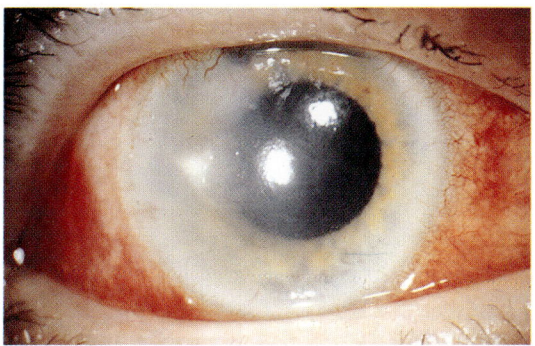

Figure 11.2 Contact lens induced corneal infiltrates with early vascularisation.

## *Corneal infiltrates* (Fig 11.2)

Small corneal infiltrates with or without overlying epithelial loss occur either at the periphery or towards the centre of the cornea.

The peripheral infiltrates are probably the result of hypoxic breakdown of the epithelium allowing bacteria access to the stroma where they set up a hypersensitivity reaction; those situated more centrally are more likely to be frankly infective. The distribution of the infiltrate is not a reliable guide to the underlying cause, however, and all such opacities should be treated with antibiotics.

### Symptoms and signs
- Discomfort to pain, photophobia, and watering
- Redness
- Discrete area(s) of anterior stromal infiltrate
- Epithelium may be intact, thickened, or have a pseudodendritic appearance
- Mild to moderate anterior chamber activity.

### Management
- Discontinue lens wear until cornea clears and epithelium becomes intact
- Intensive topical antibiotic drops
- Pseudomonas cover, for example, gentamicin forte drops
- No pad is necessary
- Review daily until clinically improved

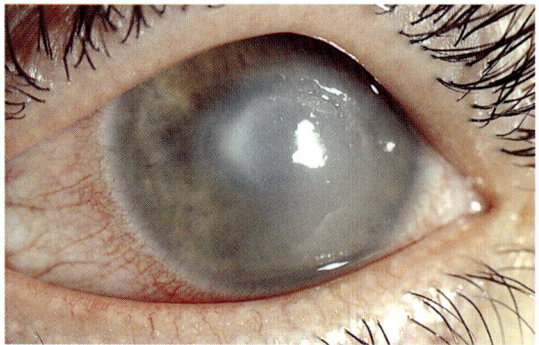

Figure 11.3   Acanthamoeba keratitis: early signs.

- Watch for corneal suppuration; if present treat as a corneal ulcer and admit to hospital.

**Acanthamoeba keratitis** (Figs 11.3 and 11.4)

This is an uncommon form of keratitis but its prevalence is increasing from the following:

- More widespread use of soft lenses
- Lack of proper hygiene
- Lack of awareness that domestic water is a potential source of infection, because *Acanthamoeba* sp. can often be found in tap water and grown from taps and sinks.

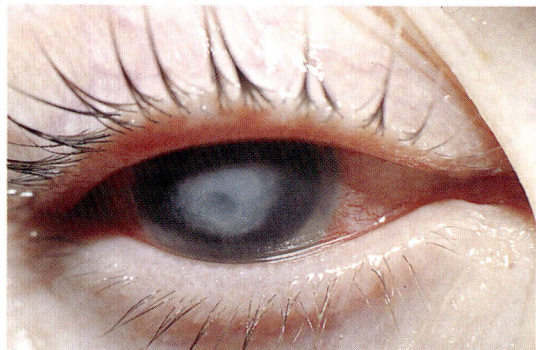

Figure 11.4   Acanthamoeba keratitis: late signs showing dense corneal scarring.

### Symptoms and signs
- Painful red eye—pain is often disproportionate to the signs
- Corneal infiltrates or ulcer
- Prominent corneal nerves from perineural infiltrates
- Unresponsiveness to antibiotics.

### Management
- High index of suspicion essential
- Early diagnosis is important because the disease is unresponsive to conventional antibiotics
- Diagnosis is from *corneal scrapings or biopsy*
- Specific therapy is with propamidine and polyhexamethylene biguanide (PHMB).

For a more detailed description of acanthamoeba keratitis and method of diagnosis see Appendix F.

## *Corneal ulcers/infectious keratitis* (Fig 11.5)

These can occur with any type of lens, but are more common with the use of disposable or extended wear lenses.

Overnight wear causes hypoxia which, if severe, leads to epithelial breakdown and allows bacteria to infect the stroma. Alternatively, there may have been a corneal abrasion or dirt under the lens which has become contaminated.

### Symptoms and signs
- Acutely painful, photophobic, sticky eye

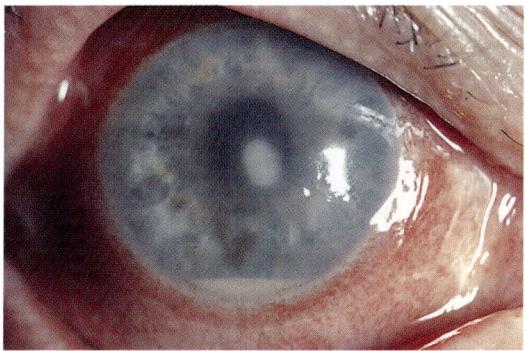

Figure 11.5  Corneal ulcer in a contact lens wearer with stromal abscess and a hypopyon.

- Conjunctival injection, tearing, and mucopurulent discharge
- Blurred vision, especially if the central cornea is involved
- Epithelial defect on fluorescein staining with some degree of surrounding corneal infiltrate
- In severe cases a corneal abscess can develop
- Check for anterior chamber activity and the presence of a hypopyon
- Corneal abscesses must be treated promptly and vigorously to avoid serious complications such as corneal perforation.

### Investigations

The following specimens must be sent to microbiology before treatment is commenced:

- The contact lenses themselves in separate labelled sterile containers for culture
- A sample of the solutions used for cleaning the lenses
- A swab of the contact lens storage case which can be cultured
- Conjunctival swab
- Corneal scrape
- If there is marked blepharitis, a lid swab.

### Management

- Admission for intensive care
- Intensive topical antibiotic treatment with a broad spectrum cephalosporin and gentamicin drops until specific sensitivities are available from the laboratory
- Regular clinical review for response

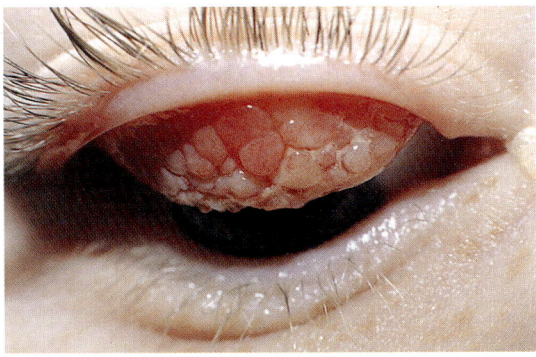

Figure 11.6 Giant papillary conjunctivitis showing the "cobblestone" appearance.

- Adjustment of the topical treatment when the results of the cultures are known
- Topical steroids may be added once the epithelium has healed.

## Giant papillary conjunctivitis (Fig 11.6)

This is a complication of prolonged lens wear or seen in patients with atopy; it is probably an immunological response to protein deposits on the lenses.

### Symptoms and signs
- Decreasing lens tolerance with irritation, itching, photophobia, and increased mucus production
- Excess mucus contamination on the lens may cause blurring of vision
- Eversion of the lid shows giant papillae with scarred apices on the upper tarsal conjunctiva
- The signs are often asymmetrical.

### Management
- Stop wearing the lenses until the papillae have resolved
- Course of topical sodium cromoglycate or weak steroids if the patient is very uncomfortable
- When contact lens wear is resumed try different lenses, for example, hard lenses or a frequent change soft lens regimen; a different solution system is also indicated, with special attention to management of protein deposition on the lens surface.

## Allergy

This is commonly an allergy to the preservatives used in contact lens solutions, for example, thiomersal, or the chemical agent.

### Symptoms and signs
- Redness, burning, and itching soon after inserting the lenses
- Examination shows mild perilimbal injection and papillary conjunctival reaction
- Signs are reversible when use of the solution or preservative is stopped.

**Management** Preservative free contact lens solutions—hydrogen peroxide systems—should be used.

### Lost/stuck lenses

Patients may be unable to remove their lenses because of pain or inexperience. The lens may be on the cornea or under the upper lid and, if soft, may be rolled up.

Often the lens is lost during a traumatic attempt at removal and gives the impression of still being lodged in the eye.

### Removal of a lens still on the cornea
#### Soft lens
- Patient sits with head tilted back
- Topical anaesthetic is instilled into the eye
- Lens pinched out between the examiner's thumb and index finger; anaesthetic is not needed if experienced.

**Hard lens** Manipulate the patient's lids such that the lid margin can be gently levered under the lens edge to displace the lens from the eye.

**Removal of lens under the upper fornix** If, on first eversion of the upper lid, no lens is found, return the lid to its normal position. Ask the patient to look down and at the same time to the extreme right and left, with the lid simply retracted upwards; this will often reveal the lens.

Failing this, instil a topical anaesthetic and double evert the upper lid using a cotton bud to sweep under the lid. Lenses that have been damaged or scratched must not be re-used and patients

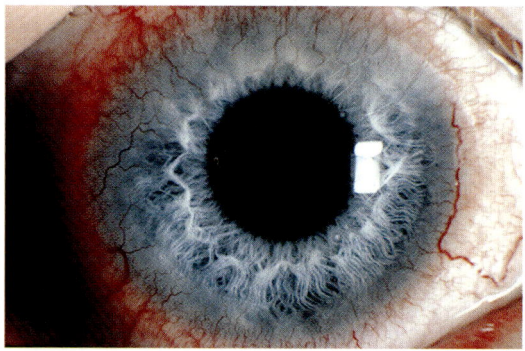

Figure 11.7  Corneal neovascularisation: superficial vessels invading the peripheral 2–3 mm of the cornea.

should be referred to their contact lens practitioner for lens renewal.

All contact lens wearers should be advised to have a spare pair of spectacles in case of problems with their lenses.

### Contact lens induced neovascularisation (Fig 11.7)

This is usually an incidental finding at a routine check up. Limbal neovascularisation probably results from the combined effect of slight hypoxia and prolonged "irritation".

#### Clinical features
- The patient is usually asymptomatic but may have unrelated symptoms
- Superficial corneal vessels within 2 mm of the limbus; they do not extend to the visual axis
- Vessels regress or become "ghosted" once the lenses are discontinued for a few weeks, with or without topical steroids.

**Management** Although new vessels are not an absolute indication to discontinue lens wear, if there are no symptoms, the patient should ideally be refitted with a more oxygen permeable lens type or the wearing time reduced.

### Other ocular problems

Although contact lenses may be associated with certain complications, it should not be forgotten that these patients are just as likely to present with other ocular conditions, for example, anterior uveitis, as those not wearing lenses.

## The use of therapeutic contact lenses

Although contact lenses can cause various problems, therapeutic soft lenses are used in the treatment of certain medical conditions. They have no refractive power and act as a "shield" for the healing epithelium. They should be used with caution but can be used in the following situations.

### Recurrent corneal erosion (see Chapter 5)
#### Indications
- Recurrences after conventional treatment of lubricating ointments, débridement, and taping of lids

- Patients with severe symptoms
- Selected vulnerable patients with epithelial problems, for example, a corneal dystrophy.

### Persistent epithelial defects

These occur following trauma, chemical injury, or infection. Indolent ulcers caused by herpes simplex virus have been healed with prolonged use of a therapeutic lens.

### Postoperative wound leak or gape

This can involve persistent leaking of a cataract section more than two weeks after surgery. Occasionally, after trabeculectomy surgery, there is excessive drainage through the bleb site and a flat anterior chamber. A large bandage lens will compress the bleb and allow the anterior chamber to re-form. More often a specially adapted Simmons' shell is needed to apply effective pressure.

### Bullous keratopathy

The use of a bandage lens in cases of bullous keratopathy (corneal decompensation resulting from excessive endothelial cell loss) in aphakia or pseudophakia is controversial. Most patients presenting acutely with this condition are, however, in pain as a result of damaged corneal epithelium and will be made more comfortable in the short term by a lens.

In patients with epithelial oedema only, visual acuity may improve greatly by having a more regular refracting surface; if there is stromal oedema acuity will remain poor.

### Corneal perforation

In general, bandage contact lenses should not be the primary treatment for corneal perforations and they are contraindicated in large wounds with gaping edges, prolapse of the iris or other intraocular contents, and infected or dirty wounds.

In cases of small corneal perforations caused by a clean sharp object, cyanoacrylate adhesive followed by placement of a bandage lens may be successful.

## Protection from trichiasis or entropion

When symptoms are severe and where it is not possible to correct the problem surgically for any reason, a therapeutic lens will be a short term solution for symptomatic relief.

# 12 Postoperative complications

With the modern trend towards day case ophthalmic surgery, patients will increasingly present with postoperative complications to the accident and emergency department. Therefore it is important to recognise and manage such complications. This chapter presents some common complications and gives an outline of the first steps in management.

## Cataract surgery

Cataract surgery accounts for 70% of all ophthalmic operations. Common or serious postoperative complications are listed in Table 12.1. Although the trend is for surgery to be

Table 12.1  Postoperative complications of cataract surgery

| Symptoms | Differential diagnosis | Onset* |
|---|---|---|
| Pain with severe visual loss | Endophthalmitis | Usually early |
|  | Severe iritis | Usually early |
|  | Malignant glaucoma | Early |
|  | Pupil block glaucoma | Early |
|  | Choroidal haemorrhage | Early |
|  | Corneal decompensation | Usually late |
| Pain with mild if any visual loss | Drop allergy | Early |
|  | Iris prolapse | Early |
|  | Suture abscess | Usually late |
|  | Protruding suture | Late |
| Painless visual loss | Posterior capsule opacification | Late |
|  | Cystoid macular oedema | Late |
|  | Retinal detachment | Usually late |
|  | Corneal decompensation | Usually late |

* Early onset=within two weeks; late onset=after two weeks.

perfomed by phacoemulsification, a significant proportion is still done by extracapsular extraction. Some of the complications are unique to one or other form of the surgery, but most will be common to both.

## Endophthalmitis

### Symptoms and signs
- Increasing pain and decreasing vision
- Lid oedema, conjunctival injection, and chemosis
- Corneal haze
- Large numbers of anterior chamber cells or hypopyon
- Vitreous cells
- Reduced or absent red reflex (Fig 12.1).

An RAPD is a poor prognostic sign. Onset is usually within a few days of surgery, but may be delayed by several weeks if the endophthalmitits is caused by low virulence organisms such as coagulase negative staphyloccoci or *Propionibacterium acnes*.

### Management

***Identification of organism*** Aqueous and vitreous samples are obtained for microscopy (for Gram and Giemsa staining) and culture on chocolate agar, blood agar and Sabouraud's plates, and liquid thioglycolate. Positive cultures are more frequently obtained from the vitreous sample.

***Intravitreal antibiotics*** The most commonly cultured organisms are coagulase negative staphylococci and *Staphylococcus aureus*. However, Gram-negative organisms, such as *Pseudomonas* sp., account for about 15% of cases. Therefore broad spectrum antibiotics are required which are most effectively delivered by intravitreal injection after the specimens have been obtained.

Suggested intravitreal antibiotics (which must be made up from preservative free solutions):

- vancomycin 1 mg in 0·1 ml
  and either
- gentamicin 0·1 mg in 0·1 ml or
- amikacin 0·4 mg in 0·1 ml.

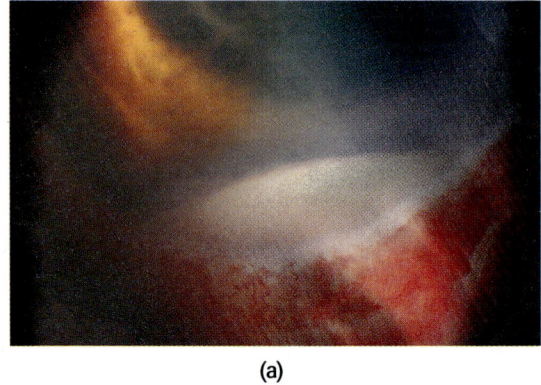

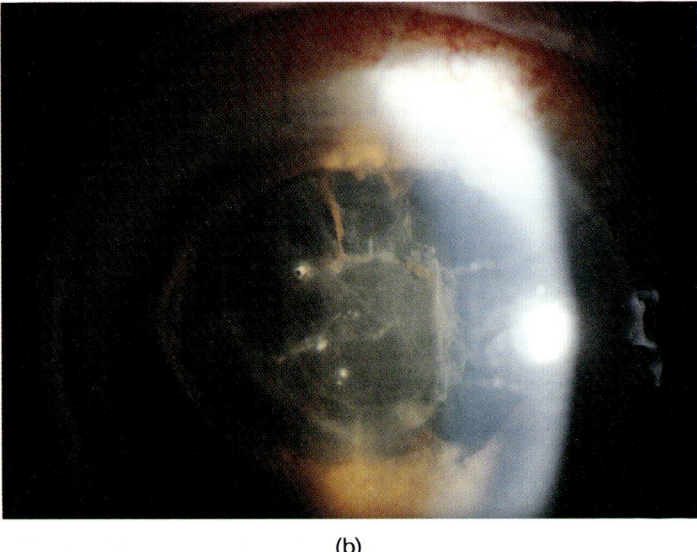

Figure 12.1   Endophthalmitis: (a) with hypopyon and (b) same eye showing plasmoid aqueous, exudates, and posterior synechiae.

**Further treatment**   This will be guided by the response to the intravitreal antibiotics, and microscopy and culture results. Topical and intravenous broad spectrum antibiotics are usually given and the pupil is dilated with atropine 1% drops three times daily. The use and timing of topical and oral corticosteroids in the treatment of endophthalmitis are not well defined.

About 50% of infected eyes will retain useful vision. The virulence of the organism is the most important prognostic factor.

## Iritis

### Severe postoperative iritis

In the early postoperative stage, it is difficult to be sure that the inflammation is sterile. A high index of suspicion for infection is needed so as not to miss a case of infection at a treatable stage.

The predisposing factors are:

- Diabetes
- Previous iritis
- Excessive manipulation at surgery
- Vitreous loss.

### Differential diagnosis
- Infection.

Table 12.2 summarises some of the useful differentiating features.

Table 12.2   Differentiation between endophthalmitis and severe iritis

| Symptoms | Iritis | Infection |
| --- | --- | --- |
| Pain | + | +++ |
| Visual acuity | Variable depending on severity | Marked deterioration |
| Cells in anterior chamber | + – ++ | +++ |
| Anterior vitreous activity | ± | + – +++ |
| Onset | Less rapid | Rapid |
| Descemet folds | Late | Early |
| Steroid response in first 24 hours | Improves | Initial improvement; progressive deterioration |
| Timing | Any time | Rarely severe after first week |

**Management** Where the distinction is impossible on clinical grounds:

- Admit for close observation and therapeutic trial with topical steroids. Assess again towards the end of the day in respect of (1) pain and (2) cellular activity.
- If in doubt, get aqueous and vitreous samples and treat as for endophthalmitis.

## Iris prolapse

Iris prolapse is associated with poor wound closure. Untreated sight limiting complications include bacterial endophthalmitis, uveitis, astigmatism, cystoid macular oedema, and epithelial downgrowth.

### Symptoms and signs
- Foreign body sensation
- Inflamed red eye in later stage
- Pupil distortion (Fig 12.2)
- Iris visible in section.

**Management** Prolapsed iris must be excised or repositioned and the section resutured. If prolapse is likely to have happened for some time or if there is severe inflammation, repositioning is inadvisable.

### Retinal detachment

The incidence of retinal detachment after intracapsular cataract extraction (ICCE) is around 2% and 1% after extracapsular cataract extraction (ECCE). Risk factors include preoperative myopia and intraoperative vitreous loss.

### Symptoms and signs
- Onset at any time following surgery, but unlikely to happen before the first postoperative visit
- The symptoms and signs of a retinal detachment are discussed on page 42.

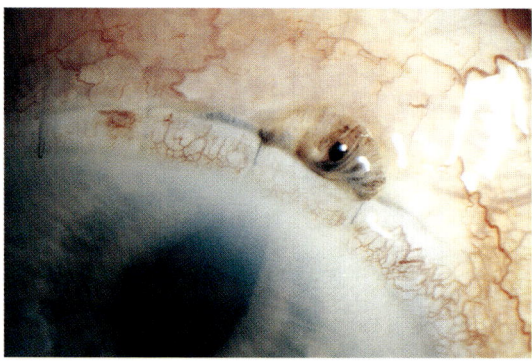

Figure 12.2 Prolapsed iris: incomplete herniation of the pigment epithelium gives the colourless stroma a jelly like appearance. Note that where the iris is not completely prolapsed, there is still iris tissue wedged between two sutures (12 o'clock).

## Management
- Surgical repair is required (see Retinal detachment, page 42)
- If the macula is still on, this should be treated as an emergency and the patient admitted to hospital for bed rest while waiting for surgery in case the macula becomes detached
- If the macula is off, surgery should be planned for the next convenient operating slot which should be in days rather than weeks.

## Corneal decompensation

The corneal endothelium is a single layer of cells the function of which is to maintain corneal clarity by pumping fluid from the stroma into the aqueous. These cells are unable to replicate and their number decreases with age. Additional loss resulting from the trauma of cataract surgery may leave insufficient cells to maintain corneal deturgesence.

Vulnerable eyes include those with a reduced number of endothelial cells preoperatively, Fuchs' dystrophy, poorly fitting intraocular lenses which abrade the endothelium, and persistent vitreocorneal contact.

### Symptoms and signs

Onset can be at any time after surgery, but is unlikely to occur in the immediate postoperative period unless there is severe physical trauma or accidental chemical injury to the endothelium.

#### *Early*
- Blurring of vision worse on waking (because lid closure prevents corneal dehydration by evaporation)
- Stromal thickening and epitheial oedema (seen as loss of bright sheen)
- Intermittent.

#### *Late*
- Sharp and severe pains
- Epithelial bullae (Fig 2.3), stromal thickening, Descemet folds, and loss of transparency.

### Management
- Hypertonic saline drops or ointment may be of benefit in early decompensation and mild oedema
- A bandage contact lens (see Chapter 11) and topical β blockers

# EMERGENCY OPHTHALMOLOGY

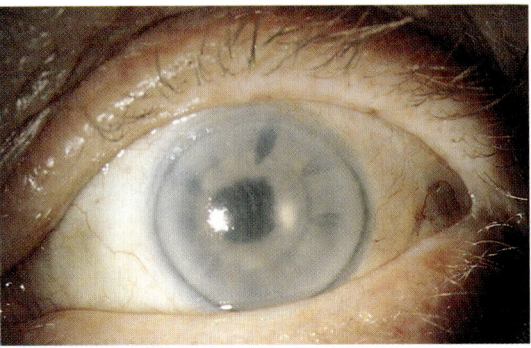

Figure 12.3   Bullous keratopathy showing mat surface and loss of sheen.

or carbonic anhydrase inhibitors for lowering the IOP may also help
- Poorly fitting intraocular lenses should be removed and any vitreous in contact with the cornea excised
- Eventually a corneal graft may be required to relieve pain and to improve vision.

## Protruding suture

The fine synthetic sutures used to close cataract incisions are almost inert and well tolerated and are commonly not removed unless they cause excessive astigmatism. However, they may either work loose or degrade and break causing irritation or giant papillary conjunctivitis.

### Symptoms and signs
- Onset often many months or several years after surgery
- Foreign body sensation often accompanied by watering and a mucus discharge
- Fluorescein staining of adherent mucus helps to identify protruding sutures
- Vessels may be seen invading the cornea from the adjacent limbus
- Irritation of the overlying tarsal plate may induce giant papillae formation.

**Management**   Involved sutures are removed at the slitlamp under topical anaesthesia. They can be cut, if necessary, with a 21 gauge needle and pulled out with suture tying forceps. Topical

# POSTOPERATIVE COMPLICATIONS

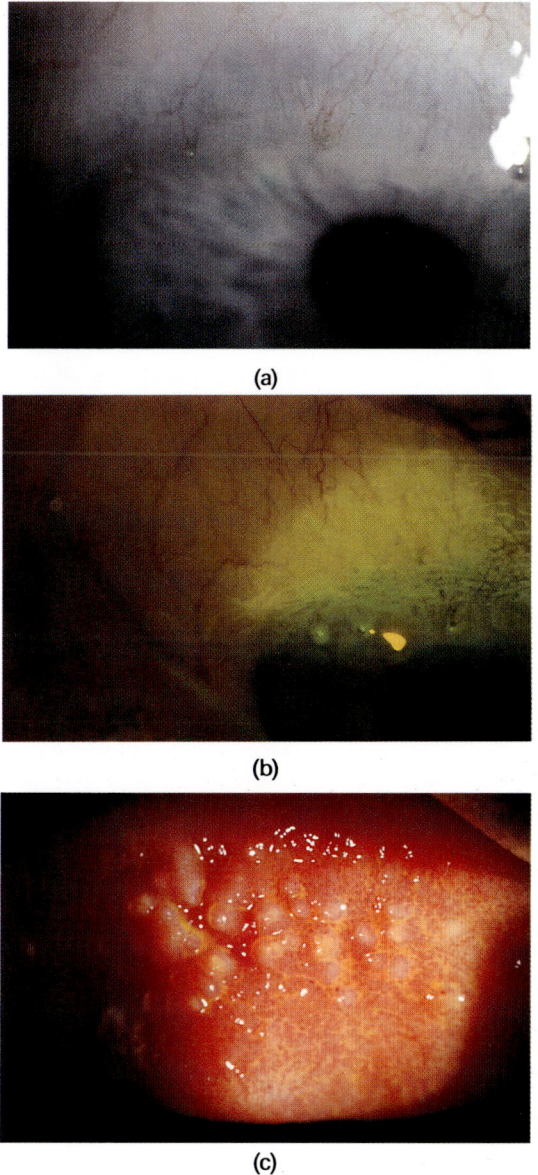

Figure 12.4 (a) Broken sutures; (b) broken suture ends and surrounding mucus stained with fluorescein (same eye); and (c) papillary hypertrophy: probably an allergic reaction to monomer release.

antibiotics should be prescribed for five days to prevent infection of the suture track, and coupled with a topical steroid in the case of papillary reaction.

### Suture abscess

Loose or broken sutures may act as an entry site for infection.

**Symptoms and signs** Similar to protruding suture (above) but:

- Pain tends to be more severe
- White infiltrate surrounds the suture (Fig. 12.4)
- There is usually an overlying corneal epithelial defect
- A reactive iritis may be present.

**Management** Identify the organism: the suture is removed and sent for culture. Scrapings of the abscess are inoculated on to culture media (chocolate agar, blood agar and Sabouraud's plates, and liquid thioglycolate) and slides for microscopy.

Treated initially with broad spectrum antibiotic drops (for example, gentamicin 1·5% drops and cefazolin 5% drops hourly).

Relieve pain from ciliary spasm and prevent posterior synechiae formation—use topical cycloplegia (for example, atropine 1% drops twice daily). When the inflammation is severe the patient is admitted.

### Drop allergy

Allergy may develop to either the prescribed drug or the solution's preservative (commonly benzalkonium chloride).

**Symptoms and signs**
- Redness, irritation, and mildly reduced vision typically develop within a few days of starting the drops.

**Management** This is by capsulotomy using an yttrium–aluminium–garnet (YAG) laser (Fig 12.5).

### Cystoid macular oedema

Cataract surgery is one of a variety of conditions that may be associated with retinal oedema, in which fluid collects in cystic spaces at the macula. With time these "cysts" coalesce, leading to

## POSTOPERATIVE COMPLICATIONS

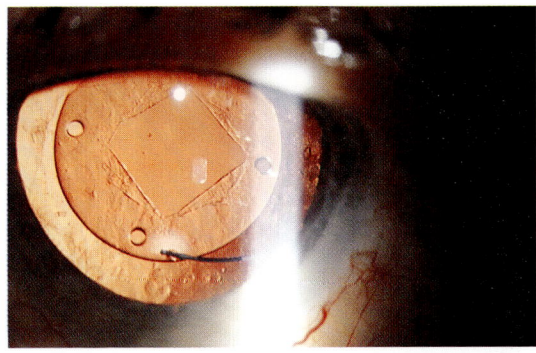

Figure 12.5  YAG laser capsulotomy showing rectangular gap from a cruciate cut. Note surrounding capsule with ground glass appearance resulting from new lens deposits.

irreversible retinal damage and a decline in central vision. Although the cause of cystoid macular oedema (CMO) is uncertain, it occurs more commonly following ICCE or rupture of the posterior capsule during an ECCE with or without vitreous loss. Persistent ocular inflammation and vitreous incarceration in the wound are also predisposing factors.

### Symptoms and signs
- Decrease in acuity occurring several weeks or months after surgery
- Occasionally causes mild ocular pain or photophobia
- Loss of the foveal light reflex
- Cystic spaces in the macula (Fig 12.6)
- There may also be evidence of ocular inflammation or vitreous strands extending to the wound.

**Management**  *Fundus fluorescein angiography* is helpful in establishing the diagnosis and in excluding other macular conditions such as age related macular degeneration. The leaked fluid characeristially shows a *petaloid* pattern centred on the fovea (Fig 12.6).

If inflammation is present, CMO may respond to topical, periocular, or oral steroids. Non-steroidal anti-inflammatory drugs and acetazolamide have also been found to benefit some cases of idiopathic CMO, but a particular patient may not respond to any of the agents. If present, incarcerated vitreous strands should be divided and vitrectomy should be considered.

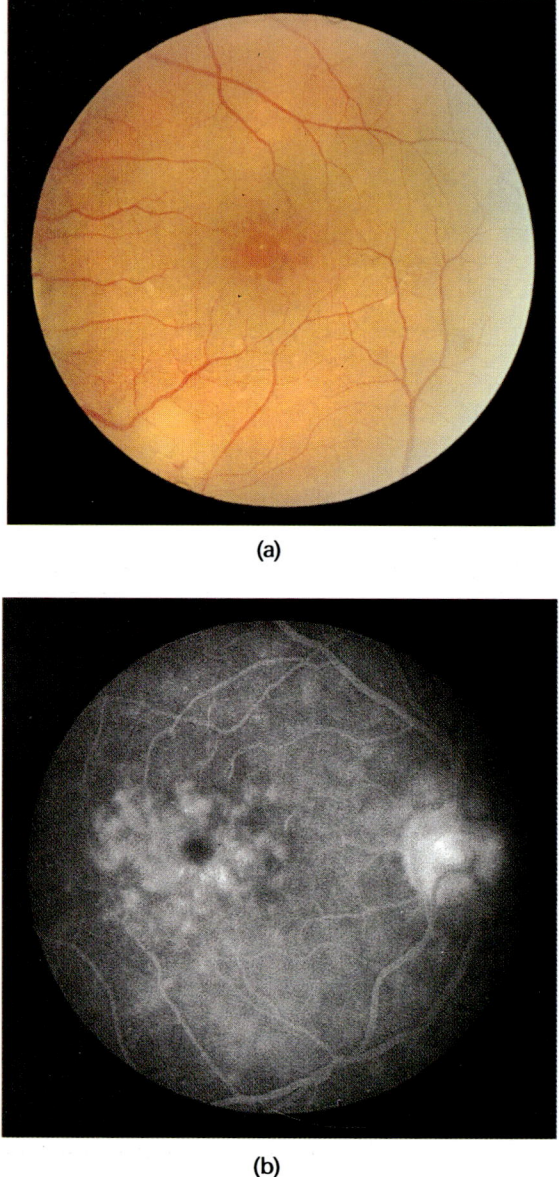

(a)

(b)

Figure 12.6  Cystoid macular oedema after uncomplicated cataract surgery showing typical petaloid appearance of oedema in late phase of fluorescein angiography.

## POSTOPERATIVE COMPLICATIONS

### Malignant glaucoma, pupil block glaucoma, and delayed choroidal haemorrhage

These can occur following any intaocular surgery and are discussed together on page 281.

## Trabeculectomy

Trabeculectomy is a drainage operation in which a guarded sclerostomy is made just behind the limbus to allow aqueous to drain directly from the anterior chamber to the subconjunctival space. Most of the early complications result from the fact that the rate of filtration cannot be strictly regulated and problems arise from excessive filtration or secondary to shallowing of the anterior chamber. A list of the common complications is presented in Table 12.3 with their probable associated symptoms. Drop allergy and endophthalmitis are described under Cataract complications.

Table 12.3  Postoperative complications of trabeculectomy

| Symptoms | Differential diagnosis |
|---|---|
| Painless visual deterioration | Hyphaema |
|  | Bleb leak |
|  | Excessive filtration |
| Pain with mild or slight effect on vision | Protruding suture |
|  | Drop allergy |
| Pain with severe reduction in vision | Endophthalmitis |
|  | Malignant glaucoma |
|  | Pupil block glaucoma |
|  | Choroidal haemorrhage |

### Leaking bleb and excessive filtration

#### Symptoms and signs
- Usually reduced visual acuity (patient may not complain)
- Usually painless (unless inflamed)
- Shallow anterior chamber with *low IOP*
- Drainage bleb may be flat or leaking
- Seidel's test positive (see Appendix B)
- Choroidal detachment (sectoral or annular) not invariable.

#### Critical signs
- Presence of a leak (Seidel's test—see above)
- Low IOP

- Choroidal detachment
- Iridocorneal contact
- Lenticulocorneal contact.

**Management** Slight shallowing of the anterior chamber is not serious, but prolonged leakage leads to complications of hypotension; iridocorneal adhesions can lead to posterior synechiae and lenticulocorneal contact results in cataract. The steps in the management are outlined in Fig 12.7.

### Malignant glaucoma, pupil block glaucoma, and delayed choroidal haemorrhage

These are rare postoperative complications which present with identical symptoms and anterior segment signs.

*Malignant glaucoma* This is caused by diverson of aqueous fluid into the vitreous cavity. The reason why this occurs is not understood, but its effect is to displace the lens and iris anteriorly thereby occluding the drainage angle and causing an acute rise in intraocular pressure. Hyperopic eyes are more vulnerable.

*Pupil block glaucoma* This arises when aqueous fluid is prevented from entering the anterior chamber by posterior synechiae or because the pupil is obstructed by an intraocular lens or vitreous. It is important to consider pupil block glaucoma even if the previous surgery included a peripheral iridectomy because the hole may have become occluded by vitreous.

*Delayed choroidal haemorrhage* This results in an accumulation of blood in the suprachoroidal space which displaces the lens and iris anteriorly.

### Symptoms and signs
- Onset within two weeks of surgery
- Pain and visual loss
- High IOP and shallow anterior chamber
- Typically the eye is also injected, the cornea hazy, and the pupil unreactive.

# POSTOPERATIVE COMPLICATIONS

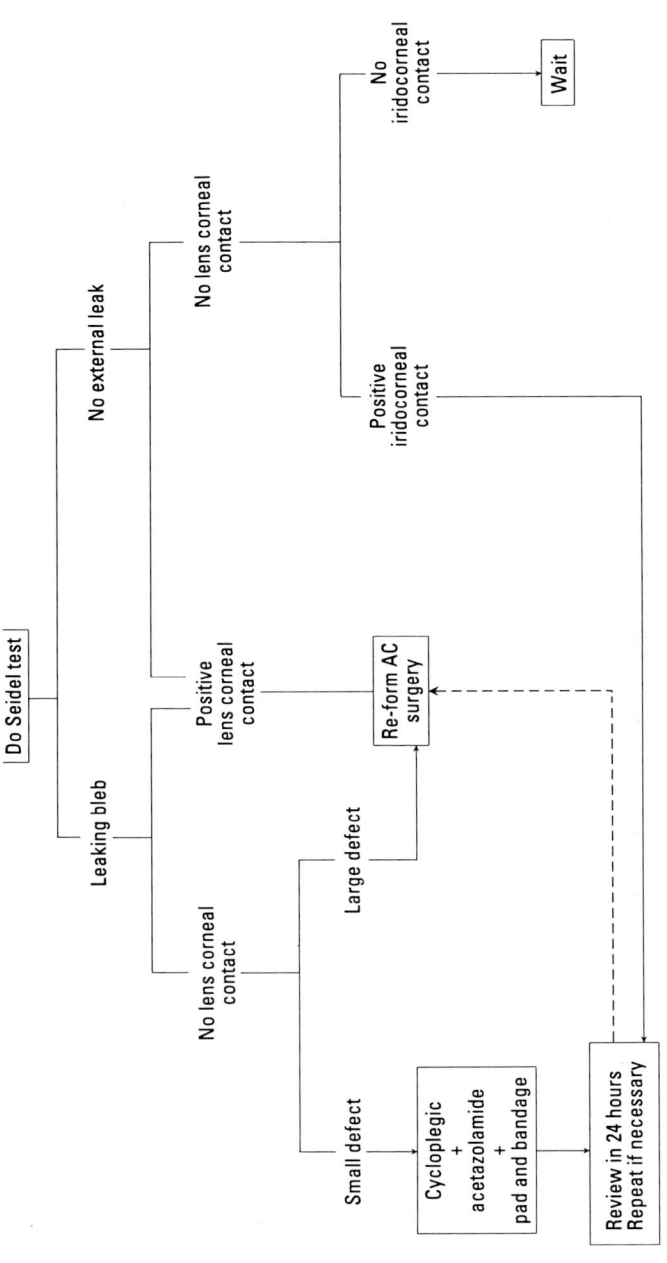

Figure 12.7 Management of shallow anterior chamber and low IOP after trabeculectomy.

### Management

***Malignant glaucoma*** Initial treatment is atropinisation to relieve the presumed ciliary block coupled with hypotensive agents and intravenous mannitol. If no response, vitrectomy and removal of the lens may be necessary.

***Pupil block glaucoma*** Treatment is to break the posterior synechiae initially by mydriatics followed by YAG laser iridotomy.

***Delayed choroidal haemorrhage*** Where possible try conservative measures and drain the blood only as a last resort.

The immediate management of all three complications is outlined in Fig 12.8.

### Hyphaema

Bleeding from either the incision site or the peripheral iridectomy is common during the immediate postoperative period.

#### Symptoms and signs
- Mild blurring to complete loss of vision according to the amount of blood in the anterior chamber
- Vision often improves if patient sits still in an upright position and allows the blood to settle
- The height of the hyphaema can be measured with the slitlamp (Fig 12.9).

***Management*** Small hyphaemas, occupying less than a third of the anterior chamber, usually reabsorb spontaneously within 2–3 days. Patients with larger hyphaemas, a raised IOP, or who are sickle cell positive should be admitted for bed rest. Occasionally they may require an anterior chamber washout if there is fear of corneal staining or if there is sustained raised pressure.

### Protruding conjunctival suture

#### Symptoms and signs
- Foreign body sensation beneath the upper lid.

***Management*** Absorbable sutures such as Vicryl will soften over a few days, so patients should be reassured that the

# POSTOPERATIVE COMPLICATIONS

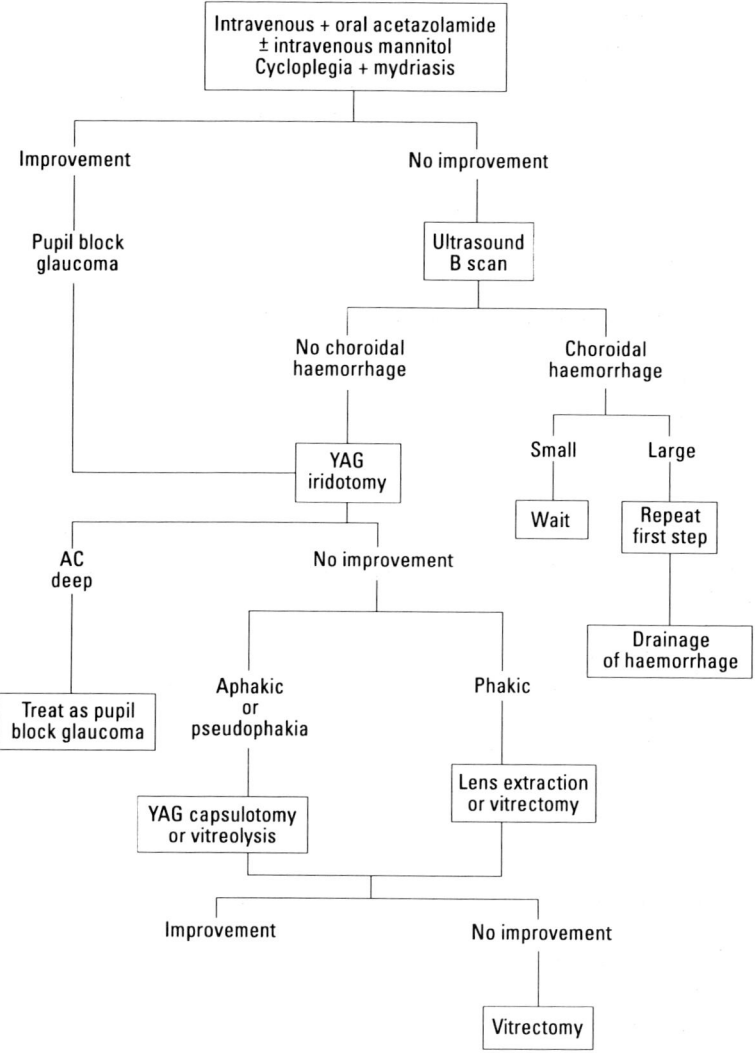

Figure 12.8 Management of shallow anterior chamber with high IOP after trabeculectomy.

discomfort will diminish. Unless pain is severe, non-absorbable sutures should not be removed for at least two weeks after surgery to minimise the risk of a bleb leak. Lubricating eye ointments may be considered as a temporising measure.

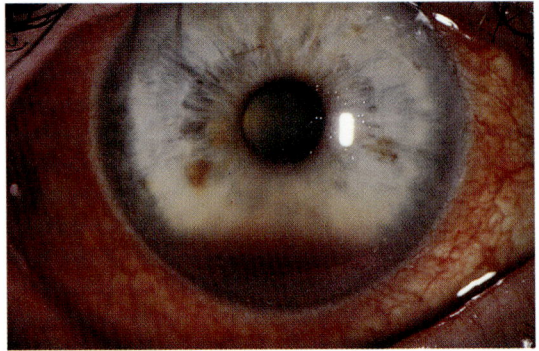

Figure 12.9  Postoperative hyphaema after trabeculectomy.

## Orbital cellulitis

Acute orbital cellulitis is rare after retinal detachment surgery, but it may occur if the explant was contaminated particularly if a Silastic sponge was used. Silastic sponges are commonly used as radial plombs.

### Symptoms and signs
- Pain, redness, chemosis, lid swelling, and proptosis
- Occasionally vitritis is the predominant sign.

**Management**  The management of orbital cellulitis is discussed in Chapter 10. It may be necessary to remove the explant.

## Anterior segment ischaemia

This complication usually presents dramatically in the early days after detachment surgery and follows an encircling procedure in which the band has been pulled too tight.

### Symptoms and signs
- Intense pain
- Chemosis and swelling of the lids and orbit
- Redness
- Cells and flare and shallow anterior chamber
- Anterior cortical lens opacities
- Clouding of the cornea
- Raised IOP.

## Management
- Pain relief
- Topical steroids
- Intravenous low molecular weight dextran
- Adjustment of encircling band or explant.

## Explant extrusion

Although sutured to the sclera at the time of surgery, explants occasionally migrate anteriorly and erode through the conjunctiva.

### Symptoms and signs
- Discomfort, redness, and discharge.

### *The exposed end of the explant*

This is usually obvious (Fig 12.10).

**Management** Extruding explants can often be removed under topical anaesthesia by gently pulling on the exposed end with a pair of forceps. Remaining small holes in the conjunctiva heal quickly without suturing. If part of the explant is still firmly attached to the sclera, it should be removed under a general anaesthetic. Following explant removal, the retinal must be examined because there is a small risk of re-detachment. Prophylactic antibiotics should be prescribed.

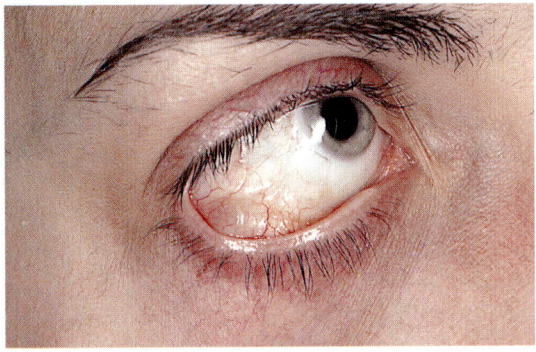

Figure 12.10   Silastic sponge emerging to surface several years after retinal detachment surgery.

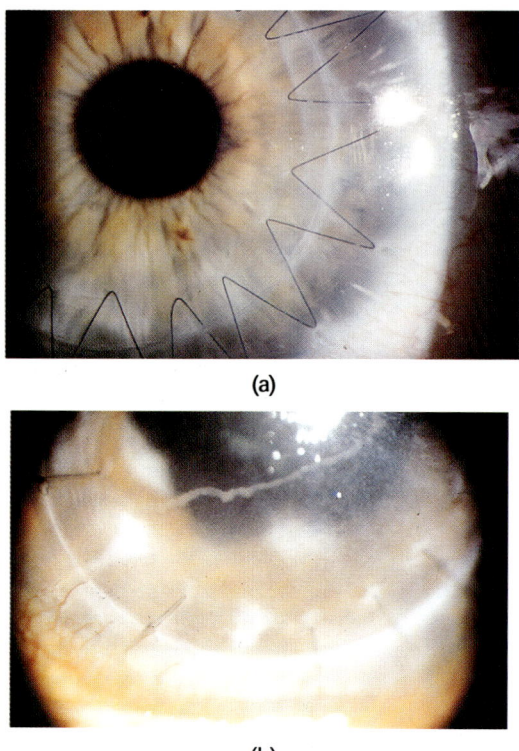

Figure 12.11  (a) Clear corneal graft, and (b) graft rejection showing Khodadoust's line.

## Corneal grafts (Fig 12.11)

### Rejection

The possibility of graft rejection must always be considered when a patient presents to the A&E department for whatever reason.

Corneal graft rejection is the most common cause of graft failure. It may occur spontaneously or be precipitated by apparently trivial postoperative complications such as a broken suture which causes inflammation and vascularisation.

### Symptoms and signs
- Progressive blurring of vision, with variable pain and redness

- Corneal signs are initially subtle and limited to a small area or to one layer:
    epithelial defects, lines, or bullae
    stromal thickening or infiltrates
    endothelial line (Khodadoust's line (Fig 12.11b) or keratic precipitates
- Other signs that may be present include injection, cells and flare in the anterior chamber, and a raised IOP.

**Management**
- Admission to hospital
- Frequent topical corticosteroid drops (for example, prednisolone drops hourly) in combination with systemic or subconjunctival steroids if the episode is severe
- Eliminate initiating factors such as a broken or loose suture, suture abscess, and other corneal infections, in particular a recurrence of herpes simplex keratitis.
- If there is coexistent infection steroid therapy may have to be reduced or deferred until it has been adequately treated.

## Loose or broken suture

Loose or broken sutures predispose to infection and rejection.

**Symptoms**
- Foreign body sensation often accompanied by watering and a mucus discharge
- Fluorescein staining of adherent mucus helps to identify protruding sutures
- Vessels may be seen invading the cornea from the adjacent limbus
- Irritation of the overlying tarsal plate may induce giant papillae formation (see Fig. 12.4).

**Management** An interrupted suture can be removed at the slitlamp under topical anaesthesia. It can be cut, if necessary, with a 21 gauge needle and pulled out with suture tying forceps. The graft–host junction should then be examined by instilling a drop of 2% fluorescein solution. Leakage of aqueous will dilute the dye, causing it to fluoresce green when observed with a blue light (the Seidel test). Small leaks are treated with a bandage contact lens and padding. Larger ones require resuturing. Continuous sutures should be removed in the operating room in case of wound dehiscence so that the means of re-suturing are immediately available.

After a suture has been removed, prophylactic topical antibiotics and corticosteroids drops should be prescribed in a reducing dose over two weeks. Patients should be warned of the possibility of rejection and advised to reattend immediately if they develop blurring of vision, discomfort, or redness.

### Suture abscess

The symptoms, signs, and management of a suture abscess are described under Cataract, page 277. The ensuing inflammation may precipitate rejection and the cornea should be monitored closely until the inflammation clears up.

## Squint surgery

### Suture granuloma

Most suture granulomata present within a few weeks of surgery, but the former use of poorly absorbable suture material means that they may also develop years later.

#### Symptoms and signs
- Irritation
- Solid red mass at the site of muscle reattachment (Fig 12.12).

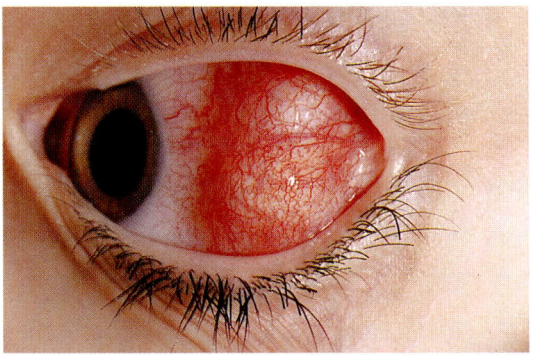

Figure 12.12 Stitch granuloma two years after squint surgery.

**Management** If the granuloma fails to resolve after Predsol 0·5% drops four times a day for two weeks it should be excised.

### Orbital cellulitis

This is an uncommon but serious complication of squint surgery.

#### Symptoms and signs
- Pain, redness, chemosis, lid swelling, and proptosis.

**Management** The management of orbital cellulitis is discussed in Chapter 10.

### Lost or slipped muslce

Partial or complete detachment of a muscle is an uncommon but serious complication.

#### Symptoms and signs
- Worsening of ocular alignment
- The affected eye is deviated away from the lost or slipped muscle and demonstrates little if any movement in the muscle's field of action.

**Management** Computed tomography or magnetic resonance imaging may help to confirm the diagnosis. The patient should be admitted for further surgery. Delay may result in fibrosis of the affected muscle and reduces further the chance of finding it for reattachment.

## Dacryocystorhinostomy and related surgery

### Wound infection

Postoperative wound infections are uncommon because of both the rich blood supply in this area and the frequent use of prophylactic antibiotics.

#### Symptoms and signs
- Pain, redness, and swelling at the incision site.

**Management** Oral antibiotics covering staphylococci and

streptococci should be prescribed. If an abscess has formed the pus should be drained by removing one or more of the sutures.

### Silicone tube displacement

Occasionally a silicone tube becomes displaced and protrudes from the punta.

#### Symptoms and signs
- Irritation of the conjunctiva or cornea giving rise to abrasion which should stain with fluorescein
- Tube visible at medial canthus.

**Management** Tubes that were inserted less than three months previously should be replaced by feeding them into the punta with a pair of forceps. Those that have been present for a longer period are normally removed. This is most easily done by cutting the tube between the punta and asking the patient to blow his or her nose.

## Eyelid surgery

The causes of pain following eyelid surgery include corneal exposure and suture irritation

### Corneal exposure

Overcorrection of a ptosis or malposition of the eyelid following entropion or ectropion surgery may cause corneal exposure.

#### Symptoms and signs
- Sore burning pain
- Punctate fluorescein staining of the exposed cornea
- Larger abrasions may result depending on the amount and duration of exposure.

#### Management
- Minor degrees of over-correction of a ptosis can be treated by massage
- Large amounts will need surgical readjustment
- Exposure resulting from other forms of lid surgery will generally require further surgical intervention.

## POSTOPERATIVE COMPLICATIONS

The immediate step is to protect the cornea with frequent applications of a lubricating ointment before corrective surgery.

### Suture irritation

Incisions through the tarsal plate are normally closed with a slowly absorbable suture such as 6/0 Vicryl. If these sutures are tied incorrectly, their ends may protrude through the tarsal conjunctiva and abrade the cornea.

#### Symptoms and signs
- Foreign body sensation
- Vertical linear abrasions of the cornea.

**Management** Involved sutures should be removed. Any resultant wound dehiscence requires resuturing.

### Wound dehiscence

Tarsorrhaphy procedures and those operations requiring a full thickness vertical incision through the eyelid are most at risk of dehiscence because the wounds are under tension. To minimise this risk, tarsorrhaphy sutures are usually tied over a bolster and left for 2–3 weeks, and vertical incision sutures are left for 10 days as compared with 5 days for other eyelid sutures. An important cause of wound breakdown is infection so that prophylaxis or early antibiotic treatment may prevent dehiscence.

**Management** Breakdown of a vertical full thickness incison requires resuturing to prevent an unsightly notch in the eyelid. If a tarsorrhaphy wound dehisces and there is threat of corneal exposure, frequent (two hourly) application of a lubricating ointment should be prescribed and the patient referred for further surgery. A pad should not be applied unless there is intact corneal sensation.

# 13 Coincidental findings

Some conditions or signs are common and one needs to recognise them to put them in their proper perspective. Sometimes they are detected when the patient presents with another complaint or they may be detected at an asymptomatic stage as a chance finding. This chapter presents a few of the common abnormalities and a brief statement about their management.

## The optic disc: common variants and abnormalities

### The normal optic disc (Fig 13.1)

A normal disc has a pink neural rim of even width which surrounds a central pit of small diameter. The vertical cup–disc (C/D) ratio is usually 0·3 or less in normal eyes but, within limits, the size of the cup is proportional to the size of the eye and may be as large as 0·7 without being pathological. The difference in C/D ratio is usually within 0·1 between the two sides so asymmetry should arouse suspicion.

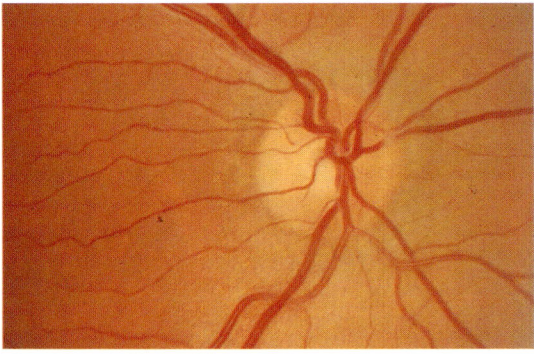

Figure 13.1  Normal optic disc.

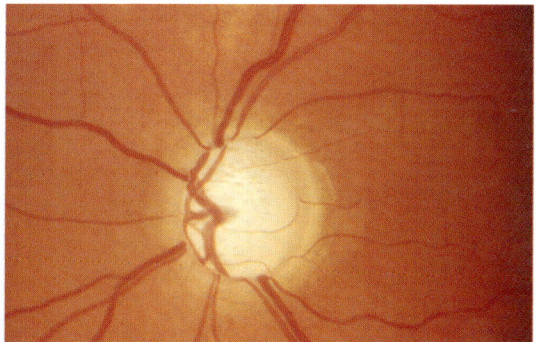

Figure 13.2 Cupping of disc in open angle glaucoma: vertical C/D ratio is >0.9; marked thinning of nerve rim, pallor of disc, and nasal shift of vessels which have to describe two right angles to "climb" out of the disc margin. There is also juxtapapillary choroidoretinal atrophy.

## Cupping of the optic disc (Fig 13.2)

Enlargement of the cup may or may not be significant. The so called physiological cupping signifies widening of the cup without loss of nerve tissue or demonstrable functional loss. There is no notching of the rim and no pallor. When the vertical C/D ratio is over 0·5, together with the loss of nerve fibres, then the cupping is pathological. Loss of nerve fibre is inferred by thinning of the neural rim, notching, increased pallor, asymmetry between the two eyes, and nasal shift of the vessels. Pathological cupping is a sign of damage caused by glaucoma in which there is raised intraocular pressure and field loss. Suspected cases should be investigated for glaucoma.

## Optic atrophy (Fig 13.3)

Pallor may be general or may affect one part of the disc more, for example, the temporal side. If unilateral, an RAPD (relative afferent pupil defect) confirms the diagnosis. Subtle loss of contrast sensitivity or colour vision precedes loss of Snellen acuity, and field loss especially to red may be an early sign. Common causes include:

- Ischaemic
- Postneuritic
- Post-traumatic
- Compressive

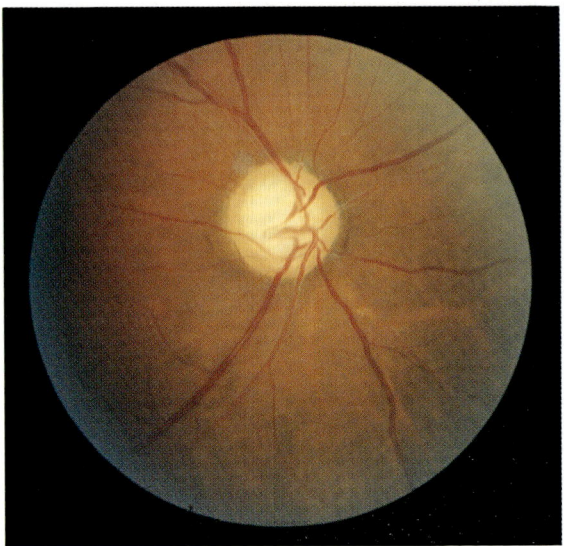

Figure 13.3  Optic atrophy: there is marked pallor but the contour of the disc is unchanged. (The retinal arterioles are coincidentally attenuated.)

- Toxic, for example, tobacco–alcohol amblyopia
- Metabolic, for example, diabetes.

A detailed history is important and if in doubt the case should be investigated.

### Tilted discs (Fig 13.4)

This congenital anomaly results in a shift of nerve fibres and the emerging vessels, usually superiorly, leaving a large inferior crescent which looks hypoplastic and lacking in nerve substance; this is frequently accompanied by a sector of hypopigmentation of the adjacent retina. There is often a matching field defect, usually in the superotemporal quadrant, corresponding to the inferonasal crescent.

Other pattern of shifts and disc colobomas will produce corresponding field abnormalities which may occasionally be bitemporal. No action is needed.

In highly myopic eyes the large globe leads to increased obliquity of the nerve as it leaves the globe and the optic disc is shelved, giving the appearance of a rim of nerve overhanging the retinal vessels shifted to the nasal side. There is often scleral

# COINCIDENTAL FINDINGS

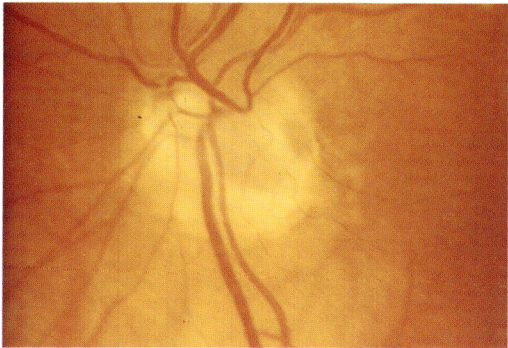

Figure 13.4   Tilted disc (see text).

baring on the temporal side and the blind spot of the visual field is enlarged.

## Optic disc drusen

Drusen (see Fig 3.4 on page 75) on the surface are seen as hyaline bodies but, if buried in the nerve head, they can mimic disc swelling. Distinguishing features are the presence of spontaneous venous pulsation and absence of congestion of the vessels of the nerve head.

A diagnostic feature is that drusen autofluoresce in blue light and can be seen or photographed using the fundus camera; they show up well on computed tomography. A visual field defect is common and should be charted as background information.

## Myelinated nerve fibres (Fig 13.5)

These are opaque nerve fibres usually radiating from the disc, although they may appear as isolated patches elsewhere. *No action is required.*

# Common macular abnormalities

## Age related macular degeneration (Fig 13.6a)

There is progressive fall out of photoreceptors with accompanying degenerative change in Bruch's membrane and the pigment epithelium. It is the most common cause of partial sight registration in the Western World, especially in the over 70s. There is no effective treatment, but the patient needs general advice and reassurance that peripheral vision will not be affected.

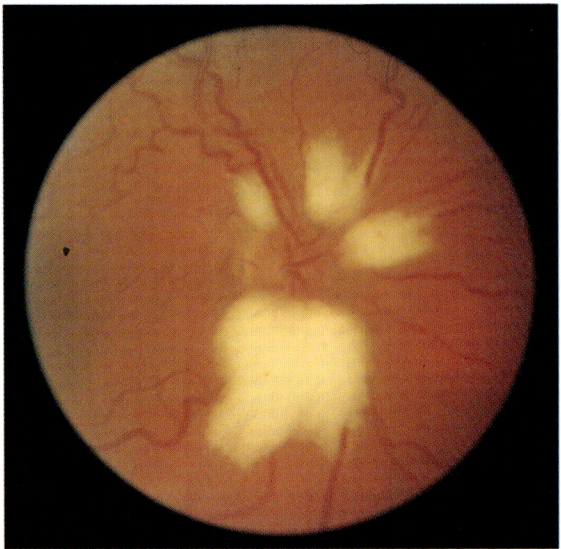

Figure 13.5  Myelinated nerve fibres: opaque fibres obscure underlying retinal details.

### Disciform macular degeneration (Fig 13.6b)

See Chapter 2.

### Diabetic maculopathy

See pages 61, 300.

## Common retinal abnormalities

### Diabetic retinopathy
*Background retinopathy.*

The following are the features of background diabetic retinopathy:

- Microaneurysms and haemorrhages or "dots and blots"
- Hard exudates
- Venous dilatation
- Cotton wool spots (Fig 13.7).

Red "dots and blots" are present in 99% of diabetic patients who have had the disease for 20 years or more. Hard exudates

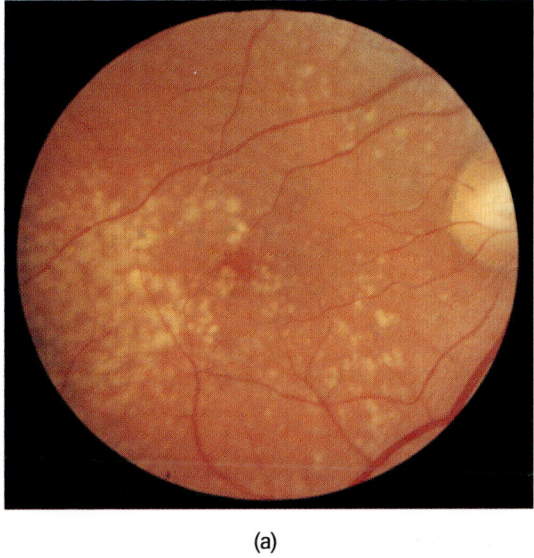

(a)

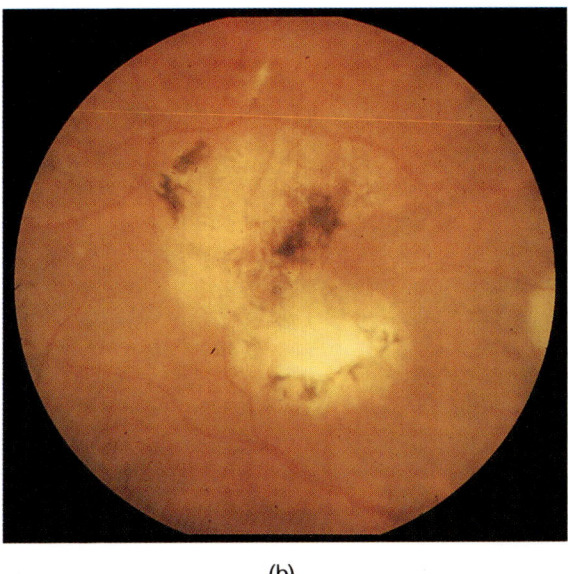

(b)

Figure 13.6 Macular degeneration: (a) hard drusen and (b) old disciform scar.

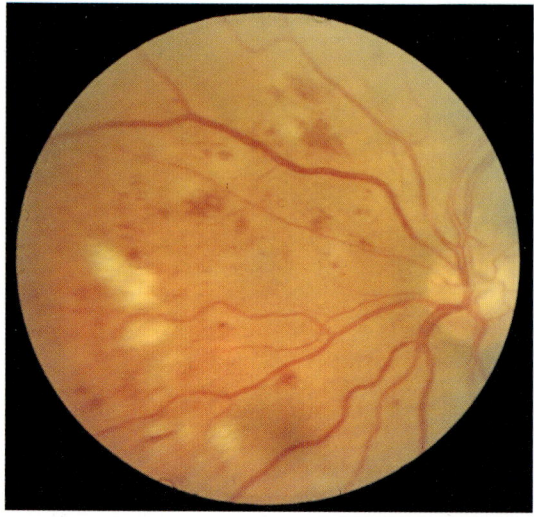

Figure 13.7 Severe background diabetic retinopathy showing "dot and blot" haemorrhages and microaneurysms, multiple cotton wool spots, and venous irregularity.

may also be present, particularly in adult onset diabetes, and indicate areas of retinal oedema.

### *Diabetic maculopathy* (Fig 13.8)

Where oedema affects the macula there will be retinal thickening and visual acuity will be reduced by varying amounts. If the macula is threatened by oedema, treatment by argon laser photocoagulation may arrest deterioration. The assumption is that adjacent microvascular abnormalities leak fluid and lipid.

Managment includes liaison between ophthalmic and diabetic clinics to improve control; this affects the severity of retinopathy.

In mild cases regular screening for sight threatening retinopathy in a primary care setting is advised. In more severe cases, where laser treatment may be required, regular follow up in a hospital setting is preferred.

### Diabetic retinopathy
### *Proliferative retinopathy* (Figs 13.9 and 13.10)

New vessels may arise from the disc or the retina or from both. Untreated they bleed repeatedly at a late stage and the

## COINCIDENTAL FINDINGS

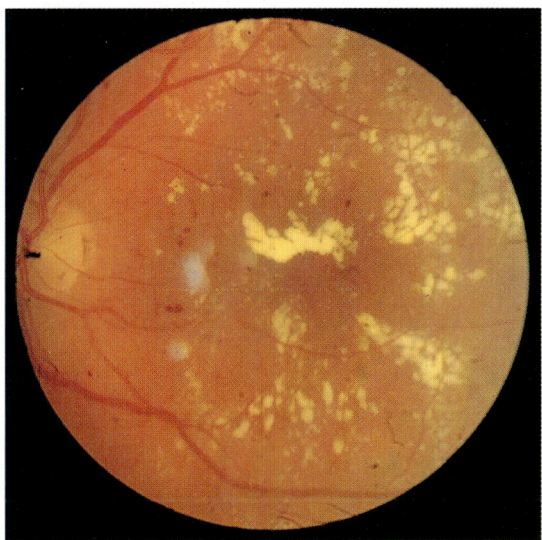

Figure 13.8  Diabetic maculopathy: macular oedema and hard exudate plaques.

accompanying fibrosis may also cause retinal detachment. Treatment by photocoagulation in the early stage is highly effective but advanced disease may need vitrectomy. Early cases

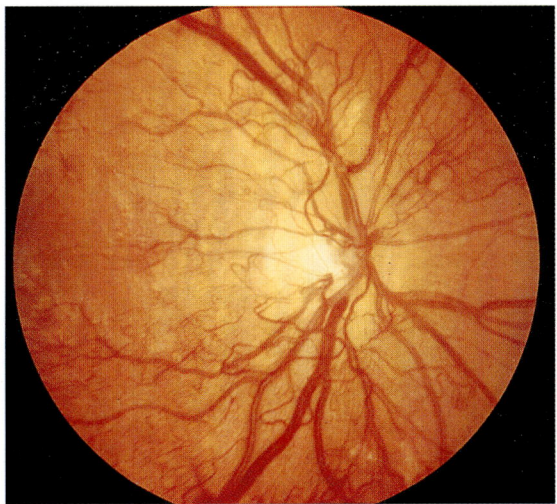

Figure 13.9  Proliferative retinopathy with a profusion of new vessels growing from the disc.

# EMERGENCY OPHTHALMOLOGY

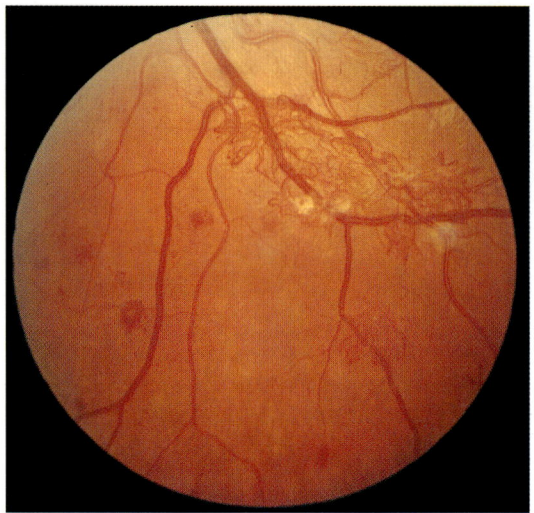

Figure 13.10  Proliferative retinopathy: a rete of new vessels arising from the inferotemporal vein

are asymptomatic and the person screening has an important role in identifying the lesions. Proliferative change is a late manifestation of diabetic retinopathy and is unknown within the first five years of the disease in insulin dependent diabetes, but its prevalence increases to 56% after 30 years. If in doubt, in patients with poor control and long duration, do fluorescein angiography. New vessels leak the dye at a fast rate.

**Pre-proliferative retinopathy** (Fig 13.11 and see Fig 13.7)

This is a loose term which, to be useful, should apply to cases with features that presage the development of proliferative change in a matter of months. These features are venous bleeding, "omega" loops, numerous cotton wool spots, and severe background retinopathy with blotchy haemorrhages. All of them denote severe ischaemia and evidence points to a neovascular factor produced by ischaemic retina which stimulates new vessel formation. These cases need close monitoring and may need laser treatment.

**Suspect angle closure glaucoma**

When the anterior chamber is very shallow (see Fig 3.1), there is a threat of acute glaucoma from angle closure. When the

## COINCIDENTAL FINDINGS

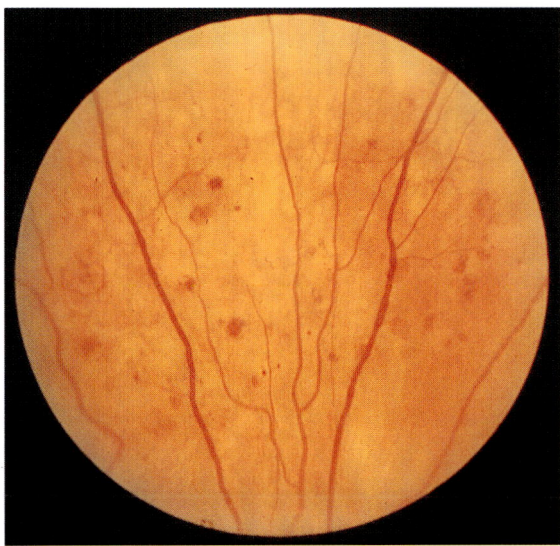

Figure 13.11 Venous beading in pre-proliferative retinopathy or early proliferative phase indicating severe ischaemia.

pressure is normal and where there is no previous history of congestive symptoms, there is little danger of an acute attack. The patient needs to be warned of the symptoms and to return if they occur, and to be advised against distant travel until provocative tests have been done to decide if prophylactic iridotomy is needed. A useful sign is to see if the iris at the temporal or nasal limbus is in contact with the cornea; if positive, the risk of a congestive attack is increased. If dilatation of the pupil is required, one should give reversal miotics, re-check intraocular pressure after an hour, and emphasise the need for re-attendance if there are symptoms of an attack.

### Raised intraocular pressure

More usually the problem arises when a patient with open angles is found to have raised intraocular pressure (IOP). A normal pressure is less than 22 mm Hg. A mildly raised IOP in the absence of optic disc cupping does not constitute an emergency. The patient should be sent on to the clinic for field plots. The IOP fluctuates and its measurement is subject to imprecision. Most clinicians would take a level of around 30 mm Hg as being significant, in that a pressure of that

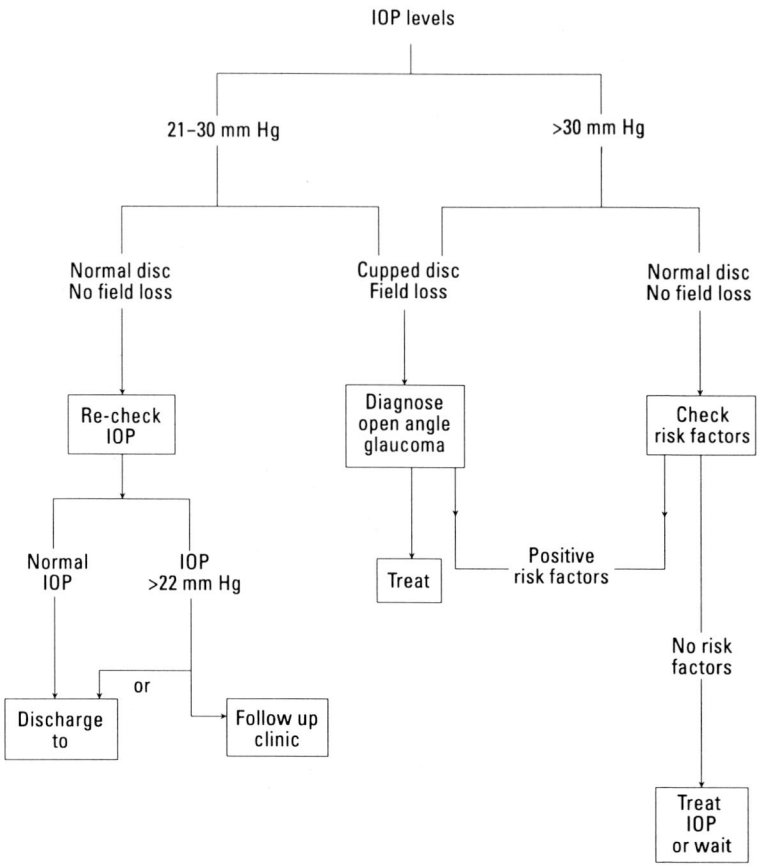

Figure 13.12 Management of suspected open angle glaucoma with raised IOP.

magnitude is unlikely to be chance variation, and treat the patient to avoid secondary problems such as vein occlusion. If the pressure is less than 30 mm Hg, and in the absence of nerve damage, a repeat check is entirely warranted to ensure repeatability.

Risk factors for open angle glaucoma are: positive family history, raised BP, smoking, asymmetry of discs, and pseudo-exfoliation.

The management of raised IOP is outlined in Fig 13.12.

# Appendices

## Appendix A   Rationale for the Bielschowsky three step test

*Normal vertical* eye movements are executed as follows:
- *Elevation* is carried out by the combined action of the superior rectus and inferior oblique
- *Depression* is by the combined action of the inferior rectus and superior oblique.

To begin with a vertical squint can be caused by any one of the eight muscles (four in each eye). Each step of the test will halve the number of suspects until one is identified by the final step.

The following description of the three step test must be read in conjunction with Table A.1 to aid comprehension.

### Step 1

Observe which eye is higher in the primary position. Confirm by the cover test if in doubt.

A vertical deviation in the primary position indicates either weakness of the elevators in the lower eye or weakness of the depressors in the higher eye.

After step 1 the number of potential contenders for the weak muscle has been reduced to four.

The fixing eye is not necessarily the unaffected eye as there may be other reasons for preferring to fix with the eye containing the weak muscle.

### Step 2

Determine if the vertical separation is greater looking to the right or left.

The rectus muscles have their maximum vertical action when the eye is in abduction, the obliques when the eye is in adduction. Take the example of a weakness of the right superior oblique: this will present with the right eye higher because it is a depressor that is at fault, but the maximum deviation will occur looking to the left because the right eye will then be in adduction.

In this instance the only other possibility is a left superior rectus (LSR) weakness. Weakness of the elevators of the left eye could also result in the left eye being lower and, as the LSR also has the principal field of action looking to the left, vertical deviation will be greater with the left eye in abduction (Table A.1).

Therefore step 2 reduces the number of contenders to two.

## Step 3

Determine whether the maximum vertical deviation of the two eyes occurs when the head is tilted to the right or left shoulder. This test makes use of the fact that, in the primary position, the chief action of the oblique muscles is torsional.

Normally, a head tilt to the right stimulates corrective intorsion of the right eye which is brought about by the right superior oblique and, to some extent, the right superior rectus, but for the left eye there will be a corrective extorsion. Extorsion is brought about chiefly by the inferior oblique and, to a lesser extent, by the inferior rectus. Head tilt to the left will bring into action a mirror image set of muscles.

Supposing there is a right superior oblique palsy, when the head is tilted to the right, the normal corrective intorsion of the eye cannot be achieved and extra effort is demanded of the right superior rectus. As the superior rectus is a weak intorter but a good elevator in the primary position, its extra action will result in greater height and increased vertical separation. Tilting the head to the left will do nothing in the case of a right superior oblique weakness because that muscle is not brought into play.

In the example above, a right superior oblique weakness will give rise to greater separation, tilting the head to the right, and an LSR weakness will produce greater deviation, tilting the head to the left.

Therefore the defective muscle can be pinpointed by seeing whether the separation is greater tilting the head to the left or right.

Although the three step test provides objective evidence of vertical muscle dysfunction, it is not infallible, particularly in cases of diplopia secondary to muscle restriction rather than weakness.

Table A.1  The three step test for vertical diplopia

| Step 1 | | | | |
|---|---|---|---|---|
| Vertical deviation in the primary position | Right eye higher ↓ | Left eye lower ↓ | Left eye higher ↓ | Right eye lower ↓ |
| Weak muscles | RSO<br>RIR | or  LIO<br>LSR | LSO<br>LIR | or  RIO<br>RSR |

| Step 2 | | | | |
|---|---|---|---|---|
| Increased vertical separation with right or left gaze | Right gaze | Left gaze | | Right Left gaze<br>gaze |
| Weak muscles | RIR<br>LIO | or  RSO<br>LSR | LSO<br>RSR | or  LIR<br>RIO |

| Step 3 | | | | | | | | |
|---|---|---|---|---|---|---|---|---|
| Increased vertical separation with right or left head tilt | Right head tilt | Left head tilt | Right head tilt | Left head tilt | Right head tilt | Left head tilt | Right head tilt | Left head tilt |
| Weak muscle | LIO | RIR | RSO | LSR | RSR | LSO | LIR | RIO |

LIO, left inferior oblique; LSO, left superior oblique; LSR, left superior rectus; LIR, left inferior rectus; RIO, right inferior oblique; RSO, right superior oblique; RSR, right superior rectus; RIR, right inferior rectus.

# Appendix B  Examination of the ocular surface

1 Start with the lid margin: chronic inflammation leads to loss of the sharp margin between the skin and the conjunctival side of the lid. Chronic inflammation also leads to scarring, telangiectasias, and distortion of the lashes.
2 The precorneal tear film: start by examining the precorneal tear meniscus between the lid margin and the cornea. Patients with dry eyes will have a poor meniscus.
3 The tear film: look for abnormal mucus, particles, and excessive lipid.
4 Tear break up time (BUT): normal tear spreads evenly on the surface of the eye and dry spots do not appear after a blink for 10–30 seconds. This is best seen with a tiny amount of fluorescein staining the tear. A short BUT is typical of sicca syndromes and patients with blepharitis.

5 The reflected beam of the slitlamp may show more than direct illumination.
6 Stains to use:
   (a) fluorescein: stains de-epithelialised surface and loss of epithelial cells; instil the stain then dilute with saline and view with the blue light of the slitlamp. Fluorescein lights up best on dilution.
   (b) rose bengal: stains inflamed surfaces and shows up damaged or dead cells; useful in distinguishing between simple loss of epithelium and active inflammation or ulceration (see Fig 5.22). Also useful in demonstrating punctate loss of epithelial cells in the sicca syndrome but bear in mind the extremely irritating nature of rose bengal. Use only in diluted form or after the eye has been anaesthetised.

## Seidel's test for wound leak

1 Instil a relatively concentrated drop of fluorescein (for example, 2% in minim form) and watch for dilution in suspected part of the wound. Escaping aqueous causes bright green fluorescence.

or

2 Moisten a strip of paper impregnated with fluorescein and apply the paper directly on to the part of the wound suspected of leaking. Escaping aqueous will cause bright fluorescence.

The choice of method is a matter of individual preference.

## Schirmer's test for dry eyes

Strips of filter paper (available in standardised form commercially) 0·5 cm wide are folded at the tip and hinged on the outer part of the lower lid. After 5 min 10–15 mm of the paper should be wetted. Normals should have more than 15 mm; 9 mm or less is suspicious and less than 5 mm is diagnostic of dry eye.

It is not an exact test and some patients can comply better with the eyes closed.

# Appendix C  Examination of the orbit

## Inspection

Look for the following:

- Vertical displacement—do both pupils lie on the same horizontal line?
- Displacement from the midline.
- Any proptosis—this is best seen from above with the patient sitting down (Naffzigger's method—see Fig 10.3). Lean over the brow until both corneas are seen, which will give a good idea of the degree of proptosis. In patients with a squint it can be very difficult to tell if there is true proptosis.
- Look for soft tissue swelling or congestion.

## Palpation

If there is asymmetry:

- Feel the bones to identify any malformations (?congenital)
- Feel the rim for masses.

## Hertel's exophthalmometry

Hertel's exophthalmometer is a device with two mirrors mounted at right angles so that one faces the cornea and the other a scale marked in millimetres. There are two foot plates, one of which is movable to fit faces of different widths. They are designed so that the foot plates rest on the lateral orbital rims to give fixed landmarks. An observer in front can see the cornea and read the scale to note the protrusion of the cornea from the lateral orbit rim.

Subsequent measurements should use the same setting to get a more reliable estimate of change.

## Auscultation

No examination of the orbit is complete without listening for bruit by placing a stethoscope over the closed lids or on the side of the temple. Acute intracavernous arteriovenous fistula will give a bruit but a dural shunt may not.

EMERGENCY OPHTHALMOLOGY

*General examination*

This includes:

- Corrected visual acuity
- Visual field—both peripheral and central (early field defect in compressive lesion is likely to be paracentral)
- Pupils for relative afferent pupillary defect
- Colour vision loss
- Eye movement: test for diplopia and muscle restriction
- Fundal examination—in addition to looking at the disc look for choroidal striae which may signify a solid lesion or thyroid eye disease.

### The pupillary light reflex

This gives the anatomy of the pupillary pathway (see Fig 1.5):

- Afferent fibres come from the retinal ganglion cells and travel along the optic nerve
- At the chiasma half the fibres decussate to the contralateral optic tract—hence afferent impulses go to the two sides
- Pupillary fibres enter the superior colliculus and synapse in the pre-tectal area
- Impulses are then relayed to the Edinger–Westphal nuclei on both sides by intercalated neurons
- Efferent fibres travel with nerve III after being relayed by the ciliary ganglion to the iris sphincter.

## The swinging light test

The anatomy of the pupillary light reflex ensures that normally, when a light is shone into one eye, both pupils react equally and that the amplitude of their response is the same whichever eye is illuminated. However, if the optic nerve of one eye is damaged the pupil responses to a light will be reduced proportionately. Thus when a light is swung from eye to eye, both pupils will constrict more when the light is shone into the undamaged eye and will dilate when the light is on the eye with the damaged optic nerve, because the eye with the damaged optic nerve will be carrying fewer nerve fibres and will have less afferent input.

## Anisocaria and its differentiation

Definition: anisocoria denotes having two unequal pupils. There are three common conditions which can produce this:

1 Physiological
2 Sympathetic paresis—Horner's syndrome
3 Parasympathetic paresis—Holmes–Adie pupil.

### *Physiological*

Some 20% of normal individuals are said to have anisocoria. The pupils will both dilate in darkness and constrict in light.

### *Sympathetic paresis*

There is no action of the dilator fibres of the iris. The lack of dilatation will be accentuated in darkness.

Accompanying signs include:

- Ptosis of about 2 mm
- Apparent enophthalmos because of narrow palpebral aperture
- Anhidrosis if the lesion is low down and involves the carotid plexus.

**Test 1: cocaine 4% to both eyes** The normal pupil will dilate but that with Horner's syndrome will remain constricted.

*Rationale:* cocaine blocks the uptake of noradrenaline at the myoneural junction, thereby prolonging its action. In sympathetic palsy, there is no free noradrenaline and hence cocaine has no effect.

**Test 2.** Instil 1% hydoxyamphetamine to test if the post-ganglionic neuron is intact. This will cause a sympathomimetic effect by bringing about the release of noradrenaline if the third order neuron is intact, when the pupil will dilate as will the normal pupil.

### *Parasympathetic paresis—the Holmes–Adie pupil*

The affected pupil is usually dilated but may be miotic (late stage). There is light near dissociation: the pupil reacts poorly or not at all to light but well to accommodation. Once contracted, the pupil dilates slowly.

Associated features include:

- Segmental palsy of iris is common
- Diminished deep tendon reflexes.

**Test.** Instil 0·1% pilocarpine—if pupil constricts then Holmes–Adie pupil is confirmed. If the pupil is dilated and unresponsive to 0·1% pilocarpine, then try 1% pilocarpine. If the pupil constricts then the patient may have palsy of nerve III (a preganglionic lesion). If there is no response then there is either sphincter damage or a pharmacological blockade, for example, atropinisation.

*Rationale:* 0·1% pilocarpine is too weak to have an action unless there is postganglionic palsy and hypersensitivity. Pilocarpine 1% will constrict a normal pupil or a preganglionic palsy.

## Appendix D   Taking an erythrocyte sedimentation rate

### Principle

When anticoagulated blood is allowed to stand undisturbed, red blood cells will normally settle out to the bottom of the tube. The ESR is the distance in millimetres that the red blood cells fall in a given time, usually an hour. The ESR is greatly influenced by the extent to which the red cells form rouleaux, which sediment more rapidly than single cells. Rouleaux formation is affected by the concentrations of fibrinogen and other acute phase proteins, anaemia, immunoglobulins, and albumin levels.

Normal values are around 0–9 mm/h in males and 0–15 mm/h in females. ESR tends to increase with age and an upper limit of normal for men could be considered as half the age plus 10, whereas for women it is half the age plus 15.

There are two basic methods used to measure an ESR: the Westergren and the Wintrobe and Landsberg method.

### *Westergren method*

This method uses a straight glass tube with a 0·05 mm bore throughout. Specially made racks with levelling screws hold the tubes firmly in an exactly vertical position. The blood sample is mixed thoroughly with an anticoagulant (trisodium citrate,

EDTA, and trisodium citrate), and then drawn up from the blood bottle into the Westergren tube to the top mark by means of mechanical suction (never suck up the blood column with the mouth). Leave the tube undisturbed in the rack for 60 min out of direct sunlight and then measure how far the blood column has fallen to the nearest millimetre. If the demarcation between plasma and red cell column is hazy, the level is taken where the full density of the blood column is definite.

### Wintrobe method

Blood should be mixed with EDTA anticoagulant, and a flat bottomed 3 mm bore tube is filled with the blood using a cannula. The tube is placed vertically in the rack and the ESR measured after an hour.

### Variants of measuring ESR

Larger bore tubes are sometimes used in A&E departments, with the ESR being measured in less than an hour as more rapid sedimentation occurs with larger bore tubes. It is important to keep the position of the tube vertical at all times as slight degrees of tilting will accelerate the ESR. Each ESR measuring device should come with instructions. Make sure you are familiar with the instructions for your particular method.

## Appendix E   Electrodiagnostics and their relevance in the diagnosis of eye problems

The nervous system generates electical impulses and, because of this, electrical patterns and potentials can be recorded along the visual pathway, detected by electrodes in preset positions.

The three common forms of electrodiagnostic measurements in clinical use are:

1 Visual evoked potentials (VEPs)
2 Electroretinograms (ERGs): flash, focal, and pattern
3 Electro-oculograms (EOGs).

### Visual evoked potential

The VEP measures the electrical response of the entire afferent visual pathway from retina to cortex, recorded by scalp electrodes. A flash of light can cause a stimulus but the response to alternating chequerboard and sine wave grating stimuli is more consistent, and this has become the standard clinical test for VEPs.

The VEP response is mostly used for studying diseases affecting the optic nerve. Unfortunately, many changes seen in the waveform are not pathognomonic, but in 90% of patients with demyelinating disorders, fragmentation and delay in the response are seen. It is also effective in demonstrating the integrity of visual pathways in hysterical blindness or malingerers. It is possible for the patient with functional blindness to produce an abnormal response by staring through or ignoring the pattern. Therefore an abnormal response in the context of a normal neuro-ophthalmic examination does not necessarily indicate organic pathology.

### The electroretinogram

The ERG measures function in the outer retinal layers. It is normal in ganglion cell, optic nerve, and higher centre visual pathology, but is abnormal in retinal photoreceptor and pigment epithelium disease. The ERG is reduced in tapetoretinal degenerations.

To obtain an ERG an electrode is placed on the cornea and the electrical response is measured in respect of a reference electrode when a flash of light is shone into a dark adapted eye.

The pattern ERG measures the ERG response to patterned stimuli (usually an alternating chequerboard as in VEP testing). The pattern ERG is reduced in inner retinal layer, optic nerve, and early macular disease.

### Electro-oculography

There is a steady potential difference between the cornea and the back of the eye. If two electrodes are placed at the inner and outer canthi, the potential difference can be measured as the eyes move from right to left. The potential difference varies in different light conditions. It reflects the presynaptic function of the retina and interaction between the retinal pigment epithelium and the photoreceptors. The EOG is decreased in retinitis pigmentosa, choroideraemia, vitamin A deficiency, toxic retinopathies, and other retinal pathology.

# Appendix F   Identification of *Acanthamoeba* spp.

## Life cycle

Acanthamoebae are small free-living amoebae found in virtually all soil and aquatic environments. Organisms are characterised by a feeding and replicating trophosoite which, under adverse conditions, can form a dormant cystic stage. Cysts are highly resistant to extremes of temperature, dessication, and disinfectants.

Once transferred to the cornea they invade through damaged epithelium and invade progressively into the stroma.

## Risk factors

Contact lens wearers account for about 80% of reported cases, affecting both hard and soft lens wearers.

Poor lens hygiene is usually at fault and there is a history of rinsing lenses in tap water instead of proper lens cleaning solutions.

A history of recent travel to tropical countries is also significant.

## Diagnosis

Successful treatment depends on early diagnosis and a high index of suspicion is required.

Inform the microbiology laboratory which needs 24 hours notice to prepare culture plates. Instruct the patient to return the next day bringing the current lenses, lens case, and all available solutions for examination and culture.

To obtain culture specimens the cornea is anaesthetised with drops and a sterile needle is used to scrape staining of the edge of a corneal infiltrate (away from the visual axis) or to remove a sheet of epithelium.

The specimen is plated on to a non-nutrient agar plate, which has been flooded with live *Escherichia coli* and is then incubated for 72 hours at 37°C.

*Acanthamoeba* sp. is identified by the presence of trophozoites.

If there is no growth the plates should be incubated for a further 72 hours at 30°C and then at room temperature.

A specimen is sent for microscopy where cysts can be stained by special techniques.

If the scapes are negative and the clinical picture suggests acanthamoeba infection, then a formal corneal biopsy is indicated.

## Appendix G Taking ocular samples for microbiology

Bacterial disease is diagnosed principally by culture of the organisms.

### Collection of the specimens

1 Do not put anything in the eye before collection which may affect results, for example, anaesthetic containing preservative.
2 Suppurative material from the conjunctiva of an infected eye should be collected from the cul-de-sac or from the inner canthus.

Swabs are commonly used for obtaining many types of cultures but they are inferior to other methods (for example, wire loop). Certain precautions need to be considered. Cotton and rayon have high absorption capacities which is useful if bacteria are in low concentrations. However, cotton swabs may contain residual fatty acids which can inhibit the growth of certain bacteria. Rayon, calcium alginate, or Dacron swabs can be used as an alternative.

Chlamydia samples are best taken by scraping the conjunctival mucosa. Wooden tipped swabs and swabs made of calcium alginate should be avoided; some cotton swabs have been toxic to *Chlamydia* sp.; Dacron or rayon material is preferred.

Samples taken directly from the surface of the cornea are best done with either a sterile platinum bacteriological loop (which can be heated in a flame and re-sterilised as the samples are taken) or alternatively the end of a sterile hypodermic needle can be used. To maximise the chances of culture, the samples should be plated out directly they are taken.

### Processing of ocular samples

1 A direct Gram stain of the material obtained should be prepared to determine the type of bacteria present. A sample of the exudate is placed on a glass microscope slide for Gram staining in the laboratory.
2 If trachoma is suspected, conjunctival scraping should be smeared onto a glass microscope slide, air dried, and fixed in

absolute methanol. Chlamydia antigen detection systems using fluorescent tagged monoclonal antibodies are 95% sensitive and the answer can be available within one hour.
3 Agar plates are used to plate out the specimens. The plate is inoculated inside the rim. The bacteriological loop is used to draw out parallel lines, for example, in an anticlockwise direction around the circumference of the dish over 2–3 clock hours from the inoculation site. The loop is then re-sterilised and the procedure repeated from the left hand edge of anticlockwise rows of parallel lines, overlapping them in a crisscross fashion. The loop is re-sterilised and the procedure repeated again. This is done four or five times in total, with the final stroke with the loop being a zig zag around the remaining circumference of the dish. Blood agar is a good general medium for growing most ocular pathogens. Chocolate agar is preferred by *Haemophilus* sp., *Moraxella* sp., and *Neisseria gonorrhoeae*. Sabaroud's medium is used to isolate fungal infections, for example, *Aspergillus* and *Fusarium* spp.
4 *Chlamydia* sp. is an obligate intracellular pathogen. Collect the specimen in specific transport medium (for example, sucrose phosphate glutamate medium) for culture in irradiated or cycloheximide treated McCoy cells for 2–3 days.
5 Viral samples need to be sent in a viral transport medium to the laboratory promptly for inoculation into cell culture. Dry swabs are not acceptable.

# Further reading

## History and examination

Huber MJE, Reacher MH. *Clinical tests. Ophthalmology.* Ipswich: Wolfe Medical Publications, 1990.
Kanski JJ. *Clinical ophthalmology*, 3rd edn. Oxford: Butterworth-Heinemann, 1994.
Miller S, ed. *Clinical ophthalmology.* Bristol: Wright, 1987.
Spalton DJ, Hitchings RA, Hunter PA. *Atlas of clinical ophthalmology.* Edinburgh: Churchill Livingstone, 1984.

## Transient and persistent visual loss

Kupersmith MJ. *Neurovascular neuro-ophthalmology.* Berlin: Springer-Verlag, 1992.
Newman NM. *Neuro-ophthalmology: A practical text.* Stamford: Apple & Lange, 1992.

## Flashing lights and floaters

Kanski J. *Retinal detachment.* Guildford: Butterworths, 1985.
Kanski J. *Uveitis: A colour manual of diagnosis and treatment.* Guildford: Butterworths, 1987.
McLeod D. The vitreous and its disorders. In: Miller S, ed. *Clinical ophthalmology.* Bristol: Wright, 1988.

## The red eye

Kanski JJ. *Clinical ophthalmology*, 3rd edn. Oxford: Butterworth-Heinemann, 1994.
Miller S, ed. *Clinical ophthalmology.* Bristol: Wright, 1987.
Spalton DJ, Hitchings RA, Hunter PA. *Atlas of clinical ophthalmology.* Edinburgh: Churchill Livingston, 1984.

Taylor D. *Paediatric ophthalmology*. Oxford: Blackwell Scientific, 1992.

## Trauma

Catalano RA. *Ocular emergencies*. Philadelphia, PA: WB Saunders, 1992.

Eagling EM, Roper-Hall MJ. *Eye injuries—an illustrated guide*. Philadelphia, PA: JB Lipincott, 1986.

## Diplopia

Beck RW, Smith AH. *Neuro-ophthalmology: A problem orientated approach*. Boston, MA: Little, Brown & Co., 1987.

Glaser J. *Neuro-ophthalmology*. Philadelphia, PA: JB Lipincott, 1990.

Mein J, Trimble R. *Diagnosis and management of ocular motility disorders*. Oxford: Blackwell Scientific, 1991.

Newman NM. *Neuro-ophthalmology: A practical text*. Stamford: Apple & Lange, 1992.

Taylor D. *Paediatric ophthalmology*. Oxford: Blackwell Scientific, 1992.

## Headache

Bajandas FJ, Klein LB. *Neuro-ophthalmology review manual*. New Jersey: Slack Inc., 1988.

Lance JW. *Mechanism and management of headache*, 5th edn. Oxford: Butterworth-Heinemann, 1993.

Newman NM. *Neuro-ophthalmology: A practical text*. Stamford: Apple & Lange, 1992.

Weatherall DJ, Ledingham JGC, Warrell D, eds. *Oxford textbook of medicine*. Oxford: Oxford Medical Publications, 1996.

## Orbital swellings

Henderson JW. *Orbital tumors*, 3rd edn. New York: Raven Press, 1994.

Sisler H, Jakobiec FA, Trokel SI. Diseases of the Ordit in *Duane's Clinical Ophthalmology*, Vol II. Philadelphia: Harper and Rowe, 1984..

## Contact lens problems

Mackie I. *Medical contact lens practice—a systemic apprach.* Oxford: Butterworth-Heinemann, 1993: Chapters 10–14.

Phillips AJ, Stone J. *Contact lenses,* 3rd edn. Guildford: Butterworths, 1989: 270–332.

Tomlinson A. *Complications of contact lens wear.* St Louis, MO: Mosby–Year Book Inc., 1992.

## Postoperative complications

Roper-Hall MJ. *Stallard's operative surgry.* Bristol: Wright, 1980.

Willshaw H. *Practical ophthalmic surgery.* Edinburgh: Churchill Livingstone, 1993.

# Index

abscess
  infective corneal 103–5, 264
  Meibomian gland 242
  suture 278, 290
*Acanthamoeba* 315–16
  diagnosis of infection 315–16
  keratitis 262–3
  life cycle 315
  risk factors 315
accommodation
  insufficiency 171, 203
  spasm 203
acetazolamide 36, 100, 194
acetylcysteine 156, 235
acid burns 153, 154, 155
acyclovir 110, 122
adenocarcinoma, lacrimal gland 248–9
adenoid cystic carcinoma, lacrimal gland 248–9
adenoviral conjunctivitis 116–17
adhesives, cyanoacrylate based contact 157
agar plates 317
age
  contact lenses 258
  macular disease and 44
  related macular degeneration 45–8, 87, 297, 299
alcohol intoxication 209
alkali burns 153, 154, 155
allergy 118–20, 225
  in contact lens wearers 120, 257, 258, 265
  drops prescribed after cataract surgery 278
alternate cover test 166
altitudinal headache 209
amaurosis fugax 66, 73
amblyopia 26
amikacin 271
Amsler grid 7
  visual field testing 10–11
anaemia 76
analgesic abuse, chronic 206
aneurysms

posterior communicating artery 181, 218
  ruptured intracranial 209–10
angioid streaks 48
angle, anterior chamber
  gonioscopic examination 18, 19
  recession, traumatic 134
  Schaffer grading system 18, 20
anisocoria 11, 311–12
  parasympathetic paresis 311–12
  physiological 311
  sympathetic paresis 311
anterior chamber
  angle *see* angle, anterior chamber
  in chemical burns 155
  paracentesis 36
  shallow, after trabeculectomy 282, 283, 285
  slitlamp examination 14–17, 97–8
anterior ischaemic optic neuropathy (AION) 28–33
  arteritic 31, 32–3
  further management 32–3
  immediate management 31–2
  non-arteritic 31, 32, 33
  prognosis 32
  symptoms and signs 29–31, 39, 42, 217
anterior segment ischaemia, after retinal detachment surgery 286–7
antibiotics
  in bacterial conjunctivitis 112
  in blepharitis 124
  in chemical burns 156
  in endophthalmitis 271–2
  in infective corneal lesions 104–5
  in penetrating trauma 152, 153
  in suture abscess 278
  in toxoplasmosis 86
antiviral agents 122
appearance, general 95, 163–4
applanation tonometry 17
arc eye 158
arteriovenous fistula, intracavernous 216, 231–2, 309

321

# INDEX

arteriovenous malformations (AVMs), intracranial 91, 208–9
arteritis, giant cell/temporal *see* giant cell arteritis
ascorbic acid 156–7
aspirin 33, 74
atopy 120
atropine 156, 272
aura 198
auscultation, globe/orbit 227, 309

bacteriological loop 316, 317
basal cell carcinoma, eyelid 242–4
betamethasone 103
Bielschowsky's head tilt test 167, 305–6, 307
biomicroscope *see* slitlamp
biopsy, temporal artery 32
blepharitis 95, 123, 124
blood pressure, raised *see* hypertension
blurring of vision 57–62
  causes 58, 59
  examination 57–8
  history 57
botulinum toxin 173–4
brainstem disease 184, 185
brain tumours *see* intracranial tumours
branch retinal artery occlusion (BRAO) 39, 40, 41–2
branch retinal vein occlusion (BRVO) 37, 38, 39–41
brightness perception, reduced 44
bruits 227, 309
bullous keratopathy 268, 275, 276
burns
  chemical *see* chemical burns
  radiation (arc eye) 158
  thermal 157–8

canaliculus, torn 140
capsulotomy, laser 278, 279
carbon dioxide retention 209
cardiovascular disease
  examination 68
  risk factors 67, 74
carotid artery disease 73–4
  chronic ocular ischaemia 195
  investigations 68
  slow flow retinopathy 70
  transient visual loss 66, 67, 73

carotid artery dissection 200, 222
carotid–cavernous fistula 227, 230–2
  direct 230–1
  indirect 216, 231–2
carotid endarterectomy 73–4
cataract 58, 60–1
  glaucoma secondary to 100, 101
  surgery, postoperative complications 268, 270–81
  traumatic 144
cavernous sinus
  pathology 184, 185, 218
  thrombosis 215–16
cefuroxime 105
cells
  anterior chamber 14, 98
    grading 16–17
  anterior vitreous 79
  inflammatory, causing floaters 83–4
  neoplastic 86
cellulitis
  orbital *see* orbital cellulitis
  preseptal 240–1
central retinal artery occlusion (CRAO) 28, 29, 35–7
central retinal vein occlusion (CRVO) 28, 33–5, 38, 72
  ischaemic 33, 34
  non-ischaemic 33, 34, 58
central serous retinopathy 51–3, 60
cerebellar disease 185
cerebrovascular accident (stroke) 73, 74, 210
chalazion (meibomian cyst) 124, 125, 241, 242, 243
chemical burns 153–7
  assessment 154–6
  classification 155–6
  further management 156–7
  immediate treatment 154
chemical conjunctivitis, in neonates 114
chemosis 96, 164, 253
cherry-red spot 29, 35
children
  conjunctival lacerations 138
  headaches 193
  ocular trauma 133
  orbital pseudotumour 229

# INDEX

orbital tumours 237–8
sixth nerve palsy 173
visual acuity testing 4, 5
chlamydial conjunctivitis
  in adults 97, 113
  microbiology 316–17
  in neonates 114, 115
choroid
  haemorrhage, delayed postoperative 281, 282–4
  neovascularisation (CNV), idiopathic 48
  rupture 136, 145–6
choroiditis 83, 84
ciliary body 18
cilioretinal artery occlusion 53–4
ciprofloxacin 105
clindamycin 86
coagulopathies 76
cocaine 311
Cogan's lid twitch sign 180
collagenase inhibition 156
coloboma 74
colour vision
  loss of 44
  measurement 6–7, 26–7
commotio retinae 136, 145
computed tomography (CT scan)
  in thyroid eye disease 235
  in trauma 149, 151
confrontation techniques, visual field testing 10
conjunctiva
  chemical burns 155
  dermolipoma/lipoma 253–4
  examination 96
  granulomata 253, 255
  laceration 138
  swellings 225, 253–5
    localised cystic 253–4
    painful 253
    painless 253–5
  in thyroid eye disease 232
  tumours 254–5
conjunctivitis 95
  allergic 117–20
    acute 118
    chronic 119–20
    hayfever 118–19
  bacterial 112, 113

  in neonates 114, 115
  chemical, in neonates 114
  chlamydial *see* chlamydial conjunctivitis giant papillary 257, 264, 265
  gonococcal, in neonates 114, 115
  herpetic 116, 117
  in neonates 114, 115
  toxic 120
  viral 106, 116–17
contact lenses 256–69, 315
  age 258
  cleansing routines 257–8
  gas permeable 257
  Goldmann single mirror 18
  "hard" 257, 259
    removal 266
  lost/stuck 266–7
  movement on blinking 259
  overwear 259–60
  problems 256–67
    allergies 119, 257, 258, 265
    causes 256–7
    common presentations 256
    diagnosis 257–9
    examination 259
    infections 104, 262–5
    management 259–67
  in slitlamp examination 17
  soft 257, 258, 259
    removal 266
    soft disposable 257
  therapeutic 267–8
  wearing schedules 258
convergence
  insufficiency 170–1, 203
  spasm 171–2, 203
  testing 165
copper, retained intraocular 147
cornea
  abrasions 141
    recurrent 106–7
  abscesses 103–5, 264
  blunt trauma 134
  chemical burns 154–5, 156
  in contact lens wearers 259
  decompensation, after cataract surgery 275–6
  erosion, recurrent 106–7, 267–8
  examination 96–7

323

# INDEX

exposure 129
  complicating lid surgery 292–3
  in thyroid eye disease 235, 236
  foreign body 138
  infections 103–5
  infiltrates, in contact lens wearers 261–2
  lacerations 139
    full thickness 139, 149
    partial thickness 139
  neovascularisation, contact lens induced 266, 267
  padding 107, 141
  perforation 148, 150, 268
  persistent epithelial defects 268
  scarring 122, 123, 156
  specimen collection 316
  thermal burns 157, 158
corneal grafts 288–90
  loose/broken sutures 289–90
  rejection 288–9
  suture abscess 290
  in trauma 152
corneal ulcers
  in contact lens wearers 263–5
  herpetic
    amoeboid 123
    dendritic 121, 122
    indolent 268
  infective 103–5
  marginal 105–6
corticosteroids *see* steroids
co-trimoxazole 86
cover–uncover test 166
cranial nerve palsies 184–5 *see also* fourth (IV) nerve palsy; sixth (VI) nerve palsy; third (III) nerve palsy
  diplopia in 160, 175
  in optic chiasm lesions 64
  painful 217–18
  risk factors 163
cryotherapy, retinal tears 82
cyanoacrylate based contact adhesives 157
cyclopentolate 141
cycloplegia 141, 143, 156
cystoid macular oedema (CMO) 278–9, 280
cysts
  eyelid 241–2

orbit 237–8
retention, eyelids 242, 243

dacryoadenitis 247, 248
dacryocystitis 116, 250–1
dacryocystorhinostomy, postoperative complications 291–2
Dalrymple's sign 233
débridement, corneal abrasions 141
dellen 107, 141
dendritic ulcers, herpetic 121, 122
depression 192, 209
dermoid cysts, orbit 237–8
dermolipoma 253–4
descemetocele 103
diabetic maculopathy 61, 298, 300, 301
  management 62, 300
diabetic retinopathy 38, 58, 61–2, 298–302
  background 298–300
  pre-proliferative 302, 303
  proliferative 61, 300–2
diplopia 159–86
  binocular 159, 160, 163–8
  causes 159–61
  definition 159
  examination 163
  frontal headache with 203
  history 161–3
  horizontal 161–2, 168–76
    causes 168
    constant 172–6
    diagnostic approach 169
    differential diagnosis 168
    intermittent/variable 170–2
  monocular 159–60, 163
  in optic chiasm tumours 64
  in orbital disease 225, 226
  painful 162, 213, 215–16, 217–18
  physiological 160–1
  test 165–6
  in thyroid eye disease 160, 176, 180, 226, 235
  in trauma 137, 146, 160, 176, 185–6
  types 159
  vertical 162, 177–86
    causes 177
    constant 180–6
    diagnostic approach 178
    differential diagnosis 177

324

# INDEX

intermittent/variable 179–80
   three step test 166–7, 305–6, 307
divergence insufficiency 172
documentation, ocular trauma 133
doxycycline 156
driving, with occluded eye 107
drugs
  causing headache 209
  causing optic neuropathy 57
drusen
  in age related macular degeneration 46, 47
  optic disc 74, 75, 297
  optic nerve head 72
dry eyes 95, 108, 125, 126
  Schirmer's test 308
dural ischaemia, referred pain from 196, 219
dyes, topical 97

ectropion 95, 129–30
  complications of surgery 292–3
electrodiagnostics 313–14
electro-oculography (EOG) 314
electroretinogram (ERG) 314
endophthalmitis 103
  postoperative 271–2
  posttraumatic 152, 153
  *v* severe iritis 273
enophthalmos 137–8, 146, 164
entropion 95, 107–8
  complications of surgery 292–3
  protective lenses 269
enucleation 152–3
episcleritis 95, 128
erythrocyte sedimentation rate (ESR) 312–13
  in giant cell arteritis 32, 68, 201
  in sixth nerve palsy 173
  variants of measuring 313
  Westergren method 312–13
  Wintrobe method 313
esophoria 166, 170
ESR *see* erythrocyte sedimentation rate (ESR) examination
  ocular surface 307–8
  orbit 309–10
  visual function 3–13
exercise/exertion induced headache 197

exophoria 166, 170
explants, extruded retinal detachment 186, 287
exposure keratitis 129 *see also* cornea, exposure
eye
  alignment/position 163–4
  skew deviation 185
eyelids
  disease 240–5
    symptoms and signs 241
  eversion 97
  examination 95
  infections 241
  itching 240, 245–6
  lacerations 139–40
  lag 232
  pain/redness/tenderness 240
  position 163–4
  retraction 164, 233
  surgery, complications 292–3
  swellings
    in lacrimal gland disease 246–7
    localised 223–4, 240–3
    in orbital disease 225–6
    painful 240–1
    painless 241–3
  thermal burns 157–8
  in thyroid eye disease 232
  tumours 241–3
    benign 241–2
    malignant 242–7, 245
eye movements
  examination 164–5
  painful 45
  transient visual loss and 67
  in trauma 137
  uniocular/ductions 165
  versional 164–5
"eye strain" 187

facial pain 220–2
  atypical 222
  differential diagnosis 219, 220
fever, headache with 192, 204
"flare" 14, 98
flashing lights *see* lights, flashing
floaters 77–87, 89
  causes 77
  examination 78, 79

325

# INDEX

history 77–8
management 81
fluorescein angiography
  in central serous retinopathy 51, 52
  in cystoid macular oedema 279, 280
fluorescein staining 97, 308
  after corneal grafting 289
  in contact lens problems 259
  in dry eyes 125
  in Seidel's test 308
folinic acid 86
follicular reaction, conjunctival 97, 113
forced duction test 167
foreign bodies
  corneal 138
  intraocular (IOFBs) 147–53
    assessment 147–8
    investigations 149, 151
    management 153
    symptoms and signs 148, 149
  subtarsal 97, 138
fourth (IV) nerve palsy 175, 183–4
  congenital 179, 183, 184
fractures
  basal skull 140–1
  orbital wall 137–8, 146–7, 186
Fuch's spot 49
fundus examination 17, 310
  in macular disease 45
  in optic chiasm lesions 64
  in red eye 98
fungal infections, cornea 103–5
fusion, acute squint after interruption 174

gentamicin 105, 271
giant cell (temporal) arteritis (GCA) 69
  anterior ischaemic optic neuropathy 31, 32–3
  central retinal artery occlusion 36–7
  diagnosis 31–2, 68, 69
  diplopia 218
  headache 192, 201
  transient visual loss 66, 67
  treatment 31, 32, 69
  *v* temporomandibular joint dysfunction 202
giant papillary conjunctivitis 257, 264, 265
glaucoma 95

acute 99–101
angle closure
  acute 99, 100–1
  chronic 195
  intermittent 66, 67, 68, 69–70
  risk factors 304
  suspect 302–3, 304
headache in 195
malignant postoperative 281, 282–4
open angle 195
phacolytic/phacomorphic 100, 101
pupil block 281, 282–4
rubeotic 100, 101, 215
traumatic 143
uveitic 100
glaucomatocyclitic crisis 194
globe
  auscultation 227, 309
  displacement *see* proptosis
  injection 164
  perforated 152–3
  retropulsion 227
glycerol, oral 101
Goldmann single mirror contact lens 18
Goldmann tonometer 17
gonioscopy 18, 19
gonococcal conjunctivitis, in neonates 114, 115
Gram stain 316
granuloma
  conjunctival 253, 255
  suture 290–1
Graves' disease 232
  ophthalmic (euthyroid) 232
Graves' ophthalmopathy *see* thyroid eye disease
greater occipital neuralgia 196, 219
grittiness 124–6

haemangioma
  capillary 236, 237
  cavernous 236, 237
*Haemophilus* sp 112
hayfever 118–19
head
  injury 183
  posture, abnormal 163, 179, 183
headache 187–210 *see also* migraine
  aggravating factors 191–2

## INDEX

in/around eye 193–7
  with red eye *see* red eye, painful
  with white eye 193, 194–7
  cluster 200, 216
  diagnostic approach 188–90
  drugs causing 192
  duration 191
  episodic 191, 197–200
  examination 192–3
  exertion/exercise induced 197
  family history 192
  frontal 191, 203–4
    with use of eyes 203–4
    without use of eyes 204
  generalised/non-specific 190, 205–10
    acute onset 209–10
    chronic 205–9
  history taking 187–92
  location 191
  nature 191
  precipitating factors 191
  "sentinel" 210
  speed of onset 191
  symptomatic classification 188
  tension 205–6
  timing of onset 191
  unilateral 189, 191
    chronic/persistent 200–2
    episodic 197–200
hemianopia
  bitemporal 24, 25, 63–4
  homonymous 24, 25, 62–3
    congruous 9
    incongruous 9
hemicrania, chronic paroxysmal 202
herpes simplex
  conjunctivitis 115, 117
  in neonates 114, 115
  keratitis 106, 121–2, 123, 268
herpes zoster, ophthalmic 109–11
herpetic neuralgia 220–1
Hertel's exophthalmometry 226, 309
Hess chart 168
heterophoria 203
  concomitant 161, 170
hippus 12
histoplasmosis syndrome, presumed ocular (POHS) 48
history taking 1–2
Holmes–Adie pupil 311–12

homatropine 143
hordeolum, internal 241
Horner's syndrome 200, 311
  red eye and 216
hydrocortisone 32, 69
hyperphoria 166
hypertension 78, 192
  headaches 206–7
  malignant 72
hyperthyroidism 232
hyperviscosity syndromes 76
hyphaema 15
  postoperative 284, 286
  spontaneous 68, 74
  traumatic 134, 135, 141–3
hypophoria 166
hypopyon 15, 104
hypoxia, contact lens-associated 259–60

ice-pick pains 197
infections *see also specific infections*
  in contact lens wearers 104, 262–5
  eyelid 241
  general systemic 192, 204
  postoperative 271–2, 291–2
  posttraumatic 147
inflammatory cells, causing floaters 83–4
inflammatory disorders
  causing floaters 84–7
  orbital 160, 186
influenza 204
infraorbital nerve lesions 137
instruments, ophthalmic 13–21
internuclear ophthalmoplegia 174–6
intracranial hypertension, benign (pseudotumour cerebri) 72–3, 207–8
intracranial pressure, raised 72–3
intracranial tumours 56, 63–4, 91
  headaches 208
intraocular pressure (IOP)
  in acute glaucoma 100–1
  after trabeculectomy 282, 283, 285
  in central retinal artery occlusion 36
  in chemical burns 155, 157
  in glaucomatocyclitic crisis 194
  in intermittent angle closure glaucoma 69
  measurement 17

# INDEX

in ophthalmic herpes zoster 110
in penetrating trauma 150
raised 303–4
in thyroid eye disease 232
in traumatic hyphaema 141–2, 143
intraocular tumours 87
IOP *see* intraocular pressure
iridectomy, surgical 101
iridodialysis 134, 135, 142, 143
iridotomy, laser 101
iris
  bombé 103
  prolapse
    after cataract surgery 273–4
    in trauma 149, 150
iritis (anterior uveitis) 84, 95, 101–3
  severe postoperative 273
  symptoms and signs 101, 122–3, 194
  traumatic 134
  *v* endophthalmitis 273
iron, retained intraocular 147
irrigation, eye 154
irritation, general 124–6
ischaemia
  anterior segment, after retinal detachment surgery 286–7
  chronic ocular 195, 217
  dural/meningeal, referred pain from 196, 219
Ishihara pseudoisochromatic plates 6–7, 26–7
itching
  eyelids 240, 245–6
  red eyes 117–20

keratic precipitates (KPs) 15, 16, 98
keratitis
  *Acanthamoeba* 262–3
  disciform 121, 122
  exposure 129 *see also* cornea, exposure
  focal 95
  herpetic 106, 121–2, 123, 268
  infectious, in contact lens wearers 263–5
keratoacanthoma 242, 245
keratoconjunctivitis
  superior limbic 234
  vernal 120
keratoconus 58

keratopathy, bullous 268, 275, 276
keratoses
  seborrhoeic 242
  senile 242
Khodadoust's line 288, 289

lacrimal gland
  disease 224, 246–50
    management 248–50
    symptoms and signs 246–7
  space occupying lesions 248
  tumours 246, 248–50
    malignant 248–9
    mixed cell 249–50
lacrimal sac
  disease 224–5
  mucocele 252
  tumour 252
laser therapy
  in acute angle closure glaucoma 101
  capsulotomy 278, 279
  diabetic retinopathy 61
  retinal tears 82
lateral geniculate body 9
Leber's optic neuropathy 56
Lees screen 168
lens
  dislocation 134, 144
  subluxation 134, 135, 144
  trauma 144
lids *see* eyelids
lights, flashing 88–91
  examination 89
  history 89
  management 90
limbus
  in contact lens wearers 259
  perforation 148
lipoma 253–4
lymphoid hyperplasia, orbital 238
lymphoma
  conjunctiva 254, 255
  lacrimal gland 250
  orbit 238

macropsia 44
macular degeneration
  age related (ARMD) 45–8, 87, 297, 299
  exudative 45, 47

## INDEX

non-exudative 45, 46, 47
disciform 298, 299
myopic 45, 49–50
macular disease 26, 44–5
common 297–8
*v* optic nerve disease 44–5
macular hole 50–1
traumatic 136, 144
macular oedema, cystoid (CMO) 278–9, 280
magnetic resonance imaging 176
magnets, foreign body removal 153
malignant tumours
eyelids 242–3, 245, 246
lacrimal gland 248–9
orbit 238–9
mannitol, intravenous 101
massage, ocular 36
medial longitudinal fasciculus (MLF) 174
meibomian cyst (chalazion) 124, 125, 241, 242, 243
meibomian gland abscess 241
melanoma, conjunctival 254
meningeal ischaemia, referred pain from 196, 219
meningitis 192, 210
metamorphopsia 44
metastatic tumours, orbit 239
microbiology, ocular samples for 316–17
micropsia 44
migraine 197–9
basilar 199
cerebral 199
classic 198
common 198
complicated 198
differential diagnosis 199
equivalents 199
flashing lights 89, 90
history taking 192
management 199
ocular/periocular pain 196–7, 219
ophthalmoplegic 198, 199
retinal 198
symptoms 90, 198
transient visual loss 67, 76
mixed cell lacrimal gland tumour 249–50

Moll, cyst of 242, 243
molluscum contagiosum 245–6
mucocele
lacrimal sac 252
orbit 238
mucormycosis 229
multiple sclerosis
internuclear ophthalmoplegia 176
optic neuritis and 54–5, 56
muscae volitantes 78, 83
muscles, extraocular
imbalance 160, 179
lost/slipped, after squint surgery 291
tethering 160
in thyroid eye disease 234
myasthenia gravis 160, 176, 179–80
ocular 179
mydriasis, traumatic 134, 144
mydriatics 102–3
myelinated nerve fibres 297, 298
myopia
in cataract 60
macular degeneration 45, 49–50
myositis, orbital 160, 176, 186, 215

Naffzigger's method 309
nasolacrimal disease 224–5, 250–2
management 250–1
painful 250–1
painless 250–1
symptoms and signs 250–1
nasolacrimal duct, congenital obstruction 114–15
neonates, conjunctivitis 114–15
neoplastic cells 86
neurological symptoms 162–3
neuromuscular disorders 160

occipital lobe lesions 9, 63
referred pain from 196
occipital neuralgia, greater 196, 219
ocular ischaemia, chronic 195, 217
ofloxacin 105
ophthalmia neonatorum 114–15
ophthalmic artery disease 73
ophthalmic instruments 13–21
ophthalmitis, sympathetic 152–3
ophthalmoplegia, internuclear 174–6
ophthalmoscopy
binocular indirect 20–1

# INDEX

direct 18–20
optic atrophy 295–6
optic chiasmal lesions 9, 63–4
optic disc
  common variants/abnormalities 294–7
  cupping 295
  drusen 74, 75, 297
  normal 294
  in optic neuritis 54, 55
  swelling 58, 72, 192
  tilted 296–7
  vertical cup–disc (C/D) ratio 294, 295
optic nerve 8
  contusion 136
  disease 26
  *v* macular lesions 44–5
  head
    bilateral drusen 72
    infiltrations 72
optic neuritis 37, 54–6, 72
  *v* optic neuropathy 45
optic neuropathy 37, 56–7
  aetiology 56–7
  anterior ischaemic *see* anterior ischaemic optic neuropathy
  Leber's 56
  retrobulbar ischaemic 217
  in thyroid eye disease 234, 235
  *v* optic neuritis 45
optic radiation 9
optic tract 9
orbit
  examination 309–10
  myositis 160, 176, 186, 215
orbital apex syndrome 185, 186, 218
orbital cellulitis 186, 227–8, 229
  after retinal detachment surgery 286
  after squint surgery 291
orbital disease 225–39
  with discomfort 230–6
  inflammatory 160, 186
  painful 225, 226, 227–30
  painless 236–9
  swellings in 223, 224
  symptoms and signs 225–7
orbital tumours 56, 160, 186, 236–9
  cystic 237–8
  malignant 238–9

metastatic 239
vascular 236–7
orbital wall blowout fractures 137–8, 146–7, 186

padding 107, 141
pain 193, 211–22 *see also* headache
  definition 211
  diplopia and 162, 213, 215–16, 217–18
  examination 214
  on eye movement 45
  facial 219, 220–2
  history taking 211–14
  in lacrimal gland disease 246–7
  nature 213
  in ocular trauma 134
  in orbital disease 225, 226, 227–30
  photophobia with 213
  red eye with *see* red eye, painful
  symptomatic classification 212
  in third nerve palsy 181
  *v* ache 187
  visual loss/disturbance with 211, 214–15, 216–17
  with white eye 193, 194–7, 216–22
palpation, orbit 309
papillae, conjunctival 97, 98
papillitis 72
papilloedema 66, 67, 71–3
papillophlebitis 34
paracentesis, anterior chamber 36
parasympathetic paresis 311–12
paratrigeminal syndrome, Raeder's 202, 216
parietal lobe lesions 9, 63
paroxysmal hemicrania, chronic 202
pars planitis (intermediate uveitis) 83, 84
perforated globe 152–3
perimetry, mechanical/computerised 11
phenylephrine 102–3
phlyctenulosis 128–9
phorias
  alternate cover test 166
  decompensating 160, 170, 179
photocoagulation, retinal 35
photophobia 94, 121–3, 213
photopsia *see* lights, flashing

330

# INDEX

phthisis bulbi 214–15
pilocarpine 100–1, 312
pingueculum 130
pinhole visual acuity 5–6, 57
pituitary apoplexy 208, 218
pituitary dysfunction 64
polymyalgia rheumatica 31–2
Posner–Schlossman syndrome 194
posterior communicating aneurysms 181, 218
posterior segment
 in blunt trauma 136
 slitlamp examination 17
posterior vitreous detachment (PVD) 77, 78–80, 89, 91
postoperative complications 268, 270–93
posture
 abnormal head 163, 179, 183
 transient visual loss and 67
prednisone, oral 32
preseptal cellulitis 240–1
presumed ocular histoplasmosis syndrome (POHS) 48
proptosis 163, 224, 226
 direction of displacement 223, 227
 examination 309
 measurement 225, 226, 309
 in thyroid eye disease 234, 236
*Pseudomonas* 271
pseudotumour
 cerebri (benign intracranial hypertension) 72–3, 207–8
 orbital inflammatory 160, 186, 215, 228–30
pterygium 131
ptosis 164
pupil
 dilation 98
 examination 98
 Holmes–Adie 311–12
pupillary light reflex 310
pupillary reaction 11–13 *see also* relative afferent pupillary defect
Purtscher's retinopathy 35
purulent discharge 112
pyrimethamine 86

radiation
 burn 158

optic neuropathy caused by 57
radiography, plain 149
Raeder's paratrigeminal syndrome 202, 216
RAPD *see* relative afferent pupillary defect
records, ocular trauma 133
red eye 92–131
 classification of causes 92
 examination 95–8
 history taking 92–4
 non-painful 93, 112–31
  with general irritation/grittiness 124–6
  with itching 117–20
  with photophobia/watering 120–3
  with purulent discharge 112–17
  with sectoral redness 127–31
 painful 93, 99–110, 193, 194, 214–16
  diplopia with 215–16
  Horner's syndrome with 216
  with little/no loss of vision 105–9
  with loss of vision 94, 99–105, 214–15
  with ophthalmic herpes zoster 109–11
 symptomatic classification 93
red reflex 19–20
refractive errors 58–60
 diplopia caused by 159–60
 headache associated with 204
rejection, corneal graft 288–9
relative afferent pupillary defect (RAPD)
 causes 26, 44, 57, 225
 detection 11–13
relative afferent pupillary response 11–13
retinal abnormalities 26, 58
 common 298–302
retinal artery occlusion
 branch (BRAO) 39, 40, 41–2
 central (CRAO) 28, 29, 35–7
retinal detachment 42–3, 87
 after cataract surgery 274–5
 management 42–3
 prognosis 43
 surgery, complications 186, 286–7
 symptoms and signs 42
 traumatic 136, 144

331

# INDEX

visual loss 28, 29, 37, 39
vitreous haemorrhage causing 38
retinal dialysis 136, 143, 144
retinal new vessels 87
retinal tears 77, 82–3, 87, 91
  traumatic 136, 143, 144
retinal vein occlusion
  branch (BRVO) 37, 38, 39–41
  central *see* central retinal vein occlusion
retinopathy
  central serous 51–3, 60
  diabetic *see* diabetic retinopathy
  Purtscher's 35
  slow flow 66, 70–1
retrobulbar neuritis 216
retrobulbar tumours 74
retroillumination 14, 15, 16
rhabdomyosarcoma 238–9
rodent ulcer 242–3, 244
rosacea 124
rose bengal 97, 126, 308

saline, irrigation with 154
sarcoidosis 78, 84–5, 249
scarring, posttraumatic 147
Schirmer's test 125, 308
Schwalbe's line 18, 19
sclera
  chemical burns 155
  rupture 136, 146
  traumatic perforation 148, 149
scleral scatter 14
scleral spur 18, 19
scleritis
  anterior 95, 108–9
    necrotising 109
    non-necrotising 109
  posterior 194–5, 216–17
scotoma 7
  negative 25, 44
  positive 25, 44
seborrhoeic keratosis 242
Seidel's test 149, 281, 289, 308
senile keratoses 242
serous retinopathy, central 51–3, 60
Sheridan–Gardiner cards 4, 5
shingles, ophthalmic 109–11
sickle cell disease 38
silicone tube displacement 292

sinus disease 204
sinusitis 196, 219
sixth (VI) nerve palsy 172–4, 175
skew deviation 185
skull fractures, basal 140–1
slitlamp (biomicroscope) examination 13–18
  anterior chamber 14–17, 97–8
  applanation tonometry 17
  direct illumination 13, 14
  ocular surface 308
  posterior segment 17
  in red eyes 97–8
  retroillumination 14, 15, 16
  scleral scatter 14
  specular reflection 13, 15
slow flow retinopathy 66, 70–1
"smoke stack" sign 52
Snellen chart 3, 4
"E" 4
specimen collection
  in *Acanthamoeba* infections 315
  in endophthalmitis 271
  infective corneal lesions 104
  microbiological 316
specular reflection 13, 15
squamous cell carcinoma, eyelid 243, 245
squamous papilloma, eyelid 242
squint *see* strabismus/squint
staphylococci 110, 271
steroids
  in allergic conjunctivitis 119–20
  in chemical burns 156
  in giant cell arteritis 32, 69
  in herpes simplex infections 122
  in iritis 103
  in ophthalmic herpes zoster 110
  in optic neuritis 54–5
  in thyroid eye disease 235
  in toxoplasmosis 86
  in traumatic hyphaema 143
sticky eyes 94, 112
strabismus/squint
  acute 174
  concomitant 161, 165, 166
  definitions 161
  incomitant 161, 164–5
  latent 166, 170
  surgery, complications 290–1

# INDEX

*Streptococcus pneumoniae* 112
stroke (cerebrovascular accident) 73, 74, 210
stye 125, 241
subarachnoid haemorrhage 209–10, 218
subconjunctival haemorrhage 95
  spontaneous 127–8
  traumatic 134, 135, 140–1, 148
subretinal neovascular membrane (SRNVM)
  in age related macular degeneration 45, 46, 47, 87
  causes 48
  management 47–8
  posttraumatic 146
sulphadiazine 86
superglue injuries 157
superior oblique muscle weakness 179
surface, ocular
  examination 307–8
  trauma 138–40
surgery
  postoperative complications 270–93
  previous periocular 186, 213
sutures
  abscess 278, 290
  broken/loose 277, 278, 289–90
  conjunctival lacerations 138
  eyelid lacerations 140
  granuloma 290–1
  irritation 293
  protruding 276–8, 284–5
  tarsorrhaphy 293
swabs 316
  conjunctival, in neonates 115
swellings 223–55
  conjunctival 225, 253–5
  examination 225
  eyelids 223, 224, 225–6, 240–5
  history taking 225
  in lacrimal gland disease 224, 246–50
  in nasolacrimal disease 224–5, 250–2
  in orbital disease 223, 224, 225–39
swinging light test 11–13, 310
sympathetic ophthalmitis 152–3
sympathetic paresis 311–12
synechiae 102–3
syneresis, vitreous 83

tarsorrhaphy sutures 293
tear
  break up time (BUT) 125, 307
  film 307
  precorneal 307
  substitutes 125
teeth clenching/grinding, nocturnal 209
temporal arteritis *see* giant cell (temporal) arteritis
temporal artery biopsy 32
temporal lobe lesions 9, 63
temporomandibular joint dysfunction 201–2
Tensilon test 180
Terson's syndrome 87
thermal burns 157–8
third (III) nerve palsy 175, 180–3
  pupil sparing 181, 182
three step test, for vertical diplopia 166–7, 305–6, 307
thromboembolic disease 66, 67, 73–4
thymoma 180
thyroid eye disease (TED) 232–6
  clinical features 232–4
  diplopia in 160, 176, 180, 226, 235
  investigations 234
  management 235–6
  pain in 215
Tolosa–Hunt syndrome 186
tonometry, applanation 17
topical anaesthesia 138
toxic conjunctivitis 120
toxicity, contact lens associated 260
toxic optic neuropathy 57
toxoplasmosis 78, 85–6
trabecular meshwork 18, 19
trabeculectomy
  leaking bleb/excessive filtration 268, 281–2, 283
  postoperative complications 281–5, 286
trachoma *see* chlamydial conjunctivitis
trauma 132–58
  advice to patients 134
  blunt 134–8
  burns 153–8
  chemical *see* chemical burns
  classification 132
  diplopia after 137, 146, 160, 176, 185–6

333

INDEX

documentation 133
non-penetrating 134–47
penetrating 133, 147–53 see also
  foreign bodies, intraocular
  assessment 147–8
  investigations 149
  management 152–3
  symptoms and signs 148–9
  preliminary assessment 133
  superglue injuries 157
  surface injuries 138–40
trichiasis 95, 108
  after chemical burns 156
  protective lenses 269
trigeminal neuralgia 221–2
tropicamide 102–3
tumours
  conjunctiva 254–5
  eyelid 241–3
  intracranial 56, 63–4, 91, 208
  intraocular 87
  lacrimal gland 246, 248–50
  lacrimal sac 252
  orbital see orbital tumours

ultrasonography 38, 149
uvea, prolapsed 149, 150
uveitis 72
  anterior see iritis
  granulomatous 84
  herpes zoster 110
  intermediate 83, 84
  posterior 83, 84

vancomycin 271
van Herrick's sign 69
vascular disease
  cranial nerve palsies 173, 182, 183, 184
  internuclear ophthalmoplegia 176
vascular events, causing flashing lights 91
vascular tumours, orbit 236–7
vasculitis 74, 109 see also giant cell arteritis
vernal keratoconjunctivitis 120
vertebrobasilar stenosis 73, 74
viral conjunctivitis 106, 116–17
viral samples 317
vision

blurring 57–62
colour see colour vision
dimming 44
distorted 44
double see diplopia
examination 3–13
visual acuity 3–6, 26
  corrected 5
  distance
    in adults 3–4
    in children 4, 5
  near 5
  pinhole 5–6, 57
  red eyes 95
visual evoked potential (VEP) 313–14
visual fields 7–11
  anatomical basis 7–9
  defects 38–57 see also hemianopia; scotoma
    absolute 7
    causes 39
    congruity 7
    examination 39
    heteronymous 7
    history 25, 39
    homonymous 7, 25
    patterns 25
    relative 7
  methods of documenting 10–11
    Amsler grid 10–11
    confrontation techniques 10
    perimetry 11
  terminology 7
visual loss 22–64
  anatomical diagnosis 22, 23
  binocular 22–5
  central 43–5
  classification 24
  examination 26–7
  history 22–5
  monocular 22–5
  in orbital disease 225, 226
  painful white eye with 216–17
  pain with 211, 214–15, 216–17
  profound 27–38
    associated symptoms 27
    causes 27
    examination 28
    onset 27
  red eye with 94, 99–105, 214–15

334

# INDEX

segmental 38–57 *see also* visual fields, defects
  causes 39
  examination 39
  history 39
  transient 65–76
    causes 65
    examination 67–8
    history 66–7
    initial diagnosis 66
    investigations 68
visual pathway 7–9, 23
vitrectomy 38, 87, 153
vitreous
  base detachment 136, 144–5
  fluid 83
  opacities 83
  in penetrating trauma 150
  posterior detachment (PVD) 77, 78–80, 89, 91

slitlamp examination 17
vitreous haemorrhage 28, 37–8, 86–7
  in diabetic retinopathy 61, 62
  management 88
  traumatic 136, 145, 152
Von Graefe's sign 234

"washing line" sign 144, 145
watering eyes 94, 121–3
Weiss ring 79, 80
Wilbrand's knee 9
wound
  dehiscence, eyelid surgery 293
  infections, postoperative 291–2
  leaks
    postoperative 268, 281–2
    Seidel's test 308

Zeiss, cyst of 242, 243

# ABC of Eyes—Second Edition
## P T Khaw, A R Elkington

*An excellent introduction to ophthalmology . . . it presents basic ophthalmology with admirable simplicity, authority and clarity.*
American Journal of Ophthalmology

The *ABC of Eyes* is already well established as the standard guide for general practitioners, nurses and medical students encountering eye problems. It provides a symptom led approach to identifying and managing all the common eye disorders encountered, whether in the GP surgery or the outpatients department. The revised second edition includes a completely updated chapter on cataracts, the latest information on refractive surgery and even more colour photographs.

ISBN: 07279 0766 2
60 pages approx
Readership: general practitioners, nurses, medical students